HANDBOOK OF ART THERAPY

Handbook of
Art Therapy

Edited by
CATHY A. MALCHIODI

THE GUILFORD PRESS
New York   London

© 2003 The Guilford Press
A Division of Guilford Publications, Inc.
72 Spring Street, New York, NY 10012
www.guilford.com

Printed in the United States of America

This book is printed on acid-free paper.

Last digit is print number: 9   8   7   6   5   4   3

Library of Congress Cataloging-in-Publication Data

Handbook of art therapy / edited by Cathy A. Malchiodi.
        p.   cm.
Includes bibliographical references and index.
     ISBN 1-57230-809-5 (alk. paper)
   1. Arts—Therapeutic use—Handbooks, manuals, etc. I. Malchiodi,
Cathy A.
   RC489.A7 H365 2003
   615.8′5156—dc21

                                                    2002012812

About the Editor

Cathy A. Malchiodi, ATR, LPAT, LPCC, is an art therapist, expressive art therapist, and clinical mental health counselor, as well as an internationally recognized authority on art therapy with children, adults, and families. She is a member of the Board of Directors of the American Art Therapy Association (AATA) and is the past editor of *Art Therapy: Journal of the AATA.* She has received numerous honors for her work, including recognition from the AATA, the Kennedy Center for the Arts, Very Special Arts, and the China Association for the Handicapped. An author of several books, including *The Art Therapy Sourcebook, Understanding Children's Drawings,* and *Breaking the Silence: Art Therapy with Children from Violent Homes,* and editor of *Medical Art Therapy with Children* and *Medical Art Therapy with Adults,* she has written more than 60 articles and chapters and has given more than 160 presentations on art therapy throughout the United States and abroad. She currently serves as editor for *Trauma and Loss: Research and Interventions,* and is on the faculty of the National Institute for Trauma and Loss and the Graduate Program in Expressive Therapies at the University of Louisville.

Contributors

Wae Soon Choi, PhD, K-ATR, Department of Rehabilitation, Taegu University, Taegu, Korea

Marcia Sue Cohen-Liebman, MA, MCAT, ATR-BC, Drexel University, College of Nursing and Health Professions, Hahnemann Creative Arts in Therapy Program, Philadelphia, Pennsylvania

Tracy Councill, MA, ATR-BC, Art Therapy Program, Lombardi Cancer Center, Georgetown University Medical Center, Washington, DC

Carol Thayer Cox, MA, ATR, REAT, private practice, Washington, DC

Robin L. Gabriels, PsyD, Department of Pediatrics, University of Colorado Health Sciences Center, and JFK Partners, Denver, Colorado

Linda Gantt, PhD, ATR-BC, Trauma Recovery Institute, Morgantown, West Virginia

Eliana Gil, PhD, Abused Children's Treatment Services, Inova Kellar Center, Fairfax, Virginia

Samuel T. Gladding, PhD, Department of Counselor Education, Wake Forest University, Winston-Salem, North Carolina

Janice Hoshino, PhD, ATR-BC, LMFT, Center for Programs in Psychology, Antioch University–Seattle, Seattle, Washington

Tomio Kakuyama, BA, Department of Rehabilitation, Kanagawa Prefectural Ashigara-kami Hospital, Kanagawa, Japan

Frances F. Kaplan, MPS, DA, ATR-BC, Department of Art Therapy, Marylhurst University, Lake Oswego, Oregon

Dong-Yeun Kim, PhD, K-ATR, Department of Rehabilitation, Taegu University, Taegu, Korea

P. Gussie Klorer, PhD, ATR-BC, LCSW, LCPC, Department of Art and Design, Southern Illinois University, Edwardsville, Edwardsville, Illinois

Marian Liebmann, MA, PGCE, CQSW, Inner City Mental Health Service, Bristol, United Kingdom

Cathy A. Malchiodi, MA, ATR, LPAT, LPCC, Department of Expressive Therapies, University of Louisville, Louisville, Kentucky; National Institute for Trauma and Loss in Children, Detroit, Michigan

Anne Mills, MA, ATR-BC, LPC, Art Therapy Program, The George Washington University, Washington, DC; private practice, Alexandria, Virginia

Debbie W. Newsome PhD, Department of Counselor Education, Wake Forest University, Winston-Salem, North Carolina

Joan Phillips, MA, MS, LMFT, LPC, ATR-BC, Department of Human Relations, University of Oklahoma, and private practice, Norman, Oklahoma

Shirley Riley, MA, MFT, ATR-HLM, Department of Art Therapy, Marital and Family Therapy Graduate Program, Phillips Graduate Institute, Encino, California

Aimee Loth Rozum, MA, ATR, Child and Adolescent Services, Hospice and Palliative Care of Cape Cod, Hyannis, Massachusetts

Diane S. Safran, MS, LMFT, ATR-BC, Attention Deficit Disorders Institute, and Learning Strategies, Westport, Connecticut

Rawley A. Silver, EdD, ATR, HLM, National Institute of Education Project, Sarasota, Florida

Susan Spaniol, EdD, ATR-BC, LMHC, Expressive Therapies Division, Graduate School of Arts and Social Sciences, Lesley University, Cambridge, Massachusetts

William Steele, MSW, PsyD, National Institute for Trauma and Loss in Children, Grosse Pointe Woods, Michigan

Lenore Steinhardt, MA, ATR, Art Therapy Training Program, The Center for Training Creative Expressive Therapists, Continuing Education, Kibbutzim College of Education, Tel Aviv, Israel; Rakefet Children's Therapy Center, Ramat Hasharon, Israel

Carmello Tabone, MA, ATR, Chestnut Ridge Hospital, Morgantown, West Virginia

Masahiro Tanaka, MA, Department of Psychological Counseling, Mejiro University, Tokyo, Japan

Madoka Takada Urhausen, MA, ATR, Intercommunity Child Guidance Center, Whittier, California

Randy M. Vick, MS, ATR-BC, LCPC, Department of Art Therapy, School of the Art Institute of Chicago, Chicago, Illinois

Judith Wald, MS, ATR-BC, Department of Therapeutic Activities, New York Presbyterian Hospital, White Plains, New York; College of New Rochelle, Graduate Division of Art and Communication Studies, New Rochelle, New York

Diane Waller, MA (RCA), ATC, DIP. Group Psych, DPhil, SRAsT, Unit of Psychotherapeutic Studies, Goldsmiths College, University of London, London, United Kingdom

Marie Wilson, MA, CSAT, CSAC, ATR-BC, LPC, Art Therapy Programs, Caldwell College, Caldwell, New Jersey

Preface

Art is a powerful tool in communication. It is now widely acknowledged that art expression is a way to visually communicate thoughts and feelings that are too painful to put into words. Creative activity has also been used in psychotherapy and counseling not only because it serves another language but also because of its inherent ability to help people of all ages explore emotions and beliefs, reduce stress, resolve problems and conflicts, and enhance their sense of well-being.

The countless individuals I have been privileged to work with over the last 20 years have repeatedly demonstrated to me how art expression is effective as both a form of therapy and a method of nonverbal communication. On the jacket of this volume, there is an image by one of these individuals, Eduardo, a remarkable man whose struggle with mental illness was helped through art therapy along with psychiatric interventions. Now in his early 30s, he had been struggling with depression and mood swings since adolescence, and was looking for answers about his condition and seeking professional help. Even though he lived more than 2,000 miles away, Eduardo sent me a letter of introduction and a large envelope with some of his drawings and paintings. He had been carefully saving his artwork for many years, and it was easy to see just how much creative expression meant to him. He neatly titled each on a small piece of notepaper meticulously clipped to the upper-left-hand corner of each artwork.

For the next month, we communicated through e-mails and letters, and I learned more about Eduardo's mental illness, his life history, and lack of success in obtaining effective treatment. On good days, he wrote articulately, describing his frustration about his depression and "his problems with thinking." On other occasions his letters were disorganized and illogical, reminiscent of a thought disorder, and seemed to be a result of manic feelings and impulses. To ensure that Eduardo received appropriate treatment, and since sufficient medical care was not available where Eduardo lived, I made arrangements for his treatment at a local neuropsychiatric hospital. Fortunately, Eduardo was willing to relocate and was able to enter one of the hospital's inpatient programs to receive an evaluation.

Eduardo was diagnosed with bipolar disorder, which accounted for his mood swings, from lethargy to mania and days of insomnia. Psychiatric treatment included finding the correct drug combination to control his mood swings and individual and group therapy to increase the psychosocial skills that he had suffered as a result of years of emotional disturbance. I was able to work with Eduardo on an individual basis during his inpatient program and later as an outpatient for many months. I helped him to continue his creative expression during his psychiatric treatment and kept the neuropsychiatric team informed about the content and scope of his artwork. As his art therapist and clinical mental health counselor, I was intrigued by the range of colors, patterns, and subjects in his images and impressed by his creative abilities, especially because he was not a trained artist. Many of his drawings and paintings were quite playful and almost childlike abstract designs (see Figure 1) while others were haunting representations of the effects of mental illness such as his recurrent insomnia and mania (see Figure 2). Some had detailed stories about fanciful characters and animals like whales that could speak or fly or had other extraordinary powers (see Figure 3; see also book jacket).

Eduardo's experiences illustrate the value of art expression as part of psychotherapy and counseling, and his case validates the benefits of visual communication. Like many individuals, his drawings and paintings served as a record of his mood swings, giving his helping professionals a clear "picture" of how he was feeling, pre- and posttreatment. His artwork also gave him a way to express what words could not during moments when his thoughts became disorganized and inarticulate. Most

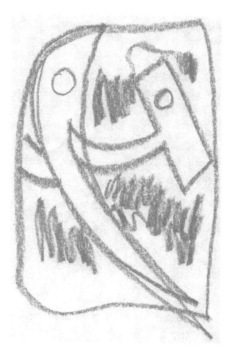

FIGURE 1. Untitled design in oil pastel by Eduardo.

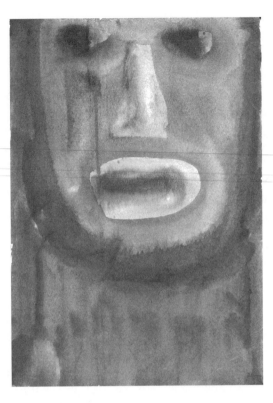

FIGURE 2. "My Insomnia," a painting by Eduardo.

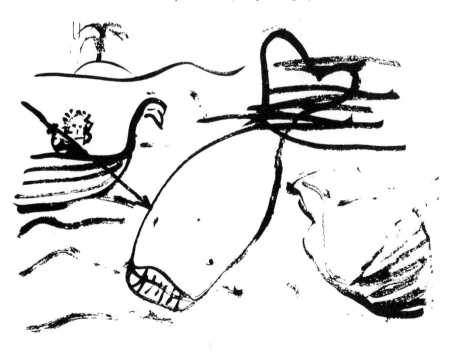

FIGURE 3. "Fisherman Hunting a Whale," an ink drawing by Eduardo.

important, in his words, it gave him a reason to "get out of bed in the morning" and "it's one of the things that helps [him] to feel free." I believe art did help him overcome his often-severe depression, find a release from his illness, and discover and nurture a sense of well-being.

What was particularly wonderful about working with Eduardo was not only being part of his journey to recovery but also once again witnessing the power of art in therapy and how it can be useful in so many aspects of evaluation and treatment. While I was the art therapist on the case, many other helping professionals also encouraged and participated in Eduardo's art therapy. For example, the staff psychiatrist asked Eduardo to complete several art-based assessments; the clinical social worker and I used Eduardo's art expressions and verbal descriptions as a way to help us design his inpatient and outpatient programs; and psychiatric nurses learned to use art as a way to help calm him when his moods were uncontrollable.

For many individuals like Eduardo, art therapy is a primary form of treatment. In his case, it provided a way to communicate and establish a relationship not only to me but also to the many other professionals who provided therapy and support that eventually led to his recovery. In other situations, art therapy may be used as an adjunct to treatment, to enhance verbal therapy through working with the client to increase self-understanding and insight. For still others, art expression may be a way to reach those whose problems have not been revealed solely through talking about them. Drawing, painting, collage, or simple sculpture may be the modalities through which a child expresses an abusive experience for the first time, an adult uncovers a forgotten trauma, or a family discloses a previously hidden secret or significant incident.

While art therapists make art expression a central part of their work, other helping professionals can easily adapt art therapy approaches and applications to their own ways of working with individuals, families, and groups. With increasing frequency, clinical counselors, social workers, play therapists, marriage and family therapists, psychologists, and psychiatrists are discovering that drawing activities and other expressive media are helpful in the assessment and treatment of people of all ages. Because art therapy permits expression of feelings and thoughts in a manner that is often less threatening than strictly verbal means, there is a level of comfort and a sense of safety sometimes not found through traditional therapy alone. Clients' feelings and experiences are transformed into concrete and tangible images, allowing both the client and the therapist to obtain a fresh view of problems, conflicts, potentials, and directions. With the advent of brief forms of therapy and the increasing pressures to complete treatment in a limited number of sessions, many therapists find art expression helps people to quickly communicate relevant issues and problems, thus expediting assessment and intervention. For this reason alone, helping professionals are increasingly using drawings and other expressive art tasks in therapeutic intervention.

This volume addresses the need for a handbook that provides a clear overview of the field of art therapy and its role in contemporary practice. Thirty chapters, written by experts within the United States and abroad, present to the reader art therapy's origins, the art and science of why art therapy works, major theoretical approaches, and the extraordinary range of clinical possibilities and applications to a variety of populations. Leading-edge topics for practitioners are also presented, including art therapy and the brain; cognitive-behavioral, solution-focused, multimodal, and other contemporary approaches; clinical applications with trauma, abuse, autism, depression, learning disabilities, medical illness, and addictions; art-based assessments; and ethics, supervision, and education specific to art therapy.

The *Handbook of Art Therapy*, an assembly of theory and approaches that will enhance therapists' understanding of how to integrate art expression within treatment, is both practical and comprehensive. It brings together the theory and practice of art therapy through numerous cases and visual illustrations of how children, adolescents, adults, groups, and families can benefit from the opportunity to experience art expression as part of their psychotherapy or counseling. It is my hope that you will be inspired by the extensive range of ideas, resources, and clinical examples in the pages that follow and deepen your own understanding of art therapy's value as a potent modality for change and growth with a variety of populations and settings.

CATHY A. MALCHIODI

Acknowledgments

This is my first attempt at an edited volume of this scope, and there are many people who helped, directly and indirectly, along the journey of compiling the book over the last 2 years. First, I thank the contributors to this book, whose chapters made it possible and whose patience and support made the process pleasurable for me. My deepest gratitude goes to you for making what I believe are significant contributions to the field of art therapy and for making my job as an editor worthwhile and personally rewarding.

I offer very special thanks to The Guilford Press for supporting this project from the initial proposal through the first drafts and onward to the final manuscript and production of the book. My heartfelt thanks are extended to Rochelle Serwator, whose editorial skills and expertise took the initial jumble of chapters and transformed them into a superbly readable text. I feel privileged each time I work with Rochelle on a book because I know that not only will I enjoy the process, I will also be immensely pleased with the final product. I also want to thank Seymour Weingarten, Paul Gordon, Kim Miller, and Anna Nelson for their help and support during various stages of bringing the book to print.

Finally, I never could have envisioned this text without the encouragement and advice of so many art therapy colleagues and mentors who have supported my work for the last 20 years. Of equal importance are all the clients—children, adolescents, adults, and families—who have taught me by example about the power and value of art therapy in personal growth, recovery, and well-being. My deepest gratitude is extended to all of you for making this book possible.

Contents

PART I

The Art and Science of Art Therapy

Art therapy is based on the idea that the creative process of art making is healing and life enhancing and is a form of nonverbal communication of thoughts and feelings (American Art Therapy Association, 1996). Like other forms of psychotherapy and counseling, it is used to encourage personal growth, increase self-understanding, and assist in emotional reparation and has been employed in a wide variety of settings with children, adults, families, and groups. It is a modality that can help individuals of all ages create meaning and achieve insight, find relief from overwhelming emotions or trauma, resolve conflicts and problems, enrich daily life, and achieve an increased sense of well-being (Malchiodi, 1998). Art therapy supports the belief that all individuals have the capacity to express themselves creatively and that the product is less important than the therapeutic process involved. The therapist's focus is not specifically on the aesthetic merits of art making but on the therapeutic needs of the person to express. That is, what is important is the person's involvement in the work, choosing and facilitating art activities that are helpful to the person, helping the person to find meaning in the creative process, and facilitating the sharing of the experience of image making with the therapist.

While other forms of therapy are effective, art therapy is increasingly being used by therapists with individuals of all ages and with a variety of populations. Not only art therapists, but counselors, psychologists, psychiatrists, social workers, and even physicians are using art expression for therapy. With the advent of brief forms of therapy and the increasing pressures to complete treatment in a limited number of sessions, therapists are finding that art activities help individuals to communicate relevant issues and problems quickly, thus expediting assessment and intervention. Even the simplest drawing task offers unique possibilities for expression that complements and, in many cases, helps a child or adult to communicate what words cannot.

The field of art therapy, while a recognized form of treatment, is still somewhat of a mystery to many professionals. Therapists who use art with their clients know that it is an effective form of intervention, but most do not know its rich history, why it works, and what its benefits and limitations are as a form of therapy and evaluation. This first section of the book provides the reader with an overview of how art therapy came to be, what we know about why it is effective, and guidelines for understanding the role of art in assessment.

In Chapter 1, Vick offers a brief history of art therapy and describes the many influences from disciplines including art, psychiatry, and medicine that guided the course and development of the field. As Vick notes, during the last five decades art therapy has grown from a modality practiced predominantly in psychiatric hospitals to become a primary form of treatment in inpatients milieus, outpatient clinics, domestic violence shelters, residential facilities, trauma units, medical settings, and community centers. Whereas people with mental illness, physical disabilities, or cognitive deficits were once the principal populations, now it is common to see art therapy applied to abuse and neglect; families or couples in distress; children with learning disabilities; people with cancer, HIV, or other serious illnesses; older adults with dementia, Alzheimer's disease, or disabilities; individuals with addictions or chemical dependencies; and bereaved children and parents. Wherever psychotherapy is used as treatment, art therapy is now a commonplace form of intervention.

Because it is a relatively new field, there is still debate on how to define art therapy. Some therapists see it as modality that helps individuals to verbalize their thoughts and feelings, beliefs, problems, and world views. By this definition, art therapy is an adjunct to psychotherapy, facilitating the process through both image making and verbal exchange with the therapist. Others see art itself as the therapy; that is, the creative process involved in art making, whether it be drawing, painting, sculpting or some other art form, is what is life enhancing and ultimately therapeutic.

In actuality, both aspects contribute to art therapy's effectiveness as a form of treatment and most art therapists subscribe to both definitions in their work. Image making does help people to communicate both through image and words and, with the guidance of a therapist, can assist individuals in expressing what may be difficult to say with words alone. We are also beginning to understand the benefits of asking clients to create drawings or other art forms in therapy. Artistic expression is an activity that involves the brain in ways that can be used to enhance therapeutic treatment and evaluation. Chapter 2 explains more about the "art therapy and the brain," how neuroscience is informing a growing understanding of art expression in therapy, and why art therapy is rapidly becoming an intervention of choice with a variety of disorders.

Many therapists wonder if art therapy is purely about interpreting the content of art expressions and clinicians new to the field often wonder what exactly art expression can tell them about the client who makes them. On occasion I am asked by a professional to analyze a child's drawing or an adult's art expression to determine whether the individual has a particular emotional problem or has experienced abuse or trauma. Images are forms of nonverbal communication and therapists often are curious if it is possible to interpret their clients' artwork. To a significant extent, art therapists are concerned with understanding the meaning of client-created artworks and research is currently being conducted in the area of art-based assessments (see

Appendix I, this volume, for more information). In Chapter 3, Kaplan tackles the is-sues inherent to art-based assessments, the role of interpretation, and what is known about the content of art expressions from research data. She offers helpful guidelines on the limitations and strengths of using art expressions in evaluation, promising trends in using drawings to understand mental conditions, and caveats for therapists who use art therapy for the purpose of interpretation.

Art therapy is an exciting, dynamic field, one which continues to evolve in terms of depth and applications. For those who are art therapists, it is a modality that is central to their work and is the basis of their world view of therapy in general. For counselors, social workers, psychologists, psychiatrists, and others, art may be a tool that is employed as an adjunct to verbal therapy. This first section introduces all ther-apists who use art activities in clinical work to the foundations of this field, familiar-izes them with how art therapists view client-created art expressions, and provides them with a basic understanding how and why art expression can enhance treatment and evaluation.

REFERENCES

American Art Therapy Association. (1996). *Mission statement*. Mundelein, IL: Author.
Malchiodi, C. A. (1998). *The art therapy sourcebook*. New York: McGraw Hill-NTC.

CHAPTER 1

A Brief History of Art Therapy

Randy M. Vick

This history of art therapy focuses on the precursory and continuing trends that have shaped the theory and practice and the literature that reflects this development. Scholarship, like history, builds on the foundations laid by others. I am indebted to the authors of four other histories that I found to be particularly useful in the preparation of this chapter. Both Malchiodi (1998) and Rubin (1999) have assembled histories based on contributing trends, as did Junge and Asawa (1994) who have provided extensive details on the personalities and politics involved in the formation of the American Art Therapy Association. My fourth primary source (MacGregor, 1989), while never intended as a book about art therapy, has proven to be an excellent "prehistory" of the field. Each of these references provided information as well as inspiration and I encourage readers to consult them for additional perspectives. Finally, it should be noted here that art therapy was not a phenomenon exclusive to the United States. Readers interested in art therapy's development in Europe should consult Waller's (1991, 1998) two books on this subject.

History is like a tapestry with each colored thread contributing not only to the formation of the image but to the strength and structure of the fabric itself. Imagine for a moment a tapestry with bobbins of different-colored threads, each adding a hue that becomes part of a new creation, and we can better understand the history of this field.

INFLUENCES FROM THE DISTANT PAST AND NEIGHBORING FIELDS

Art therapy is a hybrid discipline based primarily on the fields of art and psychology, drawing characteristics from each parent to evolve a unique new entity. But the inter-

5

weaving of the arts and healing is hardly a new phenomenon. It seems clear that this pairing is as old as human society itself, having occurred repeatedly throughout our history across place and time (Malchiodi, 1998). The development of the profession of art therapy can be seen as the formal application of a long-standing human tradition influenced by the intellectual and social trends of the 20th century (Junge & Asawa, 1994).

From the Realms of Art

Art making is an innate human tendency, so much so it has been argued that, like speech and tool making, this activity could be used to define our species (Dissanayake, 1992). In his book, *The Discovery of the Art of the Insane*, MacGregor (1989) presents a history of the interplay of art and psychology spanning the last 300 years. This history covers theories of genius and insanity, biographies of "mad" artists, depictions of madness by artists, and the various attempts to reach an understanding of the potential art has as an aid to mental health treatment and diagnosis. In 1922, German psychiatrist Hans Prinzhorn (1922/1995) published *The Artistry of the Mentally Ill*, a book that depicted and described the artistic productions of residents of insane asylums across Europe. This work challenged both psychiatric and fine arts professionals to reconsider their notions of mental illness and art (MacGregor, 1989). Even today, debate rages within the field variously titled outsider art/art brut/visionary art/folk art as experts struggle to place work by self-taught artists (some of whom have experienced mental illness) within the art historical canon (Borum, 1993/1994; Russell, 2002).

Contemporary writers from art therapy and other disciplines continue to explore the notion of art practice for the purpose of personal exploration and growth (Allen, 1995; Cameron & Bryan, 1992; C. Moon, 2002) and to reevaluate the traditional boundaries between personal and public art (Lachman-Chapin et al., 1999; Sigler, 1993; Spaniol, 1990; Vick, 2000).

Medicine, Health, and Rehabilitation

Hospitals have long served as important incubators for the field of art therapy. For better or worse, medical model concepts such as diagnosis, disease, and treatment have had a strong influence on the development of most schools of thought within Western psychotherapy, including art therapy. While psychiatry has always been the medical specialty most closely allied with the field, art therapists have worked with patients being treated for AIDS, asthma, burns, cancer, chemical dependency, trauma, tuberculosis, and other medical and rehabilitation needs (Malchiodi 1999a, 1999b). Our understanding of the interplay between biochemistry, mental status, and creativity continues to evolve and a new medical specialty, arts medicine, has recently emerged (Malchiodi, 1998). All this seems to suggest that art therapy will continue to have a role in exploring the connections between body and mind.

TRENDS IN 19TH- AND 20TH-CENTURY PSYCHOLOGY

For much of human history mental illness was regarded with fear and misunderstanding as a manifestation of either divine or demonic forces. Reformers such as Rush in the United States and Pinel in France made great strides in creating a more humane environment for their patients. Freud, Kris, and others contributed to this rehumanization by theorizing that rather than being random nonsense, the productions of fantasy revealed significant information about the unique inner world of their maker (MacGregor, 1989; Rubin, 1999). Building on these theories, many writers began to examine how a specific sort of creative product—art—could be understood as an illustration of mental health or disturbance (Anastasi & Foley, 1941; Arnheim, 1954; Kreitler & Kreitler, 1972). Other authors began recognizing the potential art has as a tool within treatment (Winnicott, 1971). Soon enough, the term "art therapy" began to be used to describe a form of psychotherapy that placed art practices and interventions alongside talk as the central modality of treatment (Naumburg, 1950/1973).

The significance psychoanalytic writers placed on early childhood experiences made the crossover of these theories into education an easy one (Junge & Asawa, 1994). Some progressive educators placed particular emphasis on the role art played in the overall development of children (Cane, 1951/1983; Kellogg, 1969; Lowenfeld, 1987; Uhlin, 1972/1984). This trend toward the therapeutic application of art within educational settings continues today (Anderson, 1978/1992; Bush, 1997; Henley, 1992).

PSYCHOLOGICAL ASSESSMENT AND RESEARCH

In addition to psychoanalysis and the rehumanization of people with mental illness, one of the strongest trends to emerge within modern psychology has been the focus on standardized methods of diagnostic assessment and research. Whether discussing the work of a studio artist or the productions of a mentally ill individual, Kris (1952) argues that they both engage in the same psychic process, that is, "the placing of an inner experience, an inner image, into the outside world" (p. 115). This "method of projection" became the conceptual foundation for a dazzling array of so-called projective drawing assessments that evolved in psychology during the 20th century (Hammer, 1958/1980). These simple paper-and-pencil "tests," with their formalized procedures and standardized methods of interpretation, became widely used in the evaluation and diagnosis of children and adults and are still employed to a lesser degree today (though often with revamped purpose and procedure). Two parallel themes from this era are the relatively unstructured methods of art assessment (Elkisch, 1948; Shaw, 1934) and the various approaches to interpreting these productions (Machover, 1949/1980).

The impact of psychoanalysis on the early development of art therapy was profound. Hammer's (1958/1980) classic book on drawing as a projective device illustrates the diversity within this area and the inclusion of two chapters on art therapy by pioneering art therapist Margaret Naumburg demonstrates the crossover of influences. Many of the more common stereotypes about art therapy (specific, assigned drawings; finger painting; and the role of the therapist in divining the "true meaning" of the drawings) can, in fact, be traced directly to this era.

Nearly all the major art therapy writers from this time developed their own methods of assessment consisting of batteries of art tasks with varying levels of structure (Kramer & Schehr, 1983; Kwiatkowska, 1978; Rubin, 1978/1984; Ulman & Dachinger, 1975/1996). Even today, the notion that artworks in some way reflect the psychic experience of the artist is a fundamental concept in art therapy.

Despite this common history, there are distinctions between the approach to assessment used in psychology and that found in art therapy. The key difference is the art therapy perspective that the making and viewing of the art have inherent therapeutic potential for the client, a position not necessarily held by psychometricians. In addition, art therapists tend to use more varied and expressive materials and to deemphasize formalized verbal directives and stress the role of clients as interpreters of their own work. Finally, art therapists are also quite likely to improvise on the protocol of standardized assessments to suit a particular clinical purpose (Mills & Goodwin, 1991).

An emerging theme in the literature is the unique role the creative arts therapies can play in the assessment and evaluation of clients (Bruscia, 1988; Feder & Feder, 1998). Contemporary developers of art therapy assessments have abandoned orthodox psychoanalytic approaches in favor of methods that emphasize the expressive potential of the tasks and materials (Cohen, Hammer, & Singer, 1988; Cox & Frame, 1993; Gantt & Tabone, 1997; Landgarten, 1993; Silver, 1978/1989).

Early art therapy researchers also looked to psychology and embraced its empirical approach for their research (Kwiatkowska, 1978). More recently, models from the behavioral sciences and other fields have been used as resources in conducting art therapy research (Kaplan, 2000; McNiff, 1998; Wadeson, 1992).

THE DEVELOPMENT OF THE ART THERAPY LITERATURE

The development of any discipline is best traced through the evolution of that field's literature. The historian's convention of artificially dividing time into segments is employed here to illustrate three phases of growth in the profession of art therapy.

Classical Period (1940s to 1970s)

In the middle of the 20th century a largely independent assortment of individuals began to use the term "art therapy" in their writings to describe their work with clients. In doing so, these pioneering individuals began to define a discipline that was distinct from other, older professions. Because there was no formal art therapy training to be had, these early writers were trained in other fields and mentored by psychiatrists, analysts, and other mental health professionals. The four leading writers universally recognized for their contributions to the development of the field during this period are Margaret Naumburg, Edith Kramer, Hanna Kwiatkowska, and Elinor Ulman. The lasting impact of their original works on the field is demonstrated by the fact that their writings continue to be used as original sources in contemporary art therapy literature.

More than any other author, Naumburg is seen as the primary founder of American art therapy and is frequently referred to as the "Mother of Art Therapy" (see Junge & Asawa, 1994, p. 22). Through her early work in the innovative Walden School, which she founded (along with her sister Florence Cane), and later in psychiatric settings she developed her ideas and, in the 1940s, began to write about what was to become known as art therapy (Detre et al., 1983). Familiar with the ideas of both Freud and Jung, Naumburg (1966/1987) conceived her "dynamically oriented art therapy" to be largely analogous to the psychoanalytic practices of the day. The clients' art productions were viewed as symbolic communication of unconscious material in a direct, uncensored, and concrete form that Naumburg (1950/1973) argued would aid in the resolution of the transference.

While Naumburg borrowed heavily from the techniques of psychoanalytic practice, Kramer took a different approach by adapting concepts from Freud's personality theory to explain the art therapy process. Her "art as therapy" approach emphasizes the intrinsic therapeutic potential in the art-making process and the central role the defense mechanism of sublimation plays in this experience (Kramer, 1971/1993). Kramer's (1958, 1971/1993) work in therapeutic schools (as opposed to Naumburg's psychiatric emphasis) allows for more direct application of her ideas to educational settings.

Ulman's most outstanding contributions to the field have been as an editor and writer. She founded *The Bulletin of Art Therapy* in 1961 (*The American Journal of Art Therapy* after 1970) when no other publication of its kind existed (Junge & Asawa, 1994). In addition, Ulman (along with her coeditor Dachinger) (1975/1996) published the first book of collected essays on art therapy that served as one of the few texts in the field for many years. Her gift as a writer was to precisely synthesize and articulate complex ideas. In her essay "Art Therapy: Problems of Definition," Ulman (1975/1996) compares and contrasts Naumburg's "art psychotherapy" and Kramer's "art as therapy" models so clearly that it continues to be the definitive presentation of this core theoretical continuum.

The last of these four remarkable women, Kwiatkowska, made her major contributions in the areas of research and family art therapy. She brought together her experiences in various psychiatric settings in a book that became the foundation for working with families through art (Kwiatkowska, 1978). Like Kramer, she had fled Europe at the time of World War II adding to the list of émigré thinkers who influenced the development of mental health disciplines in the United States. She also coauthored a short book that helped introduce the field of art therapy to the general public (Ulman, Kramer, & Kwiatkowska, 1978).

Each of these pioneers lectured widely on the topic of art therapy and served as some of the field's first educators. It was also during this period that the first formal programs with degrees in art therapy were offered (Junge & Asawa, 1994;

Levick, Goldman, & Fink, 1967). Finally, it is important not to forget the other early pioneers working in other parts of the country, such as Mary Huntoon at the Menninger Clinic (Wix, 2000), who made contributions to the developing profession as well.

Middle Years: Other Pioneering Writers (1970s to Mid-1980s)

The 1970s through the mid-1980s saw the emergence of an increasing number of publications that presented a broader range of applications and conceptual perspectives (Betensky, 1973; Landgarten, 1981; Levick, 1983; McNiff, 1981; Rhyne, 1973/ 1995; Robbins & Sibley, 1976; Rubin, 1978/1984; Wadeson, 1980), although psychoanalysis remained a dominant influence. The development of the literature was also enriched during this period with the introduction of two new journals: *Art Psychotherapy* in 1973 (called *The Arts in Psychotherapy* after 1980) and *Art Therapy: Journal of the American Art Therapy Association*, in 1983 (Rubin, 1999). The increasing number of publications, along with the founding of the American Art Therapy Association in 1969, evolved the professional identity of the art therapist, credentials, and the role of art therapists vis-à-vis related professionals (Shoemaker et al., 1976).

Contemporary Art Therapy Theories (Mid-1980s to Present)

The art therapy literature continues to grow. In 1974, Gantt and Schmal published an annotated bibliography of sources relating to the topic of art therapy from 1940–1973 (1,175 articles, books, and papers), yet Rubin (1999) notes that in that same year there were only 12 books written by art therapists, a number that crawled to 19 some 10 years later. By the mid-1980s this pace began to increase so that there are now more than 100 titles available. Rubin (1999) also speculates that art therapists may be more comfortable with an intuitive approach than other mental health practitioners because as artists they "pride themselves on their innate sensitivities, and tend to be anti-authoritarian and anti-theoretical" (p. 180).

Recently, approximately 21% of art therapists surveyed by the American Art Therapy Association described their primary theoretical orientation as "eclectic," the single largest percentage reported (Elkins & Stovall, 2000). This position is in keeping with one delineated by Wadeson (in Rubin, 1987/2001) and should not be surprising in a field that itself draws from a variety of disciplines. The next five most frequently reported models: psychodynamic (10.1%), Jungian (5.4%), object relations (4.6%), art as therapy (4.5%), and psychoanalytic (3.0%) all place a strong emphasis on intrapsychic dynamics, and this cumulative 27.6% suggests that much contemporary practice is still informed by generally psychodynamic concepts (Elkins & Stovall, 2000). In a landmark book, *Approaches to Art Therapy* first published in 1987, Rubin (1987/2001) brought together essays by authors representing the diversity of theoretical positions within the field. Perspectives from these and other relevant sources are briefly summarized here.

PSYCHODYNAMIC APPROACHES

The ideas of Freud and his followers (see Chapter 2, this volume) have been part of art therapy since the earliest days, although contemporary writers are more likely to apply terms such as "transference" and "the defense mechanisms" to articulate a position rather than employ classic psychoanalytic techniques with any degree of orthodoxy. Kramer, Rubin, Ulman, and Wilson (all cited in Rubin, 1987/2001) and Levick (1983) all use psychoanalytic language and concepts. Interpretations of the newer developments in psychoanalysis such as the theories of Klein (Weir, 1990), self psychology (Lachman-Chapin) and object relations theory (Robbins) can also be found in the art therapy literature (both cited in Rubin, 1987/2001).

With his emphasis on images from the unconscious, it was natural for Jung's concepts of analytical and archetypal psychology to cross over into art therapy (see Chapter 2, this volume). Work by Edwards and Wallace (both cited in Rubin, 1987/2001), McConeghey (1986), and Schaverian (1992) all reflect this emphasis.

HUMANISTIC APPROACHES

Elkins and Stovall (2000) suggest that only a small number of art therapists operate from a humanistic position (among humanistic, Gestalt, existential, and client centered; the highest response was to the first category with 2.9%). Yet if these approaches can be defined as sharing "an optimistic view of human nature and of the human condition, seeing people in a process of growth and development, with the potential to take responsibility for their fate" (Rubin, 1987/2001, p. 119), these figures belie a sentiment held by many art therapists (see Chapter 3, this volume).

Garai (cited in Rubin, 1987/2001) has written from a general humanistic position, Rogers (1993) and Silverstone (1997) use a person-centered model, and Dreikurs (1986) and Garlock (cited in Rubin, 1987) have adapted ideas first articulated by Alfred Adler. Other models that fall under the humanistic heading include existential (B. Moon, 1990/1995), phenomenological (Betensky, 1995), and gestalt (Rhyne, 1973/1995) approaches.

LEARNING AND DEVELOPMENTAL APPROACHES

Perhaps because they are perceived to be mechanistic, those psychological theories that emphasize learning tend to be less popular with art therapists. In the Elkins and Stovall (2000) survey, cognitive-behavioral (see Chapter 6, this volume), cognitive, developmental (Chapter 8, this volume), and behavioral received an endorsement of over 2%. Yet there are art therapy authors whose work has been informed by these theories.

Silver (2000) has written extensively on assessment using a cognitive approach, and the work of Lusebrink (1990) and Nucho (1987) is based in general systems theory. Art therapists working with children with emotional and developmental disabilities have also adapted concepts from developmental (Aach-Feldman & Kunkle-Miller, cited in Rubin, 1987/2001; Williams & Wood, 1975) and behavioral psychology (Roth, cited in Rubin, 1987/2001).

FAMILY THERAPY AND OTHER APPROACHES

A number of writers (Landgarten, 1987; Linesch, 1993; Riley & Malchiodi, 1994; Sobol, 1982) have built on Kwiatkowska's early family work, particularly in California where art therapists become licensed as marriage and family therapists. Riley (1999) also incorporates concepts from narrative therapy into her work (Chapter 5, this volume). Relational (Dalley, Rifkind, & Terry, 1993) and feminist (Hogan, 1997) approaches question the hierarchy in the client/therapist relationship and empowering the client and have also shaped contemporary art therapy practice. Publications by Horovitz-Darby (1994), Farrelly-Hansen (2001), and McNiff (1992) reflect an emphasis on spiritual and philosophical concepts over psychological theory. Franklin, Farrelly-Hansen, Marek, Swan-Foster, and Wallingford (2000) describe a transpersonal approach to art therapy. Allen (1992) called for a reversal of the perceived trend in overemphasizing the clinical orientation and encouraged art therapists to refocus on their artist identity. Writings by Lachman-Chapin (1983); Knill (1995), who espouses an expressive arts therapies approach (Chapter 8, this volume); and C. Moon (2002) reflect this studio approach to theory and practice.

CONCLUSION

Every art therapist knows there is much to be learned from the process of making an artwork as well as from standing back and viewing the finished product. The tapestry that is art therapy is not a dusty relic hung in a museum but a living work in progress. There is pleasure in admiring the work that has already been done and excitement in the weaving. It is my hope that readers can appreciate the processes and the products that have shaped this profession.

REFERENCES

Allen, P. B. (1992). Artist-in-residence: An alternative to "clinification" for art therapists. *Art Therapy: Journal of the American Art Therapy Association, 9,* 22–29.
Allen, P. B. (1995). *Art is a way of knowing.* Boston: Shambhala.
Anastasi, A., & Foley, J. (1941). A survey of the literature on artistic behavior in the abnormal: I. Historical and theoretical background. *Journal of General Psychology, 25,* 111–142.
Anderson, F. E. (1978/1992). *Art for all the children.* Springfield, IL: Charles C Thomas.
Arnheim, R. (1954). *Art and visual perception.* Berkeley: University of California Press.
Betensky, M. G. (1973). *Self-discovery through self-expression.* Springfield, IL: Charles C Thomas.
Betensky, M. G. (1995). *What do you see?: Phenomenology of therapeutic art expression.* London: Jessica Kingsley.

Borum, J. P. (1993/1994). Term warfare. *Raw Vision, 8,* 23–30.

Bruscia, K. (1988). Standards for clinical assessment in the arts therapies. *The Arts in Psychotherapy, 15,* 5–10.

Bush, J. (1997). *The handbook of school art therapy.* Springfield, IL: Charles C Thomas.

Cameron, J., & Bryan, M. (1992). *The artist's way: A spiritual path to higher creativity.* New York: Putnam.

Cane, F. (1951/1983). *The artist in each of us.* Craftsbury Common, VT: Art Therapy Publications/ Chicago: Magnolia Street.

Cohen, B. M., Hammer, J. S., & Singer, S. (1988). The Diagnostic Drawing Series: A systematic approach to art therapy evaluation and research. *The Arts in Psychotherapy, 15,* 11–21.

Cox, C. T., & Frame, P. (1993). Profile of the artist: MARI Card Test research results. *Art Therapy: Journal of the American Art Therapy Association, 10,* 23–29.

Dalley, T., Rifkind, G., & Terry, K. (1993). *Three voices of art therapy: Image, client, therapist.* London: Routledge.

Detre, K. C., Frank, T., Kniazzeh, C. R., Robinson, M. C., Rubin, J. A., & Ulman, E. (1983). Roots of art therapy: Margaret Naumburg (1890–1983) and Florence Cane (1882–1952): A family portrait. *American Journal of Art Therapy, 22,* 111–123.

Dissanayake, E. (1992). *Homo aestheticus: Where art comes from and why.* New York: Free Press.

Dreikurs, S. E. (1986). *Cows can be purple: My life and art therapy.* Chicago: Adler School of Professional Psychology.

Elkins, D. E., & Stovall, K. (2000). American Art Therapy Association, Inc.: 1998–1999 Membership survey report. *Art Therapy: Journal of the American Art Therapy Association, 17,* 41–46.

Elkisch, P. (1948). The "scribbling game": A projective method. *The Nervous Child, 7,* 247–256.

Farrelly-Hansen, M. (Ed.). (2001). *Spirituality and art therapy: Living the connection.* London: Jessica Kingsley.

Feder, B., & Feder, E. (1998). *The art and science of evaluation in the arts therapies: How do we know what's working?* Springfield, IL: Charles C Thomas.

Franklin, M., Farrelly-Hansen, M., Marek, B., Swan-Foster, N., & Wallingford, S. (2000). Transpersonal art therapy education. *Art Therapy: Journal of the American Art Therapy Association, 17,* 101–110.

Gantt, L., & Schmal, M. S. (1974). *Art therapy: A bibliography.* Rockville, MD: National Institute of Mental Health.

Gantt, L., & Tabone, C. (1997). *Rating manual for the Formal Elements Art Therapy Scale.* Morgantown, WV: Gargoyle Press.

Hammer, E. F. (Ed.). (1958/1980). *The clinical application of projective drawings.* Springfield, IL: Charles C Thomas.

Henley, D. R. (1992). *Exceptional children, exceptional art.* Worcester, MA: Davis.

Hogan, S. (Ed.). (1997). *Feminist approaches to art therapy.* London: Routledge.

Horovitz-Darby, E. G. (1994). *Spiritual art therapy.* Springfield, IL: Charles C Thomas.

Junge, M. B., & Asawa, P. P. (1994). *A history of art therapy in the United States.* Mundelein, IL: American Art Therapy Association.

Kaplan, F. F. (2000). *Art, science, and art therapy: Repainting the picture.* London: Jessica Kingsley.

Kellogg, R. (1969). *Analyzing children's art.* Palo Alto, CA: National Press.

Knill, P. J. (1995). The place of beauty in therapy and the arts. *The Arts in Psychotherapy, 22,* 1–7.

Kramer, E. (1958). *Art therapy in a children's community.* Springfield, IL: Charles C Thomas.

Kramer, E. (1971/1993) *Art as therapy with children.* New York: Schocken Books/Chicago: Magnolia Street.

Kramer, E., & Schehr, J. (1983). An art therapy evaluation session for children. *American Journal of Art Therapy, 23,* 3–12.

Kreitler, H., & Kreitler, S. (1972). *Psychology of the arts.* Durham, NC: Duke University Press.

Kris, E. (1952). *Psychoanalytic explorations in art.* New York: International Universities Press.

Kwiatkowska, H. Y. (1978). *Family therapy and evaluation through art.* Springfield, IL: Charles C Thomas.

Lachman-Chapin, M. (1983). The artist as clinician: An interactive technique in art therapy. *American Journal of Art Therapy, 23,* 13–25.

Lachman-Chapin, M., Jones, D., Sweig, T. L., Cohen, B. M., Semekoski, S. S., & Fleming, M. M. (1999). Connecting with the art world: Expanding beyond the mental health world. *Art Therapy: Journal of the American Art Therapy Association, 15,* 233–244.

Landgarten, H. B. (1981). *Clinical art therapy.* New York: Brunner/Mazel.

Landgarten, H. B. (1987). *Family art psychotherapy.* New York: Brunner/Mazel.

Landgarten, H. B. (1993). *Magazine photocollage: A multicultural assessment and treatment technique.* New York: Brunner/Mazel.

Levick, M. F. (1983). *They could not talk so they drew: Children's styles of coping and thinking.* Springfield, IL: Charles C Thomas.

Levick, M. F., Goldman, M. J., & Fink, P. J. (1967). Training for art therapists: Community mental health center and college of art join forces. *Bulletin of Art Therapy, 6,* 121–124.

Linesch, D. (1993). *Art therapy with families in crisis.* New York: Brunner/Mazel.

Lowenfeld, V. (1987). Therapeutic aspects of art education. *American Journal of Art Therapy, 25,* 111–146.

Lusebrink, V. B. (1990). *Imagery and visual expression in therapy.* New York: Plenum Press.

MacGregor, J. M. (1989). *The discovery of the art of the insane.* Princeton, NJ: Princeton University Press.

Machover, K. (1949/1980). *Personality projection in the drawing of the human figure.* Springfield, IL: Charles C Thomas.

Malchiodi, C. A. (1998). *The art therapy sourcebook.* Los Angeles: Lowell House.

Malchiodi, C. A. (1999a). *Medical art therapy with adults.* London: Jessica Kingsley.

Malchiodi, C. A. (1999b). *Medical art therapy with children.* London: Jessica Kingsley.

McConeghey, H. (1986). Archetypal art therapy is cross-cultural art therapy. *Art Therapy: Journal of the American Art Therapy Association, 3,* 111–114.

McNiff, S. (1981). *The arts and psychotherapy.* Springfield, IL: Charles C Thomas.

McNiff, S. (1992). *Art as medicine: Creating a therapy of the imagination.* Boston: Shambhala.

McNiff, S. (1998). *Art-based research.* London: Jessica Kingsley.

Mills, A., & Goodwin R. (1991). An informal survey of assessment use in child art therapy. *Art Therapy: Journal of the Art Therapy Association, 8,* 10–13.

Moon, B. L. (1990/1995) *Existential art therapy: The canvas mirror.* Springfield, IL: Charles C Thomas.

Moon, C. H. (2002). *Studio art therapy: Cultivating the artist identity in the art therapist.* London: Jessica Kingsley.

Naumburg, M. (1950/1973). *Introduction to art therapy: Studies of the "free" art expression of behavior problem children and adolescents as a means of diagnosis and therapy.* New York: Teachers College Press/Chicago: Magnolia Street.

Naumburg, M. (1966/1987). *Dynamically oriented art therapy.* New York: Grune & Stratton/Chicago: Magnolia Street.

Nucho, A. O. (1987). *The psychocybernetic model of art therapy.* Springfield, IL: Charles C Thomas.

Prinzhorn, H. (1995). *Artistry of the mentally ill.* Vienna: Springer-Verlag. (Original work published in German, 1922)

Rhyne, J. (1973/1995). *The Gestalt art experience.* Monterey, CA: Brooks/Cole/Chicago: Magnolia Street.

Riley, S. (1999). *Contemporary art therapy with adolescents.* London: Jessica Kingsley.

Riley, S., & Malchiodi, C. A. (1994). *Integrative approaches to family art therapy.* Chicago: Magnolia Street.

Robbins, A., & Sibley, L. (1976) *Creative art therapy.* New York: Brunner/Mazel.

Rogers, N. (1993). *The creative connection: Expressive arts as healing.* Palo Alto, CA: Science and Behavior Books.

Rubin, J. A. (1978/1984). *Child art therapy: Understanding and helping children through art.* New York: Van Nostrand Reinhold/Wiley.

Rubin, J. A. (1987/2001) *Approaches to art therapy: Theory and technique.* New York: Brunner/Mazel/Philadelphia: Brunner-Routledge.

Rubin, J. A. (1999). *Art therapy: An introduction.* Philadelphia: Brunner/Mazel.

Russell, C. (2002). Simply art. *Raw Vision, 38,* 36–41.

Schaverien, J. (1992). *The revealing image: Analytical art psychotherapy in theory and practice.* London: Routledge.

Shaw, R. F. (1934). *Finger painting, a perfect medium for expression.* Boston: Little, Brown.

Shoemaker, R .H., Ulman, E., Anderson, F. E., Wallace, E., Lachman-Chapin, M., Wolf, R., & Kramer, E. (1976). Art therapy: An exploration of definitions. In R. Shoemaker & S. Gonick-Barris (Eds.), *Creativity and the art therapist's identity, Proceedings of the 7th Annual American Art Therapy Association Conference* (pp. 86–96). Baltimore: American Art Therapy Association.

Sigler, H. (1993). *Breast cancer journal: Walking with the ghosts of my grandmothers* [Exhibition catalog, Rockford College Art Gallery]. Rockford, IL: Johnson Press.

Silver, R. A. (2000). *Art as language: Access to thoughts and feelings through stimulus drawings.* Philadelphia: Brunner-Routledge.

Silverstone, L. (1997). *Art therapy: The person-centered way.* London: Jessica Kingsley.

Sobol, B. S. (1982). Art therapy and strategic family therapy. *American Journal of Art Therapy, 21,* 43–52.

Spaniol, S. E. (1990). *Organizing exhibitions of art by people with mental illness: A step-by-step manual.* Boston: Boston University Center for Psychiatric Rehabilitation.

Uhlin, D. M. (1972/1984). *Art for exceptional children.* Dubuque, IA: Brown.

Ulman, E., & Dachinger, P. (1975/1996). *Art therapy in theory and practice.* New York: Schocken Books/Chicago: Magnolia Street.

Ulman, E., Kramer, E., & Kwiatkowska, H. Y. (1978). *Art therapy in the United States.* Craftsbury Common, VT: Art Therapy Publications.

Vick, R. M. (2000). Creative dialog: A shared will to create. *Art Therapy: Journal of the American Art Therapy Association, 17,* 216–219.

Wadeson, H. (1980). *Art psychotherapy.* New York: Wiley.

Wadeson, H. (Ed.). (1992). *A guide to conducting art therapy research.* Mundelein, IL: American Art Therapy Association.

Waller, D. E. (1991). *Becoming a profession: The history of art therapy in Britain 1940–1982.* London: Tavistock/Routledge.

Waller, D. E. (1998). Towards a European art therapy. Buckingham, UK: Open University Press.

Weir, F. (1990). The role of symbolic expression in its relation to art therapy: A Kleinian approach. In T. Dalley, C. Case, J. Schaverian, F. Weir, D. Halliday, P. N. Hall, & D. Waller (Eds.), *Images of art therapy: New developments in theory and practice* (pp. 109–127). London: Tavistock/Routledge.

Williams, G. H., & Wood, M. M. (1975). *Developmental art therapy.* Baltimore: University Park Press.

Winnicott, D. W. (1971). *Therapeutic consultations in child psychiatry.* New York: Basic Books.

Wix, L. (2000). Looking for what's lost: The artistic roots of art therapy: Mary Huntoon. *Art Therapy: Journal of the American Art Therapy Association, 17,* 168–176.

CHAPTER 2

Art Therapy
and the Brain

Cathy A. Malchiodi

Art therapy has historically resisted an association with science and has favored a more art-based stance in its philosophy and practice. However, recent scientific findings about how images influence emotion, thoughts, and well-being and how the brain and body react to the experience of drawing, painting, or other art activities are clarifying why art therapy may be effective with a variety of populations. As science learns more about the connection between emotions and health, stress and disease, and the brain and immune system, art therapy is discovering new frontiers for the use of imagery and art expression in treatment.

Over the last several decades, a growing body of knowledge from science and medicine has redefined mental health interventions. In 1993, Bill Moyers brought to public consciousness "mind–body medicine" in a public television series, *Healing and the Mind*. "Mind–body medicine" is a popular term used to describe an approach that views the mind as having a central impact on the body's health. Although it has received attention over the last several decades, it is not a new idea because many mind–body techniques such as meditation and yoga have been around for thousands of years. Researchers such as Benson (1975, 1996), who has investigated the "relaxation response," and Ader (2001), who is a leader in the field of psychoneuroimmunology (the integrated study of the mind, neuroendocrine system, and the immune system), and others have expanded the incorporation of mind–body methods into mainstream medicine.

Neuroscience, the study of the brain and its functions, is rapidly influencing both the scope and practice of psychotherapy and mind–body approaches. As new technologies allow researchers to scan brain and other neurological and physiological activity in the body, we are learning more about the relationship between mind and body. Damasio (1994), Sapolsky (1998), and Ramachandran (1999), among others, have described the neurological and physiological phenomena related to memory and how images conceptualized and how they affect the brain and body. Siegel (1999); van der Kolk, McFarlane, and Weisaeth (1996); and Schore (1994) have broadened the understanding of how the brain, human physiology, and emotions are intricately intertwined, the importance of early attachment on neurological functions throughout life, and the impact of trauma on memory. These findings are far-reaching, affecting how psychotherapy is being designed and delivered.

The relationship between neuroscience and art therapy is an important one that influences every area of practice (Malchiodi, Riley, & Hass-Cohen, 2001). Kaplan (2000) underscores the overall importance of scientific-mindness in the practice of art therapy, the significance of neuroscience to the field, and the relevance of mind–body unity to mental imagery and artistic activity. Ultimately, science will be central to understanding and defining how art therapy actually works and why it is a powerful therapeutic modality.

ART THERAPY AS A MIND–BODY INTERVENTION

The National Center for Complementary and Alternative Medicine (NCCAM, 2002), a division of the National Institutes of Health (NIH), has defined mind–body interventions as those which are designed to facilitate the mind's capacity to influence bodily function and symptoms. Many approaches that have a well-documented theoretical basis, such as patient education and cognitive-behavioral approaches, are now characterized as "mainstream" by NCCAM. Art therapy is considered a mind–body intervention, although it has been used mostly as a form of psychotherapy rather than an intervention that modifies physiology, symptoms, and other aspects of health (National Institutes of Health, 1994). Only recently research in art therapy is beginning to indicate why it can be used as a mind–body method (Malchiodi, 1993, 1999). For example, DeLue (1999) demonstrated the physiological effects of drawing mandalas with a group of school-age children, using biofeedback to measure skin temperature along with blood pressure and pulse monitors. Camic (1999) conducted a study using visual art and other art forms along with cognitive-behavioral techniques, meditation, and mental imagery to reduce chronic pain in adults. Others have investigated how art making complements medical treatment and supports patients' abilities to cope with symptoms and stress (Anand & Anand, 1999; Gabriels, 1999; Hiltebrand, 1999; Lusebrink, 1990).

In general, studies of mind–body interventions (including art therapy), while promising, have had some major shortcomings. For example, much of the research in this area has yet to be replicated by independent investigators. Also, there are no clearly explained reasons why some initially promising interventions have yielded conflicting results in subsequent studies. Fortunately, with the advent of increasingly sophisticated technology that has broadened an understanding of the brain and its relationship to the body, more evidence is emerging that will demonstrate why, how, and with whom mind–body interventions are effective.

NEUROSCIENCE AND ART THERAPY

How the brain functions and how it influences emotions, cognition, and behavior are important in the treatment of most problems people bring to therapy, including mood disorders, posttraumatic stress, addictions, and physical illness. Although many areas of research are relevant to the practice of psychotherapy, several areas are particularly important to art therapy. These areas include images and image formation, physiology of emotion, attachment theory, and the placebo effect.

Images and Image Formation

Common sense tells us that images do have an impact on how we feel and react. For example, just imagining biting into a lemon may cause one's mouth to pucker and seeing a favorite food may cause one to salivate. Images can create sensations of pleasure, fear, anxiety, or calm and there is evidence that they can alter mood and even induce a sense of well-being (Benson, 1975). There is solid evidence that images have a significant impact on our bodies. Simple experiments have provided evidence that even exposure to the images of nature from a hospital room window can decrease the length of stay and increase feelings of well-being in patients (Ulrich, 1984).

   Art therapist Vija Lusebrink (1990) observes that images are "a bridge between body and mind, or between the conscious levels of information processing and the physiological changes in the body" (p. 218). Guided imagery, an experiential process in which an individual is directed through relaxation followed by suggestions to imagine specific images, has been used to reduce symptoms, change mood, and harness the body's healing capacities. Art therapists and others have applied principles of mental imagery and guided imagery to work with individuals in a variety of settings. For example, Baron (1989) employed guided imagery as a part of art therapy in the treatment of individuals with cancer.

   Until relatively recently, researchers have only been able to speculate about how guided imagery works. Neuroscience is rapidly increasing the understanding of mental imagery, image formation, and the regions of the brain involved in image creation. For example, research shows that imagery we see or we imagine activates the visual cortex of the brain in similar ways. In other words, according to Damasio (1994), our bodies respond to mental images as if they are reality. He also notes that images are not just visual and include all sensory modalities—auditory, olfactory, gustatory, and somatosensory (touch, muscular, temperature, pain, visceral, and vestibular senses). Images are not stored in any one part of the brain; rather, many regions of the brain are part of image formation, storage, and retrieval.

   The increasing understanding of the brain's hemispheres and their interactions has also contributed to the understanding of mental images and art making. In the past, it was believed that the right and left brain generally had two different functions; the right brain was the center of intuition, creativity, while the left brain was thought to be engaged in logical thought and language. Some claimed art therapy's value was due to its ability to tap right brain functions, observing that art making is a "right-brained" activity (Virshup, 1978). In reality, the brain's left hemisphere (where language is located) is also involved in making art. Gardner (1984), Ramachandran (1999), and others have demonstrated that both hemispheres of the brain are necessary for art expression and evidence can be seen in the drawings of people with damage to specific areas of the brain. Researchers have also discovered connections between language and certain movements in drawing. For example, in a study using positron emission tomography (PET) scan, brain activity of individuals drawing forms in space was recorded. The results indicate that even simple drawing involves complex interactions between many parts of the brain (Frith & Law, 1995).

Images and image formation, whether mental images or those drawn on paper, are important in all art therapy practice because through art making clients are invited to reframe how they feel, respond to an event or experience, and work on emotional and behavioral change. In contrast to mental images, however, art making allows an individual to actively try out, experiment with, or rehearse a desired change through a drawing, painting, or collage; that is, it involves a tangible object that can be physically altered.

Attachment Theory

Attachment theory (Bowlby, 1969) has been used as a theoretical base for psychotherapy for many years but has more recently become a major focus of neuroscience and renewed interest among therapists. Siegel (1999) explains attachment as follows: "Attachment is an inborn system in the brain that evolves in ways that influence and organize motivational, emotional, and memory processes with respect to significant caregiving figures" (p. 67). Schore (1994) offers a neurological model for the importance of infant attachment throughout life. He notes that soon after birth the caretaker and infant develop interactions that are important to the process of affect regulation. Face-to-face contact and soothing touch are examples of ways the infant learns to respond to stimulation from people and experiences. Perry, Pollard, Blakley, Baker, and Vigilante (1995) proposes that successful attachment is critical to optimal development of specific parts of the brain. He believes that a healthy attachment between infant and caretaker sets the stage for the individual to develop the capacity to "self-regulate" stimulating experiences. Early childhood bonding is imprinted on the brain, laying a foundation for relationship patterns later in life; when trauma is present, brain imprinting is changed, but may be corrected with appropriate intervention.

Research in neuroscience is demonstrating that infancy is not the only chance a person has for healthy attachment and there seem to be ways to reshape and repair some early experiences. Art therapy is one way being explored to reestablish healthy attachments, both through therapist and client, and through encouraging healthy interactions between parent and child. Riley (2001) cites how art activities are being used in early childhood attachment programs and how simple drawing exercises can be used to resolve relational problems and strengthen parent–child bonds. She explains that the nonverbal dimensions of art activities tap early relational states before words are dominant, possibly allowing the brain to establish new, more productive patterns.

Siegel (1999) and Schore (1994) believe that interactions between baby and caretaker are right-brain mediated because during infancy the right cortex is developing more quickly than the left. Siegel also observes that just as the left hemisphere requires exposure to language to grow, the right hemisphere requires emotional stimulation to develop properly. He goes on to say that the output of the right brain is expressed in "non-word-based ways" such as drawing a picture or using a picture to describe feelings or events. According to this idea, art therapy may be an important modality in working with attachment issues, among other emotionally related disorders or experiences.

The Physiology of Emotion

It is well-known that the body is often a mirror of an individual's emotions. When we are anxious, our palms sweat or our faces may be ashen, or we may turn red when embarrassed. Images affect our emotions and different parts of the brain may become active when we look at sad faces or happy faces or mentally image a happy or sad event or relationship (Sternberg, 2001). There are also a variety of hormonal fluctuations as well as cardiovascular and neurological effects. In fact, the physiology of emotions is so complex that the brain knows more than the conscious mind can itself reveal (Damasio, 1994). That is, one can actually display an emotion without being conscious of what induced the emotion.

Trauma has received increasing attention in neuroscience because it is now believed to be both a psychological and physiological experience. There is general agreement that traumatic events take a toll on the body as well as the mind and, thus, posttraumatic stress disorder (PTSD) is defined through both psychological and physiological symptoms. Many have pointed to the true core of trauma as being physiological (Rothchild, 2000; Levine, 1997), and, as van der Kolk metaphorically notes, "the body keeps the score" of the emotional experience.

Although many parts of the brain are important in trauma, the limbic system, the seat of survival instincts and reflexes, has been given considerable attention. It includes the hypothalamus, the hippocampus, and the amygdala, which is also pertinent to understanding traumatic memory. Though the function of the limbic system will not be covered in detail here, recent findings indicate its role in the sensory memories of stressful events and trauma. These findings are revealing why art expression is a useful part of therapy, trauma debriefing, and psychological recovery. Because the core of traumatic experiences is physiological, the expression and processing of sensory memories of the traumatic event are essential to successful intervention and resolution (Rothchild, 2000; Schore, 1994). Art is a natural sensory mode of expression because it involves touch, smell, and other senses within the experience. Drawing and other art activities mobilizes the expression of sensory memories (Steele, 1997; Steele & Raider, 2001) in a way that verbal interviews and interventions cannot. Highly charged emotional experiences, such as trauma, are encoded by the limbic system as a form of sensory reality (Malchiodi et al., 2001). For a person's experience of trauma to be successfully ameliorated, it must be processed through sensory means. The capacity of art making to tap sensory material (i.e., the limbic system's sensory memory of the event) makes it a potent tool in trauma intervention. Specific drawing tasks, such as "draw what happened" (Pynoos & Eth, 1985; Malchiodi, 2001; Steele, 1997) and other related directives are proving to be effective in tapping sensory memories as well as generating narratives that can be altered through cognitive reframing techniques (Steele & Raider, 2001) to reduce long-term sequelae of posttraumatic stress.

The way in which memory is stored is also shedding light on why art therapy may be helpful to those who are traumatized. There are two types of memory: explicit memory is conscious and is composed of facts, concepts, and ideas and implicit memory is sensory and emotional and is related to the body's memories. Riding a bicycle is good example of implicit memory; narrating the chronological details of an event is an example of explicit memory. Currently, there is some speculation that PTSD, in part, may be caused when memory of trauma is excluded from explicit storage (Rothchild, 2000). Problems also result from traumatic memories when implicit memories are not linked to explicit memories; that is, an individual may not have access to the context in which the emotions or sensations arose. Art expression may help to bridge the implicit and explicit memories of a stressful event by facilitating the creation of a narrative through which the person can explore the memories and why they are so upsetting. Art activities, in this sense, may help the traumatized individual to think and feel concurrently, while making meaning for troubling experiences.

Finally, art therapy can be used to tap the body's relaxation response. Drawing, for example, is hypothesized to facilitate children's verbal reports of emotionally laden events in several ways: reduction of anxiety, helping the child feel comfortable with the therapist, increasing memory retrieval, organizing narratives, and prompting the child to tell more details than in a solely verbal interview (Gross & Haynes, 1998). Malchiodi (1997, 2001) observed in working with children from violent homes that art activity had a soothing, hypnotic influence and that traumatized children were naturally attracted to this quality when anxious or suffering from posttraumatic stress. Someday, through the use of brain scans and other technology, we may have a clearer understanding of exactly how to use art therapy to tap the relaxation response for clients of all ages who have undergone intense stress.

Placebo Effect

The power of belief, often referred to as the placebo effect, is an effective mind–body intervention that can enhance healing and well-being (Sternberg, 2001). Art therapy, like other forms of therapy or treatment, can enhance the placebo effect because it involves the individual's confidence in the therapist and therapy, a special place of healing (in this case, the art therapy room), and an activity that the person performs (drawing, painting, or other art making). These are well-known elements recognized to contribute to the placebo effect in both psychotherapy and medicine.

Benson (1996), acclaimed for his work with the relaxation response, observes that it is possible for everyone to remember the calm and confidence associated with health and happiness. Even when physically ill, individuals can access what Benson calls "remembered wellness," increasing the sense of well-being despite distress or illness. In trauma intervention, recalling memories of positive events that can reframe and eventually override negative ones is helpful in reducing posttraumatic stress, particularly if a sensory experience of remembered wellness is included. Simple art activities such as drawing a pleasant time appear to be effective because of the sensory capacity of image making to more deeply recall actual memories and details of positive moments (Malchiodi et al., 2001).

While faith in treatment is thought to be a central feature of the placebo effect, it may be other aspects heretofore unacknowledged that contribute to healing. Tinnin (1994) proposes that art therapy facilitates healing in a similar way to the placebo effect because it uses mimicry, an instinctive, preverbal function of the brain that is basic to self-soothing. An example of mimicry might be a child stroking a blanket in a way that mimics a mother's soothing to activate an internal process of self-relaxation. Art making may stimulate a similar experience and provide experiences that self-soothe and repair, as noted in the previous section. According to Tinnin, this type of experience intentionally stimulates self-healing through placebo effect. He adds that "art therapy has a unique and specific potential relative to self-healing because of the way art affects the brain" (p. 77).

CONCLUSION

Neuroscience continues to provide an ever-widening understanding of how the brain and body react to stress, trauma, illness, and other events. It also is central to understanding how images influence emotions, thoughts, and well-being and how the visual, sensory, and expressive language of art are best integrated into treatment. Using neuroscience as a point of reference explains many of the approaches to art therapy discussed in this volume. For example, the application of object relations theory is enhanced with what is currently known about attachment and cognitive-behavioral approaches are supported by an understanding of images, image formation, and the physiology of emotions.

The impact of neuroscience on all aspects of health care will literally repaint the picture (Kaplan, 2000) of how art therapy is used in the treatment of emotional and physical disorders in the future. As additional research on neuropsychology and mind–body paradigms emerge, we will undoubtedly learn more about how artistic expression helps individuals with emotional distress or physical illness and why images and image making are central to enhancing health and well-being.

REFERENCES

Ader, R. (Ed.). (2001). *Psychoneuroimmunology* (3rd ed.). New York: Academic Press.

Anand, S., & Anand, V. (1999). Art therapy with laryngectomy patients. In C. Malchiodi (Ed.), *Medical art therapy with adults* (pp. 63–85). London: Jessica Kingsley.

Baron, P. (1989). Fighting cancer with images. In H. Wadeson (Ed.), *Advances in art therapy* (pp. 148–168). New York: Wiley.

Benson, H. (1975). *The relaxation response.* New York: Avon.

Benson, H. (1996). *Timeless healing: The power and biology of belief.* New York: Scribner.

Bowlby, J. (1969). *Attachment.* New York: Basic Books.

Camic, P. (1999). Expanding treatment possibilities for chronic pain through the expressive arts. In C. Malchiodi (Ed.), *Medical art therapy with adults* (pp. 43–61). London: Jessica Kingsley.

Damasio, A. (1994). *Descarte's error.* New York: Putnam.

Delue, C. (1999). Physiological effects of creating mandalas. In C. Malchiodi (Ed.), *Medical art therapy with children* (pp. 33–49). London: Jessica Kingsley.

Frith, C., & Law, J. (1995). Cognitive and physiological processes underlying drawing skills. *Leonardo, 28*(3), 203–205.

Gabriels, R. (1999). Treating children with asthma: A creative approach. In C. Malchiodi (Ed.), *Medical art therapy with children* (pp. 95–111). London: Jessica Kingsley.

Garnder, H. (1984). *Art, mind, and brain.* New York: Basic Books.

Gross, J., & Haynes, H. (1998). Drawing facilitates children's verbal reports of emotional laden events. *Journal of Experimental Psychology, 4,* 163–179.

Hiltebrand, E. (1999). Coping with cancer through image manipulation. In C. Malchiodi (Ed.), *Medical art therapy with adults* (pp. 113–135). London: Jessica Kingsley.

Kaplan, F. (2000). *Art, science, and art therapy: Repainting the picture.* London: Jessica Kingsley.

Levine, P. (1997). *Waking the tiger.* Berkeley, CA: North Atlantic.

Lusebrink V. B. (1990) *Imagery and visual expression in therapy.* New York: Plenum Press.

Malchiodi C. A. (1993). Art and medicine. *Art Therapy: Journal of the American Art Therapy Association. 10*(2), 66–69.

Malchiodi C. A. (1997). *Breaking the silence: Art therapy with children from violent homes.* New York: Brunner/Mazel.

Malchiodi, C. A. (Ed.). (1999). *Medical art therapy with adults.* London: Jessica Kingsley.

Malchiodi, C. A. (2001). Using drawings as intervention with traumatized children. *Trauma and Loss: Research and Interventions, 1*(1), 21–27.

Malchiodi, C. A., Riley, S., & Hass-Cohen, N. (2001). *Toward an integrated art therapy mind–body landscape* [Audiotape #108–1525]. Denver, CO: National Audio Video.

National Center for Complementary and Alternative Medicine. (2002). *Major domains of complementary and alternative medicine* [Online]. Available: http://nccam.nih.gov/fcp/classify/.

National Institute for Health. (1994). *Alternative medicine: Expanding medical horizons* [#94–066]. Washington, DC: U.S. Government Printing Office.

Perry, B. D., Pollard, R. A., Blakley, T. L., Baker, W. L., & Vigilante, D. (1995). Childhood trauma, the neurobiology of adaptation and use-dependent development of the brain: How states become traits. *Infant Mental Health Journal, 16,* 271–291.

Pynoos, R., & Eth, S. (1985). Developmental perspective on psychic trauma in childhood. In C. R. Figley (Ed.), *Trauma and its wake* (pp. 193–216). New York: Brunner/Mazel.

Ramachandran, V. (1999). *Phantoms of the brain.* New York: Quill.

Riley, S. (2001). *Group process made visible.* New York: Brunner-Routledge.

Rothchild, B. (2000). *The body remembers: The psychophysiology of trauma and trauma treatment.* New York: Norton.

Sapolsky R. (1998). *Why zebras don't get ulcers.* New York: Freeman.

Schore, A. (1994). *Affect regulation and the origin of the self.* Hillsdale, NJ: Erlbaum.

Siegel D. J. (1999). *The developing mind: Towards a neurobiology of interpersonal experience.* New York: Guilford Press.

Steele, W. (1997). *Trauma response kit: Short-term intervention model.* Grosse Pointe Woods, MI: Institute for Trauma and Loss in Children.

Steele, W., & Raider, M. (2001). Structured sensory intervention for traumatized children, adolescents, and parents. *Trauma and Loss: Research and Interventions, 1*(1), 8–20.

Sternberg, E. (2001). *The balance within: The science connecting health and emotions.* New York: Freeman.

Tinnin, L. (1994). Transforming the placebo effect in art therapy. *American Journal of Art Therapy, 32*(3), 75–78.

Ulrich, R. (1984). View through a window may influence recovery from surgery. *Science, 224,* 420–421.

van der Kolk, B. A., McFarlane, A. C., & Weisaeth, L. (1996). *Traumatic stress: The effects of overwhelming experience on mind, body, and society.* New York: Guilford Press.

Virshup, E. (1978). *Right-brained people in a left-brained world.* Los Angeles: Guild of Tutors Press.

CHAPTER 3

Art-Based Assessments

Frances F. Kaplan

Most art therapists have had this experience: An acquaintance, a student, another (well-meaning) mental health professional thrusts a drawing in front of the art therapist and says, "This was done by a male/female of such and such an age. Please tell me what it means." The art therapist then usually replies, "I'm sorry, but I can't do that. I need to know about the context in which this drawing was created; I need some background information on the person who drew it; and most of all, I need to hear from the artist about what the different images in the drawing mean to him or her." The presenter of the drawing then retreats, looking a bit crestfallen and probably feeling more than a little puzzled.

Is it true that art therapists can tell nothing by simply looking at an individual drawing or other piece of art? Don't art therapists use art-based assessments to develop a treatment plan? What about all those manuals for evaluating drawings, are they completely wrong? The answers to these questions are "no," "yes," and "no," respectively. But having given these answers, I have done little to enlighten the reader. Indeed, rather like replying to the question "Have you stopped beating your husband?" with a yes or a no, these responses are misleading without further elaboration. The purpose of this chapter, then, is to examine relevant research concerning what can and what cannot be told by looking at art and to discuss what art therapists look for when they conduct art-based assessments.

WHAT ART CANNOT TELL US

Negative Evidence Concerning Projective Drawings

As a result of the body of research bearing on the validity of projective drawing tests, many psychologists and research-minded art therapists do not hold these techniques in high esteem. For example, psychologist Stuart Vyse (1997) has intimated that projective drawing techniques have no validity. Similarly, art therapist and researcher Linda Gantt has admonished us to "re-examine the assumption underlying virtually all projective drawings—that the constituent parts somehow reflect personality traits" (Williams, Agell, Gantt, & Goodman, 1996, p. 20).

It is the perennially popular Draw-A-Person (DAP) that has been most thoroughly investigated. And, as suggested by Gantt, it is the interpretation of this projective technique based on individual drawing "signs" that has come off most poorly. Sophia Kahill (1984), extending the surveys of relevant research undertaken by Swensen (1957, 1968), has profiled allegedly significant features of human figure drawings that have received little empirical support. These include placement on page, stance, perspective, erasures, omissions, distortions, transparencies, eyebrows, ears, hair, presence of sexual organs, and sex of first-drawn figure. In addition, Kahill reported that studies pertaining to other drawing features revealed either conflicting results or negative results based on a single study. Indeed, she found just one interpretive assumption—the emotional impact of color—that had received anything like convincing support.

More recent investigations and reviews have backed up Kahill's findings (Groth-Marnat, 1997; Joiner, Schmidt, & Barnett, 1996; Motta, Little, & Tobin, 1993; Smith & Dumont, 1995). Furthermore, although not as well studied as the DAP, House–Tree–Person (HTP) drawings have not fared much better in the research literature. For example, art therapist Anita Rankin (1994) reviewed psychology research and conducted a small study bearing on the validity of trauma indicators in tree drawings. Although she found some support for a relationship between multiple signs of injury (scars, broken branches, absence of leaves) and past trauma, she found little support for the conventional interpretation that one or two knotholes signify a traumatic event. Nor did she find support for the notion that the date of a traumatic event can be estimated from the position of the knothole on the trunk of the tree.

The Puzzling Popularity of Projective Drawings

Interestingly, in spite of the large volume of negative evidence, the DAP, HTP, and similar projective drawing techniques have remained popular with clinicians (Groth-Marnat, 1997; Motta et al., 1993). A number of researchers have offered explanations for this puzzling fact. Psychologists Loren Chapman and Jean Chapman (1971) have suggested that "illusory correlation" is responsible. As defined by this husband and wife research team, illusory correlation is "the tendency to see two things as occurring together more often than they actually do" (p. 20). They have also shown this phenomenon in action through a series of cleverly designed experiments. In one of their studies, college students unfamiliar with the DAP were given figure drawings with descriptive statements about the problems of the supposed artists. The students were asked to examine the drawings for features common to those with the same problems. Although there were no real relationships between the drawings and the attached statements, relationships were perceived by almost every student. Moreover, the relationships that the students saw (e.g., large head accompanies concern with intelligence) were similar to ones that experienced clinicians had reported finding in their clinical work.

The disturbing implication that not only untrained students but experienced diagnosticians tend to see what they expect has received support from a more recent study by David Smith and Frank Dumont (1995). A mixed group of 36 experienced and novice psychotherapists were asked to comment on a case file that included a drawing of a male figure. More than half of the research participants incorporated the DAP in their commentary—unaware that it had been drawn by someone other than the man described in the file. Results revealed that the trained and the untrained gave similar interpretations of the drawing, apparently influenced by their understanding of the case. For instance, a novice clinician stated, "The eyes look a little paranoid," while a professed expert remarked, "His eyes are strange and overemphasized. I think he may have . . . some paranoid suspiciousness" (Smith & Dumont, 1995, p. 301).

Finally, Zev William Wanderer (1969/1997), another researcher who investigated the DAP and found it wanting, has offered a possible explanation for the ongoing popularity of projective drawings that suggests why clinicians have found it so hard to see beyond their expectations. He conjectures: "Could the occasional, eloquent drawing provide the clinician with partial reinforcement, producing greater resistance to extinction?" (p. 313). Ruefully, I am inclined to respond in the affirmative as for years I used in my teaching just such an eloquent—and exceptional—drawing (see Figure 3.1, discussed later in the chapter).

WHAT ART CAN TELL US

The Promise of Global Ratings

About now, one might be tempted to consign all manuals for assessing artwork to the recycling bin. But wait—as I have suggested, at least some of them have merit. Certain kinds of evaluative approaches have indeed received favorable notice from researchers. For example, Smith and Dumont (1995) have summarized Swenson's (1968) findings as follows: "Of the various relationships between drawings and diagnostic criteria that have been researched, only the relationship between global measures (i.e., rating schemes that consider the drawing as a whole or a set of specific features in the drawing) and diagnoses of gross maladjustment has reached levels of statistical significance with some consistency" (Smith & Dumont, 1995, p. 299).

Although Smith and Dumont apparently meant to emphasize the limitations of drawing assessments, others have been encouraged by the inherent possibilities of global ratings. Among these are psychologists who have argued for a fresh approach to DAP research (Riethmiller & Handler, 1997; Waehler, 1997), clinicians who have constructed or discovered ratings that differentiate people with specific problems (Marsh, Linberg, & Smeltzer, 1991; Munley, 2002; Tharinger & Stark, 1990; Waldman, Silber, Holmstrom, & Karp, 1994), and art therapists who have developed standardized art-based assessments (Cohen, Mills, & Kijak, 1994; Gantt & Tabone, 1998; Silver, 1996; see also Appendix I, this volume).

The evidence is compelling, then, that global ratings have more claim to validity than sign-based interpretations. But let us examine what this means. First, it means the "projective hypothesis" is not supported. That is, the twin assumptions that constructed images represent the persons who created them and that parts of images are unconscious representations of personality traits simply do not apply in a reliable manner. Concerning tree drawings, Rankin (1994) has pointed out that the tree may represent the artist, a person other than the artist, or even just a tree. Further, Kahill (1984) has concluded that "in contrast to the hypothesis that drawing tests are revealing undisclosed aspects of personality, subjects may be aware to some extent of what the drawings reveal" (p. 273).

Second, it means that art activity can be more or less exclusively viewed as samples of cognitive and behavioral functioning. In fact, psychologist Howard Knoff (1993) states that "there are only two defensible ways, using two particular theoretical perspectives—the behavioral and the cognitive-behavioral—in which [human figure drawings] can be used" (p. 193). He goes on to explain that behavioral information can be gained from observing the individual engaged in a specific task (e.g., drawing) and that cognitive information can be obtained through discussion of the task (e.g., postdrawing inquiry). The logic of Knoff's formulation is self-evident. Furthermore, it can be extended to encompass important cognitive and behavioral information that can be gleaned from the art itself.

Consider the following. A person who is clinically depressed has little energy, poor concentration, and an overall bleak view of the world. Contrariwise, a person experiencing mania is highly energized, has euphoric feelings, and exhibits excited behavior. In addition, other clinical conditions have their own distinct patterns of symptoms that are manifested through the cognitions and behaviors of the afflicted individuals. Thus far, I have done little more than state the obvious. But also consider that because art making is a cognitive-behavioral activity, it is a reasonable assumption that the art product will provide indications of the artist's mental condition. And this is what art therapists have found (e.g., Gantt & Tabone, 1998; Wadeson, 1980): Depressed people frequently produce constricted drawings with minimal detail, little color, and static images while manic individuals tend to create drawings that are colorful, expansive, and full of movement, and so on for other major psychiatric syndromes. Further, it has been noted that once clients' symptoms abate, their artwork tends to return to normal (Swenson, 1968; Williams et al., 1996).

Third, scientific support for global measures lends credence to an aspect of drawing analysis yet to be mentioned. Aside from detecting serious but transient psychopathology, drawings can be used as rough indicators of children's level of cognitive development. There is substantial evidence that children pass through more or less predictable stages of artistic development that are age-related and that can be recognized in the formal elements of their drawings (Anderson, 1992; Golomb, 1992; Groth-Marnat, 1997; Hagood, 2002; Wadeson, 2000).

In sum, a reliable approach to evaluating art puts the emphasis on global aspects of form rather than on content, or sign, interpretation. It also views resultant evaluations as reflective of present (not past or future) functioning. Moreover, it is most useful when supplemented by observation of behavior manifested while producing the art and by comments made concerning the completed work.

Caveats

But in spite of the apparent utility of global ratings, two caveats must be tendered. To begin with, effort must be made to control for artistic training and ability. Some years ago, I took initial steps to develop a drawing rating scheme for ego development using an adult sample (Kaplan, 1991). I obtained a weak correlation between my ratings of formal drawing elements and a verbal measure of ego development. This correlation was enhanced, however, by removing from the sample those with minimal art experience. To my surprise, the influence of drawing skill on my rating scheme turned out to be my most compelling result. Other assessment researchers have also found evidence of this confounding variable (Cressen, 1975; Koppitz, 1984).

Likewise, cultural variations in artwork must be taken into account. In regard to gauging a child's level of cognitive development based on formal elements of art, art therapist Frances Anderson (1992) states that "recent studies have underscored the importance of cultural, educational and societal influences on how the child responds to art, executes art, and understands artistic endeavors. These scholars have highlighted the importance that subcultural influences (including the child's immediate family) play and the impact that schooling has on the child's ability to engage in artistic activity" (p. 138).

Successfully controlling for artistic skill and cultural influence will mean creating norms for different skill levels and different cultures and subcultures—a daunting task. Although some work along these lines has been done for specific drawing tests (e.g., Silver, 1998), we still have a long way to go. Until we have more comprehensive data, it is important to temper conclusions based on global ratings when it appears that the client does not fit the general characteristics of the population used to develop and standardize the particular rating scheme.

ART-BASED ASSESSMENTS IN ART THERAPY

What Art Therapists Look For

Up to now, the focus has been on art used as a psychological test that can be conducted by any qualified mental health professional. But there are salient differences between an art-based assessment in art therapy and a psychological evaluation employing art, and it is time to make a distinction. The differences include both the purpose and the process involved in the assessment procedure. In regard to the purpose, the art therapist is primarily gathering information to formulate an art therapy treatment plan—not to construct a differential diagnosis. Along with attempting to determine client strengths and problem areas, an art therapist uses an assessment to observe the client's reaction to a variety of art media, to discover the ways in which the client goes about completing art tasks, and to determine the client's overall suitability for art therapy treatment.

In regard to process, an art therapist generally (and ideally) offers a selection of media and requests that the client complete a series of three to five pieces of art. Directives for the art pieces vary from the highly structured such as "draw your family" to "create whatever you wish," and to the extent to which the client is able, he or she is encouraged to discuss the meaning of each piece of completed art.

In toto, this procedure provides many things for the therapist to consider. Does the client have a preference for controlled or fluid media? Does the way in which the client uses a particular medium suggest that a change of media would facilitate a desired loosening or tightening of control? Do the formal aspects of the art suggest that the client's level of psychological development is age appropriate? Does the overall form of the art suggest serious pathology? Does the content of the art (as explained by the client) indicate a capacity to think in terms of visual metaphor? What particular concerns are contained in the art content? Does the client evidence ability for creative self-expression through visual art? Answers to questions such as these provide goals for art therapy and indicate the degree to which art therapy is a treatment of choice.

A couple of examples will help to clarify this procedure. In discussing them, I touch once again on the pitfalls and possibilities of art-based assessments.

A Better and a Worse Example

In the early days of art therapy education when art therapists of my generation were trained, many art therapy students were taught the more popular projective drawing techniques developed by psychologists. In my case, these were the DAP and the HTP (already mentioned) and the Kinetic Family Drawing (KFD; Burns & Kaufman, 1972). In addition, newly minted practitioners of the time were likely to find themselves in settings in which the ideal art therapy assessment could not be conducted. Again in my case, I found myself in a psychiatric institution where I had to do group—rather than individual—assessments and only had time to collect one drawing per participant. Frequently, there was minimal (or no) time to discuss the drawings with those who drew them. I relied on the KFD—the directive for which is "draw your family doing something"—because I reasoned that it was sufficiently complex to give me maximum information.

The drawing shown in Figure 3.1 was obtained during that relatively early phase of my working life. (It is also the "exceptional" drawing mentioned previously that tended to reinforce my adherence to conventional drawing interpretations.) This drawing is a KFD produced by a man in his late 20s who was a resident in a nonpsychiatric alcohol rehabilitation program connected with the psychiatric hospital where I worked. Herein I indicate the least and most questionable of the interpretations I made based on that drawing.

Looking at the picture from a global point of view, I found something vaguely bizarre about it. It was out of the mainstream of the drawings I usually obtained from the rehab population. It was more colorful, somewhat idiosyncratically so; more detailed; and rather oddly structured, presenting what seemed to be both above- and below-ground perspectives. There was also a dark cloud that appeared to be moving toward the self-figure. (Indeed, I found out this was an intentional representation of increasing difficulties from the few words I was able to exchange with the young man who drew it.) As a result of noting these features, I speculated that the drawer was a candidate for the dual-diagnosis unit within the hospital. I was correct,

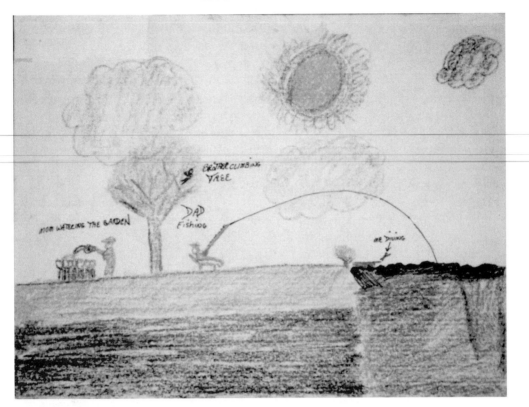

FIGURE 3.1. Family drawing by 28-year-old man (certain lines enhanced for clarity).

and a few days later, he was moved into the hospital proper, with a diagnosis of bipolar disorder in addition to his initial diagnosis of alcohol dependence.

In my write-up of the assessment, I recommended that the client receive art therapy along with his other therapies. I came to this conclusion by observing that he had used the drawing activity in a thoughtful and expressive manner and that he seemed to have some capacity for visual creativity and visual metaphor. Again, I was not wrong—although he did not use art therapy quite as well as I had hoped. Possibility, the medication and other treatments he was receiving leveled his mood to the extent that his normal defenses were restored; therefore, he felt less compelled to reveal himself through creative activity.

After this, I went seriously off the track. I reviewed the young man's hospital chart and compared the psychological testing results, social history, and chart notes to the drawing. I had a field day. For instance, his history revealed that there had been sexual abuse by his father. I then decided that the fishing pole held by the father was more than a pole (in contrast to the cigar that is "just a cigar") and that the client was about to be "caught" by his father's fishing line. I also learned from the chart that the client had described his brother as "an intellectual and we have nothing in common." Aha, I said, the brother is in a tree which suggests that from the client's viewpoint, he puts himself "above" the client. And so I proceeded, reading virtually everything I found in the chart into the drawing. I even went so far as to decide that the apparent layers in the earth under the groundline in the drawing (probable a consequence of lack of skill in rendering pictorial perspective) reflected the fact that the client lived in the basement of his parents' home!

Although it can be argued that my latter set of interpretations were plausible, they were made after I had increased knowledge of the client and can be explained by the ambiguous nature of visual imagery. Although this very ambiguity is part of what makes art images therapeutic, it also renders them problematic for assessment purposes. Advantages stem from the fact that art can stimulate a wide range of associations in the client, and assessment difficulties arise because attempts to interpret content without client input are largely guesswork. As we have seen (Chapman & Chapman, 1971; Smith & Dumont, 1995), it is quite easy to discover what one expects in drawings. And it is quite likely that this was exactly what I was doing.

Although not an example of an ideal art therapy assessment (I did not provide a variety of media, nor did I obtain more than one piece of art), the drawing shown in Figure 3.2 exemplifies a more appropriate use of an art-based assessment. The client in this case was a young woman of 23 who was seeking outpatient treatment for recurring bouts of anxiety. The directive for the drawing was again that for the KFD.

The client is pictured at the left end of the table with her parents at the right. Her younger brother and sister are behind her on the left side of the page. Whereas one

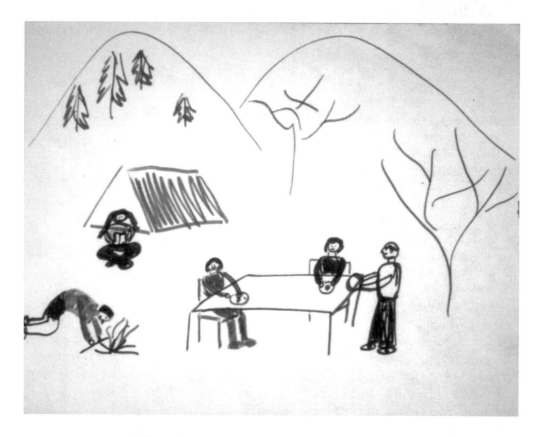

FIGURE 3.2. Family drawing by 23-year-old woman.

might speculate based on KFD interpretive guidelines that the client was at least as close to her siblings as to her parents, this was not the case. (Indeed, Motta et al., 1993, cite a study that failed to find a relationship between closeness of figures in KFDs and interpersonal closeness.) The client revealed while discussing the drawing that she felt closest to her mother and more like a parental figure in regard to her siblings. Certainly, in regard to interpersonal relations, there is no obvious indication in the drawing of the secret she disclosed—that she had recently taken a woman lover.

In any event, because this was individual treatment, there was sufficient time to discuss this drawing in depth with the client and little need for me to speculate about possible meanings. In the process of the discussion, I learned a great deal about the client and her family background. I also learned that she was willing to engage in the art-making process as part of therapy and that she had the imaginative ability to make good use of visual metaphor. A revealing instance of the latter was her response to my question, "If the trees were people, who might they be?" This prompted her to tell me about a couple of important members of her extended family who had not been previously mentioned. Beyond what the client had to tell, I concluded based on my overall impression of her drawing—and on the coherence and quality of her verbalizations—that she was not suffering from any serious pathology or cognitive deficits. Long-term, insight-oriented art therapy treatment of this client ultimately backed up my deductions.

CONCLUSION

Taken together, the studies and examples presented in this chapter supply compelling evidence that much is wrong with traditional drawing tests. On the other hand, a case has also been made that art-based assessments are an important prerequisite to art therapy or art-facilitated treatment. Significant findings can be derived from this latter type of assessment based on global features of the art and on the client's reactions to engaging in art activity. Furthermore, a wealth of information can be gathered just by discussing the art with the client. As Groth-Marnat (1997) has reported, "Some authors have . . . suggested that drawing techniques be considered not so much a formal test but rather a way to increase understanding of the client based on client/clinician interaction related to the drawing" (p. 504).

REFERENCES

Anderson, F. E. (1992). *Art for all the children: Approaches to art therapy for children with disabilities* (2nd ed.). Springfield, IL: Charles C Thomas.

Burns, R. C., & Kaufman, S. H. (1972). *Actions, styles and symbols in Kinetic Family Drawings (K-F-D): An interpretative manual.* New York: Brunner/Mazel.

Chapman, L. J., & Chapman, J. (1971). Test results are what you think they are. *Psychology Today, 5*(6), 18–22, 106–107.

Cohen, B. M., Mills, A., & Kijak, A. K. (1994). An introduction to the Diagnostic Drawing Series: A standardized tool for diagnostic and clinical use. *Art Therapy: Journal of the American Art Therapy Association, 11*(2), 105–110.

Cressen, R. (1975). Artistic quality of drawings and judges' evaluations of the DAP. *Journal of Personality Assessment, 39*(2), 132–137.

Gantt, L., & Tabone, C. (1998). *The Formal Elements Art Therapy Scale: The rating manual.* Morgantown, WV: Gargoyle Press.

Golomb, C. (1992). *The child's creation of a pictorial world.* Berkeley & Los Angeles: University of California Press.

Groth-Marnat, G. (1997). *Handbook of psychological assessment* (3rd ed.). New York: Wiley.

Hagood, M. M. (2002). A correlational study of art-based measures of cognitive development: Clinical and research implications for art therapists working with children. *Art Therapy: Journal of the American Art Therapy Association, 19*(2), 63–68.

Joiner, T. E., Jr., Schmidt, K. L., & Barnett, J. (1996). Size, detail, and line heaviness in children's drawings as correlates of emotional distress: (More) negative evidence. *Journal of Personality Assessment, 67*(1), 127–141.

Kahill, S. (1984). Human figure drawing in adults: An update of the empirical evidence, 1967–1982. *Canadian Psychology 2*(4), 269–292.

Kaplan, F. F. (1991). Drawing assessment and artistic skill. *The Arts in Psychotherapy, 18*(4), 347–352.

Knoff, H. M. (1993). The utility of human figure drawings in personality and intellectual assessment: Why ask why? *School Psychology Quarterly, 8*(3), 191–196.

Koppitz, E. M. (1984). *Psychological evaluation of human figure drawings by middle school pupils.* Orlando, FL: Grune & Stratton.

Marsh, D. T., Linberg, L. M., & Smeltzer, J. K. (1991). Human figure drawings of adjudicated and nonadjudicated adolescents. *Journal of Personality Assessment, 57*(1), 77–86.

Motta, R. W., Little, S. G., & Tobin, M. I. (1993). The use and abuse of human figure drawings. *School Psychology Quarterly, 8*(3), 162–169.

Munley, M. (2002). Comparing the PPAT drawings of boys with AD/HD and age-matched controls using the Formal Elements Art Therapy Scale. *Art Therapy: Journal of the American Art Therapy Association, 19*(2), 69–76.

Rankin, A. (1994). Tree drawings and trauma indicators: A comparison of past research with current findings from the Diagnostic Drawing Series. *Art Therapy: Journal of the American Art Therapy Association, 11*(2), 127–130.

Riethmiller, R. J., & Handler, L. (1997). Problematic methods and unwarranted conclusions in DAP research: Suggestions for improved research procedures. *Journal of Personality Assessment, 69*(3), 459–475.

Silver, R. (1996). *Silver Drawing Test of Cognition and Emotion* (3rd ed.). Sarasota, FL: Ablin Press.

Silver, R. (1998). *Updating the Silver Drawing Test and Draw A Story manuals: New studies and summaries of previous research.* Sarasota, FL: Ablin Press.

Smith, D., & Dumont, F. (1995). A cautionary study: Unwarranted interpretations of the Draw-A-Person Test. *Professional Psychology: Research and Practice, 26*(3), 298–303.

Swensen, C. H. (1957). Empirical evaluations of human figure drawings. *Psychological Bulletin, 54*, 431–466.

Swensen, C. H. (1968). Empirical evaluations of human figure drawings: 1957–1966. *Psychological Bulletin, 70*(1), 20–44.

Tharinger, D. J., & Stark, K. (1990). A qualitative versus quantitative approach to evaluating the Draw-A-Person and Kinetic Family Drawing: A study of mood- and anxiety-disorder children. *Psychological Assessment, 2*(4), 365–375.

Vyse, S. A. (1997). *Believing in magic: The psychology of superstition.* New York & Oxford, UK: Oxford University Press.

Wadeson, H. (1980). *Art psychotherapy.* New York: Wiley.

Wadeson, H. (2000). *Art therapy practice: Innovative approaches with diverse populations.* New York: Wiley.

Waehler, C. A. (1997). Drawing bridges between science and practice. *Journal of Personality Assessment, 69*(3), 482–487.

Waldman, T. L., Silber, D. E., Holmstrom, R. W., & Karp, S. A. (1994). Personality characteristics of incest survivors on the Draw-A-Person Questionnaire. *Journal of Personality Assessment,* *63*(1), 97–104.

Wanderer, Z. W. (1969/1997). Validity of clinical judgments based on human figure drawings. In E. F. Hammer (with contributors), *Advances in projective drawing interpretation* (pp. 301–315). Springfield, IL: Charles C Thomas.

Williams, K. J., Agell, G., Gantt, L., & Goodman, R. F. (1996). Art-based diagnosis: Fact or fantasy? *American Journal of Art Therapy, 35*(1), 9–31.

PART II

Clinical Approaches
to Art Therapy

This section provides the reader with an overview of major approaches and methods employed in practice. As with psychotherapy and counseling, art therapy has used a variety of theoretical models and has followed multiple paths in its development. Because art therapy is a synthesis of many disciplines—art, psychology, medicine, and education—these approaches have emerged from multiple perspectives over the last 50 years.

Although numerous approaches to art therapy have been identified (Rubin, 2001), not all these models were included in this section for several reasons. First, although almost every possible theoretical model has been applied to art therapy, not all approaches are adequately reflected or fully articulated in contemporary art therapy literature. Some have only been briefly cited, whereas others have been proposed or delineated by a single practitioner and are not widely used. Approaches with identifiable methods, strategies, and techniques were also favored over those that are more philosophical in nature as well as models that are most frequently used in counseling and psychology. Finally, though there are many approaches to art therapy, the focus of this volume is on those models used in contemporary applications rather than those that have been described in literature of a more historic nature.

In Chapter 1, Vick summarized the number of art therapists using various approaches to art therapy according to the most recent membership survey by the American Art Therapy Association (Elkins & Stovall, 2000). Not surprisingly, a high percentage of respondents indicated that they are "eclectic" in their approach to art therapy; that is, most art therapists use more than one model or theory in their work, dependent either on the client, presenting problems, and/or setting. In addition, the survey did not include data from counselors, social workers, psychologists, and others who may use art therapy or art-based approaches in treatment. Selekman (1997), Freeman, Epston, and Combs (1997), and Gladding (1992) are examples of the growing use of art therapy within marriage and family therapy, counseling, and psychology. Thus, it is difficult to say which approaches are most used and under what circumstances.

From the available data and from reviewing the contemporary art therapy literature, psychoanalytic and analytic theories (Chapter 4) still significantly influence the way that many art therapists practice and form the basis from which almost all art therapy approaches grew. When art therapy first appeared as form of psychotherapy in the mid-20th century, it was rooted in psychoanalysis, the dominant paradigm at the time. The idea of art expression as a reflection of the art maker's unconscious was a natural fit with the central concepts of both psychoanalytic and Jungian analytic theory that stressed the importance of the individual's internal world. Object relations theory (also described in Chapter 4) evolved from psychoanalysis and also has been used as a framework for understanding the therapeutic value of art expression as a mirror of internal object relations.

Humanistic theories of psychotherapy (Chapter 5) emerged in reaction to many of the ideas proposed by psychoanalytic models, introducing concepts of self-actualization and personal potential. Ideas such as Maslow's peak experience that encompassed theories of creativity supported art therapy's underlying principle that the creative process of art making is life enhancing for all individuals (American Art Therapy Association, 1996). Person-centered, Gestalt, existential, and the more contemporary outgrowth of transpersonal therapy all support a belief in the person's creative resources to achieve insight and wellness and have been synthesized within approaches to art therapy.

As psychotherapy began to explore the areas of information processing, cognition, and human behavior, cognitive-behavioral models of treatment rapidly developed. Cognitive-behavioral approaches of Albert Ellis, Aaron Beck, and, later, Donald Meichenbaum were adapted to art therapy (Chapter 6), reflecting the idea that making images of negative behavior or anxiety-producing thoughts could be helpful in inducing change. Images, according to this approach, are recognized as not only reflections of feelings but also cognitive representations that can be modified to help the person eliminate or reduce stress, fear, or other troublesome emotions.

This section also introduces examples of approaches that reflect art therapy's integration of newer psychotherapy theories. Solution-focused and narrative theories (Chapter 7) are representative of two contemporary approaches to psychotherapy that underscore the role of the individual in treatment as a collaborator with the therapist in creating solutions to presenting problems. Art expression is used within these models as a way to help clients make visible their world views and use creative expression to imagine positive changes to problem-laden stories. Whether or not these specific approaches will be embraced by increasing numbers of therapists and stand the test of time remains to be seen. However, they are approaches that reflect the current trends in brief therapy and the demands on all clinicians to accomplish treatment goals in a limited number of sessions.

The developmental approach to art therapy (Chapter 8) is somewhat related to cognitive-behavioral models because of its emphasis on understanding normal human growth, cognition, and behavior throughout the life cycle. This approach's foundations include the developmental aspects of normal artistic expression during childhood and the cognitive levels of development proposed by Piaget. Although most often applied to work with children, the principles and overall approach are used by many practitioners in both therapy and assessment of individuals of all ages.

Finally, an expressive arts therapies (also referred to as multimodal) approach is described in Chapter 9, a model based on the concept of using all the various art forms—art, music, dance, drama, and creative writing—in therapy. While this contemporary approach is gaining recognition in treatment, expressive arts therapy has been linked to the traditions and cultural precedents of world healing practices that include the application of all the arts (McNiff, 1981). This model offers unique opportunities for self-exploration and emphasizes that all the arts can be used in an integrative way to enhance therapy.

Some art therapists believe that art therapy should have its own theory and be an approach, in and of itself, rather than relying on other frameworks of therapy. As we learn more about the "science" of art making and image formation (as discussed in Chapter 2), the connections between art and health, and changes in the brain as a result of exposure to images and art expression, a free-standing theory of art therapy may very well emerge.

Many of the approaches in this section naturally employ concepts from several theories; for example, a transpersonal approach often uses humanistic, Jungian, and even mind–body principles in practice whereas a developmental approach might include some cognitive-behavioral elements or the inclusion of other modalities such as music or movement. Most clinicians who use art therapy in their work believe that dimensions of the individual are overlooked if a therapist is restricted to a single theory or way of working. Although it is possible to use an eclectic approach to art therapy, it does not mean that simply choosing techniques from various frameworks leads to sound therapeutic treatment. In all circumstances, they must be used in response to the person's needs and specific objectives for growth and change.

As we see in the pages that follow, all approaches to art therapy have a powerful capacity to tap elements of experiences, thoughts, and emotions that verbal therapy alone cannot. This ability to capture through visual image the internal world of feeling, sensations, perceptions, and cognitions makes art therapy, whether from a psychoanalytic, humanistic, developmental, or other approach, a unique, creative, and effective way to work with clients of all ages.

REFERENCES

American Art Therapy Association. (1996). *Mission statement.* Mundelein, IL: Author.

Elkins, D. E., & Stovall, K. (2000). American Art Therapy Association, Inc.: 1998–1999 Membership survey report. *Art Therapy: Journal of the American Art Therapy Association, 17,* 41–46.

Freeman, J., Epston, D., & Combs, G. (1997). *Playful approaches to serious problems.* New York: Norton.

Gladding, S. (1992). *Counseling as an art: The creative arts in counseling.* Alexandria, VA: American Counseling Association.

McNiff, S. (1981). *The arts in psychotherapy.* Springfield, IL: Charles C Thomas.

Rubin, J. (2001). *Approaches to art therapy.* New York: Brunner-Routledge.

Selekman, M. D. (1997). *Solution-focused therapy with children.* New York: Guilford Press.

CHAPTER 4

Psychoanalytic, Analytic, and Object Relations Approaches

Cathy A. Malchiodi

As noted in Chapter 1, the contemporary practice of art therapy emerged primarily from psychiatry in the first half of the 20th century. The impact of both Freudian psychoanalytic and Jungian analytic theory on the development of art therapy was profound, and, to some extent, all art therapy approaches grew from these foundations. Psychoanalytic personality theory continues to be a strong thread in the field of art therapy in general, and the work of Sigmund Freud and Carl Jung has been incorporated not only in psychoanalytic and analytic approaches to art therapy but also within the conceptual framework of many art therapy methodologies.

In this relatively short discussion it is impossible to capture the diversity of these psychodynamic influences on art therapy and to describe all the ways they have been incorporated in clinical practice. The main focus of this chapter instead provides a brief overview of major concepts in Freudian, Jungian theory, and object relations that influenced art therapy; contributions within the field of art therapy to psychoanalytic and analytic approaches; the role of the psychoanalytic principle of transference in art therapy; and basic principles and techniques used in psychoanalytic, analytic, and object relations approaches to art therapy.

PSYCHOANALYSIS AND PSYCHOANALYTIC PERSONALITY THEORY

Sigmund Freud's views are the foundation for most theories of psychotherapy and undoubtedly have been a major influence on the development of art therapy in the

20th century and continue to be up to the present day. Freud observed that many patients' most meaningful remarks were descriptions of visual images; in his first case of child analysis he reported on drawings in the case of Little Hans (1905) and later in the classic case known as "the wolfman" (1918). Freud's discovery that dreams have meaning was also key to the foundation of psychoanalytic approach to art therapy. He noted, "We experience it [a dream] predominantly in visual images . . . part of the difficulty of giving an account of dreams is due to our having to translate these images into words. 'I could draw it,' a dreamer often says to us, 'but I don't know how to say it' " (1916–1917, p. 90). This statement served as an inspiration for the emergence and consequent development of art therapy as a treatment modality.

Perhaps Freud's greatest contribution is his concept of the unconscious. Dream, as well as slips of the tongue, material derived from free association and projective techniques, and symbolic content of psychotic symptoms were considered by Freud to be evidence of the unconscious. His theory of the unconscious influenced the development of psychoanalytic approach to art therapy as well as the development of projective drawing techniques that emphasized the emergence of unconscious material through images. Freud's theory of ego defense mechanisms, particularly sublimation which has been related to artistic expression (Kramer, 1993), also influenced the course of the psychoanalytic approach to art therapy. Freud's daughter, Anna, also had an impact on art therapy. Although her father did not direct his patients to draw, Anna used art and other expressive activity in her work and recognized art expression as an aid in treatment because children could not engage in adult free association.

ANALYTIC PSYCHOLOGY

Carl Jung had different ideas about the symbolic role of images than Freud. In contrast to Freud, he used art as a method of self-analysis and his personal experience as the foundation for his thinking about the importance of imagery in analysis. Jung believed that if a patient relied on the therapist to interpret a dream or fantasy, the patient would remain in a state of dependence on the analyst. Jung (1934) invited his patients to paint, noting that "the aim of this method of expression is to make unconscious content accessible and so bring it closer to the patient's understanding" (p. 182).

Jung's ideas about treatment developed partially from his belief that one must establish a dialogue between the conscious and unconscious in order to achieve psychic equilibrium. He believed one way this balance could be achieved was through tapping the transcendent qualities of symbols such as those in art and dreams. Jung considered symbols to be unifiers of opposites within a single entity and as natural attempts by the psyche to reconcile inner conflicts and to achieve individuation. He endeavored to work with an individual's images to reveal hidden possibilities and thereby help the person find meaning and wholeness in life.

Jung believed that all humans shared a collective unconscious and universal archetypes common to all cultures. Archetypes underlie fairy tales, myths, and rituals and are also recognizable in dreams and art. In reality, they do not take on form but are the fundamental element of images, the content of the image rather than the image itself. Jung understood from his own experiences and those of his patients that art making was useful method of tapping the healing aspects of archetypes. Along with analysis he thought images helped his patients to become aware of the archetypes in their lives and to bring them to consciousness.

THE DEVELOPMENT OF PSYCHOANALYTIC AND ANALYTIC APPROACHES TO ART THERAPY

Several figures in the field of art therapy emerged in the second half of the 20th century who paved the way for the integration of psychoanalytic and analytic theories with art therapy. The most notable perhaps was Margaret Naumburg (1966) who used spontaneous drawings within the framework of psychoanalysis. She coined the term "dynamically oriented art therapy" to describe her belief that the unconscious can be communicated through symbolic expression. Naumburg noted that art expression made it possible for a person to place unconscious material directly into an image, whereas in psychoanalysis, visual experiences must be transformed into verbal communication. "Art therapy recognizes that the unconscious as expressed in a patient's phantasies, daydreams and fears can be projected more immediately in pictures than words" (Naumburg, 1966, p. 3).

Naumburg, whose training included both Freudian and Jungian approaches, subscribed to the Freudian concept of free association, encouraging the image maker to verbally provide descriptions of spontaneous art created. Although Naumburg did not agree with the psychoanalytic practice of putting subjective experiences into words, she did consider the individual's verbal associations to be important. However, she chose no specific theory for interpreting art expressions and suggested that the person's free associations were key to understanding images created in therapy and catalysts to change and growth.

Edith Kramer (1979, 1993) truly blended Freudian personality theory within art therapy with her work with children, emphasizing the importance of sublimation and other defense mechanisms derived from Freud. Through the experience of sublimation Kramer believed that a synthesis of content and form was achieved by transforming emotional material into fully formed images. Judith Rubin (1978, 1987), an art therapist who was trained in classic psychoanalytic technique, expanded the notion that a psychoanalytic understanding of the patient is enhanced through the use of art expression as therapy. Her work with children and adults synthesized Freudian theory with developmental principles and the creative process. Others who explored and integrated psychoanalytic principles in their clinical work include Milner (1957, 1969), the interplay of analysis, creativity, and artistic process; Levick (1983), art expressions as reflections of defense mechanisms; and Lachman-Chapin (2001), art therapy and self-psychology. Winnicott (1971) also provided a unique contributions to psychoanalytic understanding of art and play therapy with children; Winnicott's ideas are discussed later (scribble technique) and in Chapter 10 (art and storytelling).

British art therapists have been more active in integrating Jungian analytic principles with art therapy. Schaverien (1992), among others, has extensively explored analytic psychology's role in the art therapy process, providing the most comprehensive examination to date of the function of image making in analysis. Edwards (1987), a British art therapist trained in Jungian analysis, proposed an integration of analytic theory and art therapy. Others who have influenced the development of Jungian-based art therapy include Wallace (1975, 1987), an artist and analyst who combined active imagination and art expression; Keyes (1983), who blended Jungian principles with more humanistically based therapies such as transaction analysis and Gestalt therapy; Allan (1988), who combined Jungian principles with counseling principles in his work with children; and Kellogg (1978), who explored mandala drawings in relation to Jung's collective unconscious (see Appendix I, this volume, for more information on mandala drawings as a form of assessment). More recently, transpersonal approaches to art therapy have incorporated Jungian philosophy with transpersonal psychology and spiritual practices (Franklin, Farrelly-Hansen, Marek, Swan-Foster, & Wallingford, 2000; Malchiodi, 2002) and archetypal art therapy has been identified as an integration of archetypal psychology, analytic psychology, and art therapy (McConeghey, 2001). These approaches emphasize the central importance of imagery in psychotherapy and archetypal material that emerges through art expression and dreams is regarded as the major transformative potential of the psyche.

CONCEPTS INFLUENCING PSYCHOANALYTIC AND ANALYTIC APPROACHES TO ART THERAPY

Several concepts intrinsic to Freudian psychoanalysis and Jungian analytic psychology have influenced psychoanalytic and analytic approaches to art therapy. These include transference as the basis of analysis and treatment, spontaneous expression as material from the unconscious, and the analytic techniques of amplification and active imagination.

Transference

Transference is considered to be an important part of psychoanalysis and, in Freudian theory, the examination of transference is regarded as the basis of treatment. Simply defined, transference is the client's unconscious projection of feelings onto the therapist. These projections, which originate in repressed or unfinished situations of one's life, are thought to be the essence of therapy, and the success of treatment is dependent on their accurate analysis.

Transference is also important in art therapy but has been the subject of debate because art therapy provides a unique set of circumstances with regard to transference (Agell et al., 1981). Naumburg (1966) subscribed to the idea of transference; she believed that it occurred in both art and verbal exchange and that the image maker developed an emotional connection to not only the therapist, but also the art expression. Naumburg thought that patients' attachment to the art work gradually replaced their dependence on the therapist and that the therapist could encourage this autonomy by avoiding interpretation. In this way, the person would "discover for himself what his symbolic pictures mean to him" (p. 3).

Rubin (1978, 2001) also supported the idea of transference in art therapy but noted that it might be expressed differently than in traditional psychoanalysis. A therapist taking a psychoanalytic stance generally finds it important to remain impartial because neutrality is considered key to the development of transference. But by including art expression in therapy the therapist cannot be totally neutral because the role demands behaviors that influence transference. For example, Rubin notes that when the therapist gives supplies for art making the therapist may be seen as a nurturer and the client may naturally react to therapist, perceiving him or her as either sufficient or insufficient, depending on transference of past relationships with others to the art therapy session. Clients may also reflect transference through their actions with art materials, and regression, anger, anxiety, or other emotions related to a person's life experiences may emerge in the creative process of image making.

Some individuals use art expression as a way to directly communicate transferential reactions to the therapist. For example, a 6-year-old girl who was abandoned by her mother created what she called an "angry picture" of me in reaction to a play therapy session with her I missed because of illness (Figure 4.1). She felt uncomfortable expressing herself with words and may have feared punishment for her feelings, but art provided a less threatening way to convey both the experience of her mother's abandonment of her and the therapist's missing the session, another form of abandonment. Because of the interactive nature of art therapy, which often involves the provision of materials and the giving of assistance, a client may use art expression to project feelings about the therapist; there may also be countertransference on the part of therapist because of taking on the role of nurturer and provider in therapy.

Schaverien (1992) has extensively examined the transference relationship within the framework of what she calls "analytical art psychotherapy." According to Schaverien, images are not merely illustrations of transference but reflect elements of transference that can be amplified within the therapeutic context. Transference, according to Schaverien, is not necessarily reflected in all art expressions; she distinguishes between "diagrammatic images" (those which are merely descriptive) and "embodied images (those which contain deeper symbolic meanings). Schaverien maintains that transference is truly reflected only in embodied images, although all art expressions may convey some aspect of it upon examination with the help of the therapist.

The context in which the art expression is created is also thought to influence the degree of transference to the therapist. For example, an individual may create images to bring to therapy; in this case, the therapist may be able to take a more traditional approach to analyzing client transference to the therapist. Naumburg often had the person make artworks outside the session and then bring them to therapy; the art expressions, like dreams or fantasies, could then become objects of analysis and free association during the session with the analyst. In contrast, in most contemporary art therapy contexts, the client creates the art expression in the presence of the therapist.

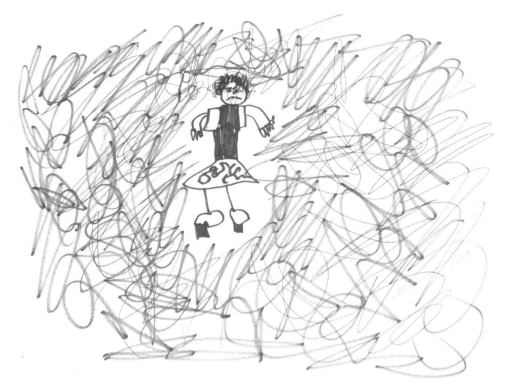

FIGURE 4.1. "Angry picture" by 6-year-old girl who felt abandoned by the therapist.

Many art therapists consider this circumstance to have a profound influence on the true development of transference. When a client makes art in the presence of the therapist, it is believed that promotion of transference in art therapy inhibits the therapeutic efficacy of the art process and that art therapy is actually at odds with the development of transference in the traditional sense (Allen, 1988). Kramer (1979, 1993) echoes this belief and favors encouraging a therapeutic alliance as opposed to transference to the therapist. However, most therapists agree that some degree of transference is always present because of the projective nature of art expression and the relationship between client and therapist.

Spontaneous Expression

Psychoanalytic and analytic approaches to art therapy are strongly linked to the idea that spontaneous art expression provides access to the unconscious. Spontaneous art expression is any image making which is nondirective; that is, the person is simply requested to make a drawing, painting, or sculpture of anything he or she wants to and may also be invited to choose freely whatever materials he or she wishes to use. The purpose of spontaneous expression, like free association, is to help clients express what troubles them as freely as possible (Rubin, 2001).

In the psychoanalytic approach, as well as many other approaches to art therapy, the therapist's role is to facilitate an interpersonal relationship that encourages the individual to create spontaneous images and to discover personal meaning in one's expressions. While image making may be spontaneous, the therapist is expected to explain art media (such as how to use drawing or painting materials) to individuals who are inexperienced in art expression. This might even include a brief demonstration of how to use a chalk pastel or paintbrush, or even a technique such as the "scribble" (described in more detail later). Emphasis, however, is on art expression as symbolic communication rather than necessarily an aesthetic product, which promotes the idea that all expression is acceptable and is intended to encourage more free communication of conflicts and emotions.

While therapists working from a psychoanalytic or analytic stance see spontaneous expression as central to the process of art therapy, some practitioners believe that it is particularly helpful in specific situations. Furth (1988) and Bach (1966, 1990), who favor a Jungian analytic approach to understanding art expressions, believe that spontaneous expression is most useful when an individual is undergoing a significant life event such as an emotional crisis, physical illness, or the process of dying. They underscore the capacity of extemporaneous expression to reveal not only unconscious material but also the psyche's intuition and the individual's internal curative potential. Like Jung, both Furth and Bach observe that spontaneous art expressions are containers of repressed emotions as well as sources of transformation.

While it is believed by both psychoanalytic and analytic practitioners that spontaneous expression has an important place in revealing the unconscious, it is also observed by some that more active direction on the part of the therapist is necessary for change to take place. Kramer (1993), who uses a psychoanalytic framework in her work, notes that art therapy should include not only spontaneous expression but also the more time-consuming process of fully formed art expression. Furth (1988), in his analytic work with children and adults with life-threatening illnesses, found that projective drawing tasks (such as requesting a drawing of a house, tree, and person) and other therapist-directed activities were just as revealing of unconscious material as impromptu drawings and had potential to enhance the course of therapy.

One method that has been used as a catalyst for spontaneous expression is the "scribble technique" (Cane, 1951; Naumburg, 1966). Although it is used in many different approaches to art therapy, it is most often associated with the psychoanalytic approach. When creating impromptu images is difficult for an individual, introducing the scribble technique often helps the person to generate images and, subsequently, to project thoughts or feelings through art expression. In its simplest form it involves drawing a series of scribbled lines on paper and then looking at those lines to see shapes, figures, or objects that can be further articulated with details and color to define them. Free association is part of the process in two distinct ways: (1) it presents the possibility of freely associating images to what one sees in the scribble and (2) after completing the activity, the individual may verbally associate thoughts, feelings, and experiences with the images that were created within the scribble.

Winnicott (1971) developed a variation of the scribble technique, the "squiggle game," as a way to establish rapport with children as well as a tool to encourage creative expression. He would introduce the activity as follows: "Let's play something. I know what I would like to play and I'll show you. This game that I like playing has no rules. I just take my pencil and go like that . . . (do squiggle blind). You show me if that looks like anything to you or if you can make it into anything, and afterwards you do the same for me and I will see if I can make something of yours" (Winnicott, 1971, pp. 62–63).

In a similar vein, I use "scribble chase" (Luesbrink, 1990) to engage the child or adult in free expression. To start this "game," I ask the individual to chose a crayon or chalk and I choose one in a different color. Then I say, "Now I am going to take my crayon and scribble all over the paper. But while I am scribbling I want you to use your crayon to chase my crayon around the page." After completing this scribble I ask the person to look at the drawing, look for shapes or images, and use drawing materials to add details to make one or more pictures using the scribbled lines as inspiration. The following vignette provides an example of how this technique was used with a child who was traumatized by violence in his community:

Case Example

Seven-year-old Bobby was a witness to a shooting on a street in the neighborhood in which he lived; a classmate of his was accidentally shot and killed in gang-related gunfire just a few blocks from Bobby's home. Although there was some trauma debriefing for Bobby and other children who witnessed or heard about the incident, Bobby became noticeably withdrawn and depressed in the weeks after the death of his classmate. His interest in school and friends diminished and his teacher reported that he was often caught "day dreaming" in class. His parents became worried about his dramatic change in behavior and brought him in to see me for an evaluation.

When Bobby sat down in my art and playroom he seemed disinterested in the toys and games and sat with his eyes looking down into his lap. I asked him if he liked to draw and he mumbled a quiet "yes," still not looking at me. I said that I had a game that involved drawing that I thought he would be good at and placed a large piece of white paper on the desk at which we both sat. The scribble chase turned out to be a good choice because it allowed Bobby to look at the paper rather than me for the time being. It also allowed him to participate without too much verbal communication and for me to take a neutral, observing stance.

Bobby followed my scribble on the paper for about a minute; I then asked him to look at the scribble we made and to use the drawing materials to make a picture out of the lines. Bobby spent the next 20 minutes of the session carefully creating a series of pictures from the scribble, including a car running over a person and a fire consuming a building (Figure 4.2). It was easy to see that he was focused on themes of danger and destruction and like many children who are exposed to violence, he was carrying terrifying images in his head but had had no way of communicating them. He used the activity to "free associate" thoughts and feelings through images that communicated his fears, conflicts, and, possibly, even desires to harm others as a result of his own anxieties. For Bobby, the activity served as a useful way to capitalize on projection as a way for him to safely express his feelings until he was ready to discuss his experiences more directly.

In subsequent sessions Bobby worked on more "scribble chases" as well as spontaneously creating images without direction from me. I let Bobby work on his own for several sessions, mostly quietly observing his process and images until one day he began to verbalize what he called "bad feelings" of fear, worry, or guilt about the shooting he had witnessed. In our last session about 11 weeks after the initial meeting, Bobby reported that he felt "better" and he was happy that he could talk to his parents about his "bad feelings" when he was apprehensive or sad. His parents also reported that he was socializing with his friends again and that, in general, his demeanor had greatly improved.

This brief example demonstrates how the scribble technique can be used as a way to encourage spontaneous expression and capitalize on projection when the individual may find verbal communication impossible. Finding images within the scribble and then naming the images offered Bobby a way to convey thoughts and feelings without talking about the traumatizing experience directly. Because the scribble technique complements the psychoanalytic principles of projection and free association, it has also become the basis of some art-based evaluations, including procedures developed by Ulman (1992) and Kwiatkowska (1978).

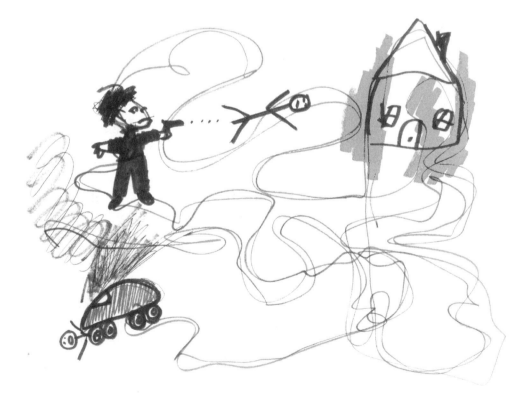

FIGURE 4.2. Images found in a scribble by 7-year-old Bobby after death of a classmate.

Amplification and Active Imagination

Amplification is strictly an analytic approach. It was originally a method of dream interpretation developed by Jung in which a dream image or motif is enlarged, clarified, and given a meaningful context by comparing it with similar images from mythology, folklore, and comparative religion. According to this process, an image cannot be interpreted by its content alone; it also must be considered in terms of what the content might symbolize and the symbol itself must be given a meaningful context. Jung believed that amplification establishes the collective context of a dream, enabling it to be seen not only in its personal aspect but also in general archetypal terms which are common to all humanity. In other words, each element in an image may be a representation of the person's life and current circumstances as well as a representation of archetypal symbols.

Amplification is different than free association in that it implies "sticking with the image" by viewing it from all facets (McConeghey, 2001). A simplified example may be helpful to illustrate this point: in free association to a drawing of a shoe, a person might say "shoe, foot, closet, clothes, bedroom," using the original image to stimulate connections between each successive association. In amplification, the person would be encouraged to stay with the original image of the shoe, perhaps saying "shoe, foot, shoe, sandal, shoe, stocking," remaining as close to the original image as possible.

In general, there are two different approaches to amplification: subjective and objective (in Keyes, 1983). In objective amplification, the analyst collects themes from mythology, religion, and other sources to illuminate the symbol. In other words, if a person related a dream about a poor relationship with her mother and meeting a man in an underground place, the analyst might relate the myth of Demeter and Persephone's descent into the underworld, a story that reflects a similar theme. In subjective amplification, the individual uses the technique of "active imagination" to find associations to the symbol. Active imagination is a method described by Jung (1916) as a way to release creativity within the individual by using fantasy and dreams as the primary mode of healing. It is the dynamic production of inward images in which the individual is encouraged to observe those images (Jacobi, 1942). While making art is believed by art therapists to be one form of active imagination, it can also be the creation of mental images.

Von Franz (in Keyes, 1983) describes active imagination in the following four stages:

1. Emptying one's mind in a similar way to meditation.
2. Allowing images to enter one's field of attention and focusing on them without holding on with too much concentration or allowing images to pass by without observation; this balance between relaxation required to allow images to emerge and the tension necessary to attend to the images can be difficult to achieve and may require both patience and practice.
3. Recording what has been seen in writing or in an art form such as paint, to give form to the experience.
4. Reflecting on the messages received from the experience.

Art expression, in and of itself, is considered by many practitioners to be a form of active imagination. The images that arise from the process of spontaneous drawing, painting, or sculpting provide material that one can amplify through "sticking with the image" or continuing exploration through active imagination. In the following brief example, active imagination is illustrated through Jungian-based art therapy with a young woman, Jenna.

Case Example

Jenna was in her late 20s at the time she started therapy for depression and problems with her social relationships as a result of her dark mood. She also was struggling to break free from her mother who whose dependence on Jenna prevented Jenna from developing her own autonomy. Jenna did not feel that she was artistic but had kept a drawing and writing journal prior to entering therapy and wanted to continue using her journal as part of treatment. After several sessions I asked her if she would like to learn some techniques that she could apply to her journal work, particularly her interest in drawing. I explained the process of active imagination to her as a way to generate mental images, helped her to practice it during the session, and asked her to try it several times on her own before coming to the next session. I also suggested that if she wanted to, she could make a drawing in her journal of the images she saw during active imagination.

Jenna's first "active imagination" images were of a dark tunnel at the end of which a star emerged (Figure 4.3). She recorded what she remembered of her initial active imagination experiences as follows: "At first I can only see darkness and then I realize that I am looking through a tunnel. Below me there is water, but I can't see it because it is so dark. Ahead there seems to be a distant light so I decide to try to walk down the tunnel to reach it. The light seems faint, like a small, white light. As I get closer, it seems to reflect on the walls of the tunnel. I begin to see that it is five-pointed star with many different colors in it, and although it shines strongly, I can see all the patterns in it. Suddenly, I feel that I can go no farther and give up trying to see anymore."

In subsequent sessions she used the star image as a starting point for art expression, both during our meetings and at home when she continued her active imagination exercises. By "sticking to the image" Jenna was able to amplify her own meanings for her images through writing about them and by using them to develop more drawings. Her artwork and active imagination experiences eventually reflected a slow transformation from depression to more positive feelings about the future and to understanding how she could change her relationship with her mother to one in which she could feel more autonomy. Simultaneously, the star image moved from its original dark surroundings and eventually appeared as a multipointed star alone in the sky (Figure 4.4).

Jenna's therapy was conducted over the course of several months, and fortunately, she was committed to staying with the process of active imagination, drawing, and writing, despite severe bouts of depression on many days. Active imagination requires that the person be ready and able to undertake the process of self-examination and expression. In other words, the client must become actively involved in therapy

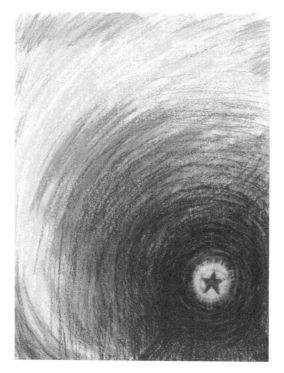

FIGURE 4.3. Jenna's active imagination drawing of a star at end of dark tunnel.

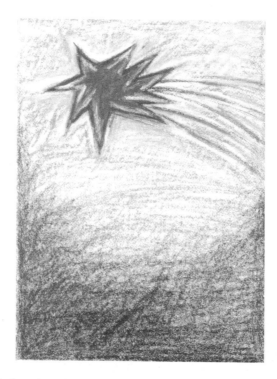

FIGURE 4.4. Jenna's active imagination drawing of a multipointed star drawing.

and be willing to remain committed to staying with the images that emerge over what may be a long period. Jenna was ready to make that type of commitment and her active imagination work revealed a story of transformation and recovery through both words and images. With the help of the therapist, she was able to sustain this process and find meaning for her images in relation to her life.

Jung's technique of active imagination has been adapted by McNiff (1994), referred to as "dialoguing with the image," and others. These adaptations, as well as the original process of active imagination described by Jung and his followers, help the person and the therapist consider images created in therapy in a nonreductive way, as opposed to judging them through the lens of psychoanalytic theory. In Chapter 20 (this volume), Steinhardt provides a more detailed example of the process of Jungian analysis through the visual process of sandplay, illustrating both amplification and active imagination.

OBJECT RELATIONS

Object relations is a theory that is considered to be a contemporary trend of psychoanalytic theory (Corey, 1996). Therapists who subscribe to an object relations approach to treatment believe that humans have an innate drive to form and maintain relationships and it is through our relationships with people around us that shapes our personality. Once formed, personality can be modified, but we tend to seek out others who reaffirm these early relationships. Object relations are interpersonal relationships that shape an individual's current interactions with people, both in reality and in fantasy (Corey, 1996). This theory provides a framework for understanding the ways clients superimpose early relationships and experiences on present relationships. Helping clients with issues of separation and individuation, dependence and independence, and intimacy are intrinsic to this approach.

The term "object" is at the center of object relations theory. Freud believed that an object was a person, thing, or mental representation through which one is gratified, while his student, Melanie Klein (1964) observed that it was someone (usually the mother) onto whom the child projects desires, wishes, or other powerful emotions. The concept of attachment is also at the foundation of object relations. Initially, a child is joined with mother, experiencing bonding along with good and bad aspects of that attachment; the task is to successfully separate from mother and eventually, with maturity, to take in all aspects, both good and bad, and develop autonomy. Recently, the concept of attachment found in object relations has taken on renewed interest in the work of Bowlby (1969), Karen (1998), and others with the goal in treatment of repairing developmental deficits that may have resulted from early relationships.

In the field of art therapy, Robbins (1987, 2001) is best known for an object relations art therapy approach to treatment. In his work with adults with psychiatric problems, he observes that art can contain, organize, and mirror internal object relations and the interplay between therapist, client, and art product. Art expression, an activity of early childhood, can be used at any age to reflect unfinished stages of development. Observing and facilitating art expression in therapy can help to amplify unresolved interpersonal issues that may need to be addressed in treatment.

Henley (1991,1992) has developed an object relations approach in his work with children with developmental, emotional, and other disabilities. He notes that individuals with developmental disabilities, including autism and mental retardation, and those with physical disabilities such as deafness or blindness, may lack a sense of self and may experience difficulties in relating to others. These individuals are well suited to an object relations approach because early attachments may be impaired or not fully developed. Because object relations plots a developmental sequences of maturation and attachment to objects, it complements the art process encourages sensory stimulation, object formation, and interaction with both therapist and the art product.

Art adds a dimension to therapist–client interactions because it creates a setting in which individuation and separation can be witnessed, practiced, and mastered through creative experimentation and exploration. By its very nature, offering art materials is often perceived as a form of nurturing by providing the opportunity for creative expression, encouraging attachment to the therapist.

CONCEPTS INFLUENCING AN OBJECT RELATIONS APPROACH TO ART THERAPY

Transitional Space and Transitional Objects

Two concepts in object relations theory that are of particular interest to art therapy are Winnicott's (1953) concepts of "transitional space" and "transitional objects." Transitional space is an intermediate area of experience where there is no clear distinction between inner and outer reality. Art making and play activity are considered transitional spaces because they are ways that children bridge subjective and objective realities and practice attachment and relationship to the world around them. The art process, including the presence of the therapist who facilitates and guides creative expression, is considered to be somewhat of a holding environment within which object relations can emerge and develop.

The term "transitional object" has been used by Winnicott to describe an actual object, such as a blanket or stuffed toy, that is important to the child because it represents something beyond what it actually is. Art products can become transitional objects which may become imbued with meaning beyond what they are in reality. For example, a drawing or painting made by a child who is dependent on the therapist for support may become a transitional object in the absence of the therapist, defusing separation anxiety. In a similar vein, an adult may make a clay figure of a parent who abandoned her as a child, symbolically evoking that person and the unresolved trauma of separation. Henley (1992) notes that the art product functions as a transitional object because it supports self-relationship and empowerment and encourages connection with the therapist who facilitates the creative expression.

Mahler's Stage Theory of Object Relations

Many object relations theorists see psychological problems as expressions of being "stuck" in a certain stage of development. Treatment encourages resolution through relationship with the therapist. Mahler (1968; Mahler, Pine, & Bergman, 1975), Winnicott (1965), and others believed that successful attachments between mother and infant influenced relationships throughout life. Mahler et al. (1975) outlined stages leading to separation and individuation that have been used in art therapy with an object relations approach. She developed theories that placed importance on the making attachment between mother and child. Each stage has different character- istics and developmental tasks that must be accomplished. The first stage, "normal autism," is a blissful existence that begins when the child is *in utero* and continues until shortly after birth. Mahler calls the subsequent stage of bonding "symbiosis," a time during which the child bonds with the mother and cannot conceive of being a separate entity. At approximately 5 to 6 months of age the child begins to develop a sense of self-awareness and differentiation, which Mahler called the "hatching stage." It is shortly after this stage that the child begins to practice "separation/indi- viduation" from the mother. Finally, "object constancy" occurs around age 3, when others, including mother, are seen as more fully separate from the self.

Mahler's stages have been used as a framework for understanding clients' work in art therapy where art making is seen as mirroring and facilitating interpersonal communication and potential difficulties with object relations. For example, Henley (1992) shares the following brief case example of a young man with Down syndrome who had a profoundly enmeshed relationship with his mother and sister: "his figura- tive imagery was consistently in the state of merging. One of his pictures depicted the two figures literally tied in a symbiotic union, with each face mirroring each other. Throughout this young man's art therapy program, focus was on facilitating separa- tion and building self-concept and a sense of empowerment that was not so depend- ent upon the females in his family" (p. 234). Object relations theory was used by Henley to provide a structure for assessing the child's relationships to significant oth- ers and establishing a treatment plan with the goal of resolving attachment problems and encouraging autonomy.

In his work with adults, Robbins (2001) sums up an art therapy approach to ob- ject relations, noting that the therapist must use the art process to communicate: "I am with you, will help you and teach you, but I am also separate and must promote in you, regardless of your pleasure or pain, your own independence and autonomy" (p. 64). This statement underscores that object relations theory is a helpful construct in organizing art therapy and understanding the client's presenting problems with early attachments in mind. The images created in therapy reflect past relationships while interactions between therapist and client support and enhance the process of individuation.

CONCLUSION

The advent of psychoanalysis early in the 20th century provided a natural catalyst for the emergence of the idea of art therapy and offered a conceptual framework complementary to the potential of art expression in psychotherapy. Equally, Jung's belief in the inherent healing power of images and art making fueled the analytic approach to art therapy and techniques such as amplification and active imagination, providing ways to work with and understand images created in therapy. Object relations, a more contemporary development of psychoanalytic theory, has provided a way of thinking about client's responses in art therapy, reflecting early attachments and current relationship issues. Although most contemporary practitioners do not take a strictly psychoanalytic, analytic, or object relations approach to art therapy, elements of these philosophies are present in many contemporary art therapy approaches to treatment. Together, these theories have formed the bedrock for the subsequent development and advances of art therapy as a method of client communication and therapeutic change.

REFERENCES

Agell, G., Levick, M., Rhyne, J., Robbins, A., Rubin, J., Ulman, E., Wang, C., & Wilson, L. (1981). Transference and countertransference in art therapy. *American Journal of Art Therapy, 21,* 13–24.

Allan, J. (1988). *Inscapes of the child's world.* Dallas, TX: Spring.

Allen, P. (1988). A consideration of transference in art therapy. *American Journal of Art Therapy, 26,* 113–118.

Bach, S. (1966). *Spontaneous paintings of severely ill patients.* Basel, Switzerland: Geigy.

Bach, S. (1990). *Life paints its own span.* Zurich: Daimon.

Bowlby, J. (1969). *Attachment and loss.* New York: Basic Books.

Cane, F. (1951). *The artist in each of us.* Craftsbury Common, VT: Art Therapy.

Corey, G. (1996). *Theory and practice of counseling and psychotherapy.* Pacific Grove, CA: Brooks/Cole.

Edwards, M. (1987). Jungian analytic art therapy. In J. Rubin (Ed.), *Approaches to art therapy* (pp. 92–113). New York: Brunner/Mazel.

Franklin, M., Farrelly-Hansen, M., Marek, B., Swan-Foster, N., & Wallingford, S. (2000). Transpersonal art therapy education. *Art Therapy: Journal of the American Art Therapy Association, 17*(2), 101–110.

Freud, S. (1905). *Analysis of a phobia in a 5-year-old boy* (Vol. 10). London: Hogarth Press.

Freud, S. (1916–1917). *Introductory letters on psychoanalysis* (Vol. 12). London: Hogarth Press.

Freud, S. (1918). *From the history of an infantile neurosis* (Vol. 17). London: Hogarth Press.

Furth, G. (1988). *The secret world of drawings.* Boston: Sigo.

Henley, D. (1991). Facilitating the development of object relations through the use of clay in art therapy. *American Journal of Art Therapy, 29,* 69–76.

Henley, D. (1992). *Exceptional children, exceptional art.* Worcester, MA: Davis.

Jacobi, J. (1942). *The psychology of C. G. Jung.* London: Routledge & Kegan Paul.

Jung, C. G. (1916). *The transcendent function, CW 8.* Princeton, NJ: Bollingen [reprinted 1960].

Jung, C. G. (1934). *Mandala symbolism.* Princeton, NJ: Princeton University Press.

Karen, R. (1998). *Becoming attached: First relationships and how they shape our capacity to love.* New York: Oxford University Press.

Kellogg, J. (1978). *Mandala: Path of beauty.* Clearwater, FL: Association for Teachers of Mandala Assessment.

Keyes, M. (1983). *Inward journey: Art as therapy.* La Salle, IL: Open Court.

Klein, M. (1964). *Contributions to psychoanalysis.* New York: McGraw-Hill.

Kramer, E. (1979). *Childhood and art therapy.* New York: Schocken.

Kramer, E. (1993). *Art as therapy with children.* Chicago: Magnolia Street.

Kwiatkowska, H. Y. (1978). *Family therapy and evaluation through art.* Springfield, IL: Charles C Thomas.

Lachman-Chapin, M. (2001). Self-psychology and art therapy. In J. Rubin (Ed.), *Approaches to art therapy* (pp. 66–78). New York: Brunner-Routledge.

Levick, M. (1983). *They could not talk and so they drew: Children's styles of coping and thinking.* Springfield, IL: Charles C Thomas.

Lusebrink, V. (1990). *Imagery and visual expression in therapy.* New York: Plenum Press.

Mahler, M. (1968). *On human symbiosis and the vicissitudes of individuation.* New York: International Universities Press.

Mahler, M., Pine, F., & Bergman, A. (1975). *The psychological birth of the human infant.* New York: Basic Books.

Malchiodi, C. A. (2002). *The soul's palette.* Boston: Shambhala.

McConeghey, H. (2001). *Art and soul.* Dallas, TX: Spring.

McNiff, S. (1994). *Art as medicine.* Boston: Shambhala.

Milner, M. (1957). *On not being able to paint.* New York: International Universities Press.

Milner, M. (1969). *The hands of the living god.* New York: International Universities Press.

Naumburg, M. (1966). *Dynamically oriented art therapy: Its principles and practice.* New York: Grune & Stratton.

Robbins, A. (1987). *The artist as therapist.* New York: Human Sciences Press.

Robbins, A. (2001). Object relations and art therapy. In J. Rubin (Ed.), *Approaches to art therapy* (2nd ed., pp. 54–65). New York: Brunner-Routledge.

Rubin, J. (1978). *Child art therapy.* New York: Van Nostrand Reinhold.

Rubin, J. (2001). *Approaches to art therapy.* New York: Brunner/Mazel.

Schaverien, J. (1992). *The revealing image.* London: Routledge.

Ulman, E. (1992). A new use of art in psychiatric diagnosis. *American Journal of Art Therapy, 30,* 78–88.

Wallace, E. (1975). Creativity and Jungian thought. *Art Psychotherapy, 2,* 181–187.

Wallace, E. (1987). Healing through the visual arts: A Jungian approach. In J. Rubin (Ed.), *Approaches to art therapy* (pp. 95–107). New York: Brunner/Mazel.

Winnicott, D. (1953). Transitional objects and transitional phenomena. *International Journal of Psychiatry, 34,* 89–97.

Winnicott, D. (1965). *The maturation processes and the facilitating environment.* New York: International Universities Press.

Winnicott, D. W. (1971). *Therapeutic consultations in child psychiatry.* New York: Basic Books.

CHAPTER 5

Humanistic Approaches

Cathy A. Malchiodi

Humanistic psychology is known as the "third force of psychology" and emerged as an alternative to psychoanalytic and behavioral approaches. The following models, among others, encompass humanistic psychology: existential therapy (Frankl, 1963; May, 1953, 1961), person-centered therapy (Rogers, 1951, 1961), and Gestalt therapy (Perls, 1969; Passons, 1975; Zinker, 1978). Maslow (1968) was also instrumental in developing the humanistic trend in psychology, proposing the ideas of self-actualization and personal potential. He criticized Freud, observing that Freud paid too much attention to hostility, aggression, and neuroses and too little attention to humans' capacity for love, creativity, and joy.

The humanistic approaches to art therapy developed both in reaction to psychoanalytic approaches to art therapy and as a result of the human potential movement of the 1960s and 1970s. Art therapist Josef Garai (1987) conceived an overarching humanistic approach to the practice of art therapy based on three principles: "1) emphasis on life-problem solving; 2) encouragement of self-actualization through creative expression; and 3) emphasis on relating self-actualization to intimacy and trust in interpersonal relations and the search for self-transcendent life goals" (p. 189). According to Garai, the goal of a humanistic approach to art therapy is not so much to eliminate anxiety, unhappiness, or other emotions but to assist the individual in transforming them into authentic expressions through art modalities. His observation is consistent with the values of humanistic psychology and, in particular, reinforces the centrality of creativity as a means of experiencing and actualizing human potential as a healing agent.

This chapter introduces three humanistic approaches to art therapy—person-centered, Gestalt, and existential—and a fourth approach that emerged in part from humanistic philosophy—transpersonal. All these approaches share a respect for the client's subjective experiences as expressed through art and each trusts the individual to make positive and constructive choices. All emphasize concepts such as personal freedom, choice, values, responsibility, autonomy, and meaning. Each proposes that the individual and the therapist work together to explore imagery and creativity and supports the uniqueness of each individual's attending to each moment in order to fully understand oneself.

EXISTENTIAL APPROACH

The idea of existentialism began as a philosophy and then was later adopted by the fields of psychology and psychiatry. Frankl (1963), a noted figure in existential theory, embraced the concepts of personal freedom, meaning, and the search for values. A core belief in his work is the "will to meaning"; Frankl felt that therapy should be aimed at challenging individuals to find meaning and purpose in life. Bugental (1987) later echoed this idea, noting that the central concern of therapy is to help the individual examine how he or she has answered life's existential questions and to begin to live authentically.

Rollo May (1961) is a key figure bringing existential theory into the practice of therapy and is important to the development of an existential approach to art therapy because of his ideas on creativity (May, 1976). May (1976) saw creativity as a struggle against disintegration and as a means to bring into existence "new kinds of being" (p. 22). Although he did not propose the use of art in existential therapy, he supports the idea that it takes "courage to create" and the creative process is an expression of the self and the dilemmas of human existence. Clark Moustakas (1959) and May (1976) believed that creativity is central to mental health and used the concept of creativity in existential therapy.

The conceptual framework developed by Frankl, Bugental, May and others became the basis for an existential approach to art therapy. Art therapist Bruce Moon (1995) proposed a theory for the application of existential principles to art therapy, based on art expression as a personal search for meaning and creativity as an important component of health. An existential approach to art therapy can best be described as a philosophy that influences how a therapist practices, rather than a defined model with specific techniques. A therapist applying this theory to clinical work is guided by existential ideas and themes that individuals universally experience, such as love, joy, suffering, and the quest for personal meaning.

Because existential values grew out of an intense consciousness of the tragic and noble in human potential, an existential approach emphasizes liberating the individual from fears and anxieties and helping the person to live life to the fullest. Creative work is believed to be part of this and offers the experiences of free choice and the opportunity to make sense of what often seems senseless or meaningless. The process of art making within the therapeutic relationship serves as a metaphor for the existential dilemmas and art making may lead a person toward a state of mindfulness (B. Moon, 1995).

Taking an existential approach to art therapy includes addressing the following through the process of art making and therapeutic exchange: (1) the capacity for self-awareness; (2) freedom and responsibility; (3) creating one's identity and establishing meaningful relationships with others; (4) the search for meaning, purpose, values, and goals; (5) anxiety as a condition of living; and (6) awareness of death and non-being (adapted from Corey, 1996). The practitioner adopting an existential approach strives to understand deep human experience and to help the individual make sense of existence. Questions such as "Who am I?", "Who have I been?", and "Where am I going?" are the focus of an existential model.

As with other humanistic approaches, existential art therapy is considered to be a shared journey and the person finds meaning for images that result from this encounter. Interpretation is only relevant in as much as the individual interprets artistic expression and the creative process. The therapist models authentic behavior—not only in the verbal exchange but also through artistic expression. For example, selectively disclosing thoughts and personal experiences as well as sharing one's own artistic expression may become the basis for the therapeutic relationship and for existential themes to be explored.

Art therapist Bruce Moon shares the following case example of an existential approach (adapted from B. Moon, 1995, p. 90):

In the studio I watched Rob put the finishing touches on a painting of heavy chains and a huge key lock, on a black background. Rob said, "That's the way it is. The older I get, the more chains are wrapped around me." Rob sees no possibility that he is free to chose his path. He sees no possibility that he is responsible for his life. Needless to say, he is not free from the circumstances of his existence, either cultural, sociological or psychological.

The therapeutic task with Rob is one of empowerment. As we journey together in therapy, I pay close attention to his self-destructive self-limiting. I celebrate those moments when he owns his choices. Watching him paint, being with him as he struggles with beginning, offers a marvelous opportunity to explore with him his attitude toward the limits of his life in metaphor:

BRUCE: You choose black as your background.
ROB: Yes; it's rather dismal, isn't it?
B: It looks dark and heavy.
R: I guess it has to be that way.
B: But you could have painted it red or blue or yellow.
R: No, it had to be black.
B: (*pointing to the paint cabinet*) I see a jar of pink, even.
R: What are you trying to say?
B: Only that you choose black.
R: It has to be.
B: No, we have other colors.
R: What's your point?
B: That you choose.
R: All right, damn it, I choose.

Moon's therapeutic goal is an existential one: By using the art process as a metaphor for choice and free will, Rob has the opportunity to own his choice and thus has the possibility to make other choices. Moon underscores Rob's dilemma of being a victim by responding with ideas that he is free to choose and that he holds the ultimate power to choose. The art process serves as stage for therapist–client dialogue about existential issues of freedom to choose, will to meaning, and the search for purpose, values, and goals.

PERSON-CENTERED APPROACH

The goal of person-centered therapy is to assist people in becoming more autonomous, spontaneous, and confident (Rogers, 1951, 1969). People find the resources within themselves to solve problems and heal and recover. The therapist provides a growth-promoting atmosphere in which the individual can reach full potential and trusts the person has an internal capacity to become well.

A person-centered approach to art therapy, like the existential approach, focuses on the individual's ability to find personal meaning. The process involved is not so much a process of reparation but of becoming (Rogers, 1969). An important aspect of this approach is the belief that people are capable of expressing rather than repressing their own maladjustments and moving toward a more healthful way of life. The client–therapist relationship capitalizes on creative art expression as a means of harnessing personal resources to change and grow.

Play therapy, which often involves some form of creative art expression, has clearly embraced the person-centered approach because of its versatility and its nondirective stance. Person-centered approaches in experiential work with children have been richly described in the work of Axline (1964) and Landreth and Sweeney (1999). Child-centered play therapy facilitates a process in which the therapist trusts the inner person to make the "journey of self-exploration and self-discovery" through creative expression (Landreth & Sweeney, 1999, p. 39) and uses Rogers's principles of self-realization and self-actualization.

A person-centered approach to art therapy, viewed through the lens of the philosophy of Carl Rogers, underscores two principles in particular:

Active and Empathetic "Seeing"

According to Rogers (1969), active and empathetic listening is the ability of the therapist to provide full attention to the person and to actively enhance the person's feeling of being full heard and deeply understood. This process involves reflection of thoughts and feelings and clarification and summarization of what transpires during the session. In the case of art therapy, it is also the therapist's ability to provide full attention to that person's creative process and images—in other words, active and empathetic "seeing." In a person-centered approach, the therapist communicates to the person that he or she is seeing and understanding correctly what the person is expressing through art. This is not interpretation of the work but carefully asking questions to help the therapist understand and comprehend what the person is communicating through art. For example, after asking a child to "tell me about your drawing," the therapist may say to the child that "the little boy in your drawing feels sad because he is all alone at home and he wants his mother to come home and play with him." The purpose of a person-centered approach is to gradually reflect the contents of the art expression to the person and to receive clarification from the art maker.

A person-centered approach integrating art expression within therapy provides the added benefit of allowing the therapist to "see" what the person feels and thinks, in addition to hearing a verbal account. Rogers asserts that when therapists can grasp the client's private world and understand it as the person sees its, constructive change is most likely to occur. Art expression adds another dimension that enhances the person's ability to communicate and provides the therapist with an additional modality for understanding the client.

Acceptance

Acceptance refers to unconditional, positive regard for the individual by the therapist (Rogers, 1969). In a person-centered approach to art therapy, unconditional, positive regard for the person's art expressions is central to the experience. The therapist trusts the abilities of the person to move in positive directions and offers an atmosphere in which art expression is accepted without judgment. It is important to convey that creative work does not need to be aesthetic or beautiful, but that the purpose is to express and release thoughts and feelings through the modality. Person-centered art therapy also avoids evaluation and interference with the creative process to encourage self-direction, self-evaluation, and responsibility in treatment.

Natalie Rogers (1997), an expressive arts therapist and the daughter of Carl Rogers, is recognized as a major proponent of the person-centered approach to art therapy. Although her approach involves not only visual art, but all art forms, she does provide groundwork for the theory and practice of person-centered art therapy. A case vignette from the work of Natalie Rogers (1999) provides an example of how person-centered principles are applied to practice.

> If the facilitator intends to lead an individual in an exercise to stimulate art or movement expression and self-awareness, then he or she has the task of helping that individual talk about it. Knowing that the artist takes a risk in sharing that previously unknown aspect of the self, the facilitator needs to treat the product with great respect.
>
> It is important to me that we truly hear and respect the artist's personal experience. Therefore, I always ask the artist to speak first, giving her feelings, meanings, and interpretations of the piece. To offer feedback before hearing what it represents to the artist is to rob that person of their fresh, spontaneous reaction to the work. If we wish to create an environment for the client's self-direction and self-insight, it is necessary to honor her experience.
>
> After inviting the individual to share thoughts and feelings about her art, I ask "Do you honestly want my reactions?" If so, I offer my congruent feelings in statements that make it clear that these are my projections on her art. I do not interpret a person's art.

There is a fine line, an important nuance, between making congruent personal responses and interpreting another's work. I am owning my reactions when I preface my feedback with, "When I look at your art, I feel. . . . Or, in witnessing your painting, I felt . . . ." Giving feedback in this manner is very different from saying, "This art shows how depressed you are, or how chaotic your life is." . . . Telling a person in a declarative way what her art means takes away the sense of self-knowledge. (p. 122)

Natalie Rogers echoes the concepts developed by her father more than 40 years ago. However, she also demonstrates the power of art expression to enhance a person-centered approach, illustrating through her work how individual creativity is indeed a powerful tool in self-realization and self-actualization.

GESTALT APPROACH

Gestalt therapy is an experiential approach that, like other humanistic approaches, emerged in reaction to psychoanalysis. The word "Gestalt" refers to the whole form or configuration which is greater than the sum of its parts. The aim of a Gestalt approach is to encourage and insist on responsible, honest, direct, and authentic communication between the person and therapist. As in existential and person-centered approaches, therapy is a mutual exploration of feelings and thoughts between client and therapist. The therapist is also part of the overall "Gestalt" and is considered part of the whole configuration.

Gestalt therapists encourage active participation and enactment by the individual, believing that through sensory–motor activation, there is recognition and clarification of problems. The experiential nature of Gestalt therapy led to the integration of art activities and several individuals have contributed to the development of a "Gestalt art therapy" theory. Joseph Zinker (1977), a Gestalt therapist and sculptor, promoted the multimodal use of creative expression (meaning using many art forms and modalities; see Chapter 9, this volume) based on Gestalt theory. He believed that the art expression is therapeutic because it allows people to know themselves as a whole person in a short time, and being able to perceive the whole is consonant with the idea of the Gestalt. Violet Oaklander (1978) developed a Gestalt approach to work with children and families through art, play, and other sensory modalities. Art therapist Mala Betensky (1973) combined phenomenological approaches with Gestalt principles to develop a way for the therapist and client to determine what was present in the image.

Of all therapists who have used Gestalt principles in their clinical work, art therapist Janie Rhyne is best known for developing the idea of the "Gestalt art experience." Rhyne studied with Gestalt therapist, Fritz Perls (1969), known for his work at Esalen in the 1960s; Perls experimented with techniques that later formed some of the basis for Rhyne's ideas integrating art therapy. Rhyne (1995) sums up Gestalt art therapy as an experience of focusing on the active movement in the art expression; encouraging clients to consider forms and patterns of their visual messages and to actively perceive what is going on in lines, shapes, textures, colors, and movements;

and evoking in clients a sense of how their forms can express personal meaning. Art expression allows individuals to know themselves as a whole person; in a sense, the art expression is a "gestalt" of that person within that moment. The creative process of art making is seen as valuable in helping the person become a more fully integrated human being. Rhyne observed that Gestalt art therapy addresses the entire range of personal expressiveness, including visual, sound, body language, and verbal communication. This is reminiscent of an expressive arts therapy approach described in detail in Chapter 9 (this volume).

Thompson-Taupin (1976) explains some of the principles of Gestalt art therapy in the following brief example, called the "line game":

> The line game is played by tacking a large sheet of paper on the wall and having on hand a basket of crayons or pieces of chalk of various colors. One person at a time is "it." That person comes up to the paper and is told, "Select a color and draw a line or shape." That being done, he is told, "Now another with different color." I usually ask the person to make the sound or movement of each line or shape. Other group members are encouraged to mimic and get into the spirit of how each line feels to the person who is "it." At this point, many choices are open. One possibility is the "gestalting" of the two lines or shapes by "it." Another is to say to "it." Now use the people in the group to be your lines and dramatize what is going on. You are the director of the play for the next few minutes—and you can also be one of the characters. It's your show. (p. 113)

A Gestalt art therapy or "art experience" is appropriate for people who are capable, active, and committed to realizing and achieving their own potential. They are generally self-directed and self-motivated; the therapist facilitates the session, but it is the person who is ultimately responsible for meeting goals and making self-evaluations. The Gestalt art therapy approach can be useful with individuals; it has also been successfully employed in groupwork (Rhyne, 1995), capitalizing on group interaction as a catalyst to self-exploration.

TRANSPERSONAL APPROACH

A transpersonal approach to art therapy has emerged from the humanistic approaches described in the previous section and also incorporates the belief that what is beyond the self is important to the person's well-being. As described by Boorstein (1996), "Transpersonal psychology . . . recognizes the yearning for spiritual unfolding as one of the givens of human growth and development" (p. 5). This fourth force in psychology was officially founded by Maslow (1968), Sutich (1969), and others and concerns itself with both the development of the self and the urge to push beyond the boundaries of the self in other areas of consciousness. The transpersonal approach to art therapy strives to address mind, body, and spirit through a combination of art expression, humanistic principles, mind–body concepts, and spiritual practices such as contemplation and meditation.

Franklin, Farrelly-Hansen, Marek, Swan, and Wallingford (2000) note that Carl Jung was perhaps the first practitioner of a transpersonal approach to art therapy because he believed that individuation process required the exploration and integration of the spiritual dimension as expressed through the imagery of dreams and art (Jung, 1964). Florence Cane (1951) who developed the "scribble technique" (see Chapter 2, this volume), combined art activities with meditative awareness, also articulating theories that became the basis for a transpersonal approach to art therapy. Later, Garai (1976), who pioneered the humanistic approach to art therapy, also explored how art expression led to self-transcendence, and Joan Kellogg (1978) noted the value of artistic expression in accessing transpersonal aspects of the self through mandala drawings. Others have connected art expression with spirituality (Allen, 1995; Malchiodi, 2002; B. Moon, 1997; C. Moon, 1989), linked it to models of shamanic healing (McNiff, 1981), and have looked at the relationship between spiritual beliefs and the practice of art therapy (Chickerneo, 1993; Farelly-Hansen, 2001; Feen-Calligan, 1995; Horovitz-Darby, 1994).

Many of the concepts on which the transpersonal approach to art therapy is based are reflected in humanistic approaches to treatment. For example, much of transpersonal work is similar to the person-centered approach that maintains the person's intrinsic ability to achieve growth and health. The teaching of meditation is consonant with Carl Rogers's idea of staying in the moment with the person and empowering the individual to take charge of personal change and self-realization. Emphasis on questions such as "Who am I?" and "What is the meaning of life?" reflect an existential component in transpersonal art therapy. Mind–body techniques integrated within the transpersonal framework mirror current thinking about imagery as treatment (Achterberg, 1985) and are inclusive of physical symptoms as expressions of transpersonal aspects of the self.

A therapist working from a transpersonal approach to art therapy would address the person's needs to improve other areas of life such as relationships or life satisfaction, but this approach also includes recognizing spiritual emergencies (Grof & Grof, 1989) such as emotional crises, serious illness, or death. Art expression is seen as a way to explore that which is "beyond the self" and as a process to access to nonordinary states of consciousness. The following brief example illustrates some transpersonal approaches to working with an adult whose experience with cancer caused her to confront spiritual beliefs and the possibility of death.

Case Example

Anna, a 45-year-old woman who was recently diagnosed with breast cancer, came to my practice because of recurrent anxiety about her illness and what she called "a feeling of not knowing who I am or where I am going anymore." Recently, she had been driving home on a local freeway and had a major panic attack that was so intense she pulled over to the side of the road, hyperventilating to the point of fainting. A passerby stopped and, upon seeing Anna's rapid breathing, took her to a hospital emergency room where she was treated for anxiety and released later that day.

According to Anna, the intense panic attack brought her to therapy because she "felt like her body and soul were cracking in half." Although her anxiety was being treated with medication, Anna felt the need to try some alternative techniques to cope with her feelings and thought that art expression and imagery work might be helpful to her. During our initial meetings I taught her some simple meditation practices and suggested that she meditate at home on a regular basis to reduce stress. I also thought it might be helpful to keep a drawing journal and explained to her how drawing mandalas—images within a circular format—can be relaxing and could be helpful to decreasing her anxiety, in addition to meditation.

Meditation followed by mandala drawing helped Anna to gradually express issues relevant to her distress, such as fears of death and loss of hair (Figure 5.1) due to the chemotherapy. More important, it provided Anna with a way to relax and transcend her illness, at least momentarily. Anna reported that meditation and drawing allowed her to overcome pain and nausea, but most important, they made her feel again "like a whole person" and someone "who was not a cancer victim, at least for a little while." Eventually, this experience of feeling whole transcending the self was reflected in a change in her mandala images from images representative of the experiences of illness to ones reflective of her growing sense of inner calm and balance (Figure 5.2).

Although we worked on many issues related to Anna's anxiety and her personal search for identity and meaning during the course of therapy, the crisis she experienced in both "body and soul" was important to address. We both felt that her current panic attacks might in some way be related to the trauma of being diagnosed with cancer and the subsequent surgery and chemotherapy that quickly followed the diagnosis. Anna observed that "everything happened so fast, I did not have time to think, feel, or grieve." I asked Anna to represent feelings in her body with color and

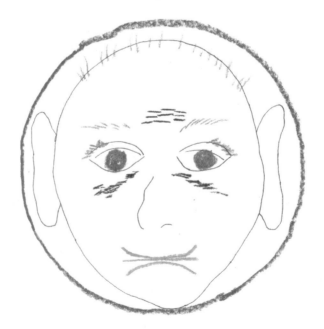

FIGURE 5.1. Anna's drawing of herself, representing fears of cancer and death.

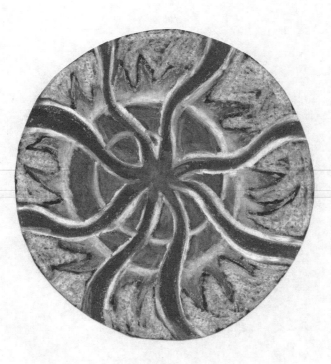

FIGURE 5.2. Mandala drawing by Anna.

imagery when her doctor told her that she had cancer. To facilitate the process, I offered Anna three simple body outlines to color, asking her to complete one to represent where she felt "hearing the diagnosis" (Figure 5.3A); the second one, what her body felt like "after the surgery" (a lumpectomy to remove an isolated tumor; Figure 5.3B); and the third one, to indicate how and where she felt "the most intensity of her panic attacks" (Figure 5.3C).

Anna's drawings revealed a pattern she felt all three experiences. It was not surprising that she chose to use color in the area of the chest to describe her breast surgery; however, in two other drawings, Anna was surprised to see that her chest was the place she felt the shock of hearing her diagnosis and the intensity of panic attacks and that these images were somewhat similar to the one of her surgery. In subsequent sessions, we worked with additional body outlines to help Anna choose colors and images that she could use in meditation to soothe the parts of her chest and body that felt discomfort, particularly the panic that interfered with her life.

While Anna used art expression and imagery in many ways during the course of therapy, she most enjoyed the mandala drawing and continued to keep a drawing journal of images she created after meditation. At our last session, Anna brought in a mandala drawing (Figure 5.4) that she said represented an "epiphany" she had the morning after a wonderful dream. In that dream she was climbing up a mountain; to either side of her were all her friends either waving or lending a hand as she made her

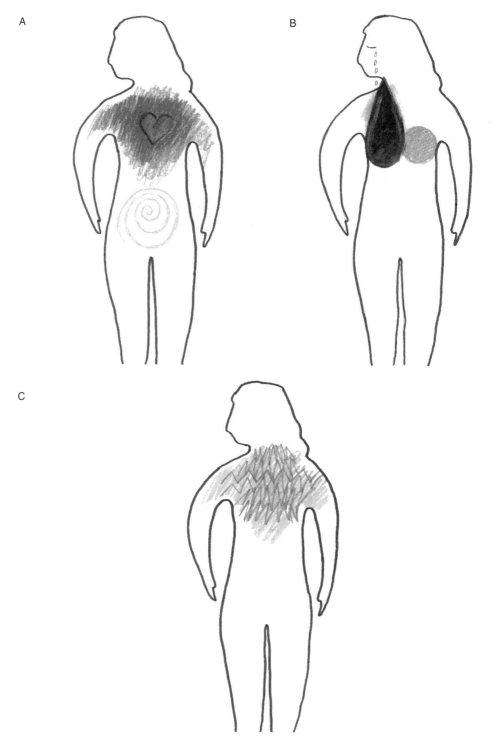

FIGURE 5.3. Three body drawings by Anna: (A) "Hearing the diagnosis"; (B) What her body felt like "after the surgery" (a lumpectomy to remove an isolated tumor); (C) How and where she felt "the most intensity of her panic attacks."

climb. What was most surprising to her as she climbed the steep slope was that she did not feel tired, only energized as she continued her hike. Anna said the ending of the dream was almost indescribable in words; when she reached the top of the mountain, she witnessed a brilliant light that enveloped her in warmth and comfort. The dream ended and she woke up with a sense of joy and peace she had not experienced for many months.

Anna's dream image and mandala drawing represented a feeling that she found within herself as a result of renewed energy but at the same time experienced "beyond" herself. It exemplifies the "peak experience" Maslow wrote about in his explorations of human potential. Like many cancer patients, Anna's diagnosis, surgery, and chemotherapy profoundly changed her life: They brought on an emotional crisis and, in a sense, a spiritual emergency, forcing her to reevaluate her life and what living life meant to her. A transpersonal approach to art therapy helped Anna to experience ways to use art expression to eventually alleviate her anxiety; offered a way to make sense of the crisis of diagnosis, surgery, and medical treatment; and provided a modality to creatively cope with the impact of illness on body, mind, and soul.

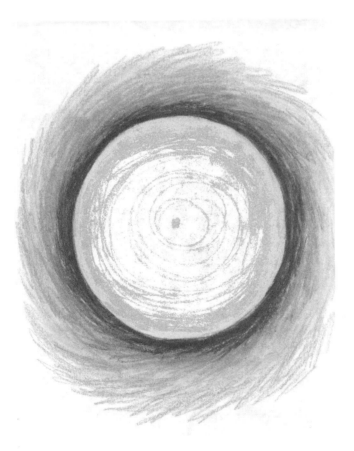

FIGURE 5.4. Anna's mandala of an "epiphany" she had after a joyful dream that left her with a sense of peace.

CONCLUSION

Humanistic approaches to art therapy range from examining life's existential meaning through the metaphor of art to more active, experiential techniques of Gestalt art therapy to the more contemplative methods such as those employed in transpersonal work. Unconditional regard, human potential, free will, self-actualization, and self-transcendence are concepts that complement the application of art expression in therapy because each underscores an element of the creative process. The common ground that connects these approaches is a respect for the person's central role in the therapeutic process, an acceptance of all artistic expression as a will to meaning, and the belief in the individual's ability to find wellness through creative exploration.

REFERENCES

Achterberg, J. (1985). *Imagery in healing: Shamanism in modern medicine.* Boston: Shambhala.

Allen, P. (1995). *Art as a way of knowing.* Boston: Shamhbala.

Axline, V. (1964). *Play therapy.* Boston: Houghton Mifflin.

Betensky, M. (1973). *Self-discovery through self-expression.* Springfield, IL: Charles C Thomas.

Boorstein, S. (Ed.). (1996). *Transpersonal psychotherapy.* Albany: State University of New York Press.

Bugental, J. (1987). *The art of the psychotherapist.* New York: Norton.

Cane, F. (1951). *The artist in each of us.* Craftsbury Common, VT: Art Therapy.

Chickerneo, N. (1993). *Portraits of spirituality in recovery.* Springfield, IL: Charles C Thomas.

Corey, G. (1996). *Theory and practice of counseling and psychotherapy* (5th ed.). Pacific Grove, CA: Brooks/Cole.

Farrelly-Hanson, M. (2001). *Spirituality and art therapy: Living the connection.* London: Jessica Kingsley.

Feen-Calligan, H. (1995). The use of art therapy in treatment programs for spiritual recovery from addiction. *Art Therapy: Journal of the American Art Therapy Association, 12*(1), 46–50.

Frankl, V. (1963). *Man's search for meaning.* Boston: Beacon.

Franklin, M., Farrelly-Hansen, M., Marek, B., Swan-Foster, N., & Wallingford, S. (2000). Transpersonal art therapy education. *Art Therapy: Journal of the American Art Therapy Association, 17*(2), 101–110.

Garai, J. (1976). New vistas in the exploration of inner and outer space through art therapy. *The Arts in Psychotherapy, 3,* 157–167.

Garai, J. (1987). A humanistic approach to art therapy. In J. Rubin (Ed.), *Approaches to art therapy* (pp. 188–207). New York: Brunner/Mazel.

Grof, S., & Grof, C. (1989). *Spiritual emergency: When personal transformation becomes crisis.* Los Angeles: Tarcher.

Horovitz-Darby, E. (1994). *Spiritual art therapy: An alternate path.* Springfield, IL: Charles C Thomas.

Jung, C. G. (1964). *Memories, dreams, and reflections.* London: Routledge & Kegan Paul.

Kellogg, J. (1978). *Mandala: Path of beauty.* Clearwater, FL: Association for Teachers of Mandala Assessment.

Landreth, G., & Sweeney, D. (1999). The freedom to be: Child-centered group play therapy. In D. Sweeney & L. Homeyer (Eds.), *The handbook of group play therapy* (pp. 39–64). San Francisco: Jossey-Bass.

Malchiodi, C. A. (2002). *The soul's palette.* Boston: Shambhala.

Maslow, A. (1968). *Toward a psychology of being.* New York: Van Nostrand Reinhold.

May, R. (1953). *Man's search for himself.* New York: Dell.

May, R. (1961). *Existential psychology.* New York: Basic Books.

May, R. (1976). *The courage to create.* New York: Norton.

McNiff, S. (1981). *The arts and psychotherapy.* Springfield, IL: Charles C Thomas.

Moon, B. (1995). *Existential art therapy.* Springfield, IL: Charles C Thomas.

Moon, B. (1997). *Art and soul: Reflections on an artistic psychology.* Springfield, IL: Charles C Thomas.

Moon, C. (1989). *Art as prayer.* Unpublished presentation at the 20th annual conference of the American Art Therapy Association, San Francisco.

Moustakas, C. (1959). *Psychotherapy and children.* New York: Harper.

Oaklander, V. (1978). *Windows to our children.* Moab, UT: Real People Press.

Passons, W. (1975). *Gestalt approaches in counseling.* New York: Holt, Rinehart & Winston.

Perls, F. (1969). *Gestalt therapy verbatim.* Lafayette, CA: Real People Press.

Rhyne, J. (1995). *The Gestalt art experience.* Chicago: Magnolia Street.

Rogers, C. (1951). *Client-centered therapy.* London: Constable.

Rogers, C. (1961). *On becoming a person.* Boston: Houghton Mifflin.

Rogers, C. (1969). *Freedom to learn.* Columbus, OH: Merrill.

Rogers, N. (1997). *The creative connection: Expressive arts as healing.* Palo Alto, CA: Science and Behavior Books.

Rogers, N. (1999). The creative connection: A holistic expressive arts process. In S. Levine & E. Levine (Eds.), *Foundations of expressive arts therapy* (pp. 113–131). London: Jessica Kingsley.

Thompson-Taupin, C. (1976). Where do your lines lead? Gestalt art groups. In J. Downing (Ed.), *Gestalt awareness* (p. 113). New York: Harper & Row.

Zinker, J. (1978). *Creative process in Gestalt therapy.* New York: Brunner/Mazel.

CHAPTER 6

Cognitive-Behavioral Approaches

Aimee Loth Rozum
Cathy A. Malchiodi

Art therapy is an active form of therapy. Clients are engaged in physical manipulation of materials and in thinking about their problems in new ways. Representing a conflict or feeling in a pencil drawing, collage, or clay sculpture allows clients literally to see their problems from all sides. At a basic level, making an image concretizes and externalizes a problem. Specific questioning by the therapist can guide the client in this process, so the problem is explored verbally and nonverbally.

Although art therapy has often focused on emotional experiences, some therapists have integrated more cognitively based constructs into their work with children and adults. Camic (1999) used cognitive-behavioral therapy based on the work of Turk, Meichenbaum, and Genest (1983) along with arts therapies to develop a treatment program for pain management. Camic's rationale was based on the use of creative arts and imagery to distract his clientele from their pain, using these modalities as a reinforcement for pain reduction. Rosal (1992, 1993, 2001) describes a variety of cognitive-behavioral approaches in the individual and group treatment of children and adults. Steele and Raider (2001) employ drawing and cognitive reframing techniques to help children recall and process traumatic events (see Chapter 11, this volume); similarly, Malchiodi (2001) uses specific drawing tasks and questions to assist children in crisis to depict their experiences, with the goal of reframing emotions and negative thoughts and reducing the sequelae of posttraumatic stress.

Image making can be integrated with cognitive-behavioral therapy to improve efficacy of the treatment. This chapter discusses the major concepts of cognitive treatment and offers suggestions for using art expression within the framework of cognitive-behavioral techniques. To introduce the theory and practice of "cognitive-behavioral art therapy," a brief overview of cognitive-behavioral theory and principles is provided to describe and illustrate how these techniques can be used within the context of art therapy.

COGNITIVE-BEHAVIORAL THERAPY

Cognitive-behavioral therapy encompasses several different approaches, including rational-emotive behavior therapy (REBT; Ellis, 1993), cognitive-behavioral modification (Meichenbaum, 1977, 1985), and cognitive therapy (Beck, 1987; Ellis & Grieger, 1996). The central notion in all these approaches is that it is not events per se but rather the person's assumptions, expectations, and interpretations of events which are responsible for the production of negative emotions (Beck & Emery, 1985; Clark, 1989). It is these negative emotions that cause people to feel depressed and anxious and can lead to full-blown emotional disorders. According to cognitively based theories psychological distress is largely a function of disturbances of cognitive processes and changing cognitions can produce desired changes in affect and behavior.

The basic goal of cognitive-behavioral therapy is to help the client identify the false and negative rules and assumptions governing actions and then find ways to replace or restructure assumptions with more realistic and positive rules and expectations. Beck's techniques, Meichenbaum's stress inoculation, and Ellis's REBT deal primarily with the elimination of symptoms. A collaborative relationship between the client and therapist is at the foundation of this approach and treatment is generally time-limited and psychoeducational in nature.

Cognitive frameworks for treatment recognize two levels of disturbed thinking. First, dysfunctional assumptions and rules are those ideas and beliefs we hold about ourselves, how we live, and how we influence individuals and situations around us. For example, when a situation triggers these rules and expectations, a depressed or anxious person responds with repetitive negative thoughts. These are referred to as "automatic negative thoughts" or "negative self-talk," because they are produced without effort or intention in response to a specific situations (Hawton, Salkovskis, Kirk, & Clark, 1989). Personal beliefs and expectations about situations are organized into "constellations" which are triggered when we are placed in a specific situation (for instance, public speaking, driving a car, or making a decision). Beck (1976) describes this constellation of rules and assumptions as "schema." A cognitive schema is a code by which people decipher and evaluate their experiences and behaviors and those of others. When a schema is organized around a negative or unrealistic rule, all experiences are filtered through this punitive filter and individuals begin to see the world as unsafe and themselves as unworthy, untalented, and unlovable.

Meichenbaum (1977, 1985) defines cognitive-behavioral therapy through the lens of stress inoculation which not only includes the principles of self-talk and schema but also emphasizes the skills in developing "coping self-statements." Such statements help the individual prepare to meet stress and include: "Don't worry. You can meet this stress successfully"; "One step at a time; you can handle the situation"; and "Relax. You are in control. Take a slow, deep breath." The overall goal is to develop positive self-statements and internal images that reduce negativity and enhance successful performance.

Cognitive-behavioral therapy is a highly directive and structured approach that requires the clinician to play an active and educational role in the therapy. In most cases, the goal of treatment is to eliminate or drastically reduce symptoms in 6 to 20 sessions as well as give the client the tools to remain symptom-free. As mentioned earlier, the key components in cognitive-behavioral therapy are the identification, restructuring, and/or elimination of negative thoughts, teaching the client to control the autonomic responses that usually attend feelings of anxiety and panic, and to use these skills to remain symptom free.

IMAGE MAKING AND COGNITIVE-BEHAVIORAL THERAPY

While art therapy is based on the use of imagery in treatment, cognitive-behavioral therapy is about language. Clients are taught to track, verbalize, and record negative thoughts in writing. Lists are made, charts are completed, and emotions ranked on scales to determine severity and monitor progress. It is a highly intellectual method, dealing with logic and cognition and questions and answers. So how does one use a nonverbal technique such as image making within such a structured therapeutic agenda?

The first barrier to using art in cognitive-behavioral therapy is the client's assumptions and expectations about being "artistic"; therapists reading this chapter also may have to confront similar personal assumptions and expectations. "Art" is a loaded word and when asked to make a picture most people will experience the triggering of a universal responses: "I can't draw." "I have no talent." "I will embarrass myself." "I will fail." The best way to avoid these responses is to jettison the use of the term "art" altogether. The term "image" is far less controversial and is actually a more accurate word for what will be produced in a cognitive-behavioral session. The client will be making concrete representations or images of negative schema, anxiety-producing cognitions, and negative self-talk. These images can be powerful representations of the workings of the mind and the interior life of the person. Asking an individual to make an image about his or her depression or anxiety makes the individual feel less inadequate and paralyzed than asking him or her to make "art." This is the one of the first acts of cognitive restructuring in treatment and it is used to illustrate how the client will be restructuring other negative schema and assumptions.

While much of cognitive-behavioral therapy has traditionally involved verbal and written exercises, there is a tradition of using mental imagery as a method of practicing new emotional patterns. Clients are asked to visually imagine themselves thinking, feeling, and behaving the way they would like to think, feel, and behave (Maultsby, 1984). Ellis (1993) observes that if we keep practicing such imagery several times a week for a few weeks, we reach a point where we are no longer upset by events that trigger negative feelings or self-talk. Meichenbaum's (1985) cognitive-behavioral modification techniques have also incorporated mental imagery to reduce stress and as a means of self-help.

Because cognitive-behavioral therapy is an approach that involves collaboration between client and therapist, it is well suited to the context of image making for several reasons. First, developing successful strategies for change in cognitive-behavioral therapy involves the input of the client in determining the course of the treatment. In an approach that includes image making, the client is offered the opportunity to collaborate with the therapist in designing creative activities to support and enhance behavioral change. Also, cognitive-behavioral therapy is action oriented; that is, the client must be willing to put time and energy into treatment, both within the therapeutic hour as well as through work outside the session. Image making as part of therapy requires the client to be an active participant in the process of change and recovery and to commit oneself to "hands-on" strategies through drawing, collage, or other media.

INITIAL SESSIONS

When using a cognitive-behavioral approach to art therapy it is best to introduce the image making to the client as soon as possible, usually by the second session (assuming the first session is spent explaining cognitive-behavioral treatment, establishing goals, and gathering information). One way to do this is to replace a verbal directive with an imaginal one. For instance, rather than asking a client to list things that contribute to depression, the therapist might ask the client to make an image presenting a problem that contributes to depression. To be able to guide the client through an analysis of the image and the problem, it is helpful for the therapist to prepare a list of questions used in cognitive-behavioral work such as:

- What is the problem?
- What does the image tell the viewer about the problem?
- What thoughts came up during the making of the image?
- What thoughts are you having now?

Introducing image making within the early sessions allows clients to practice this form of expression before they attempt it outside the session. Visual strategies are involved in some forms of cognitive-behavioral therapy; for example, the use of a chalkboard to chart negative thoughts and track dysfunctional schema is a common practice (Emery 1989; McMullin, 2000). Seeing one's negative thought in "black and white" can be a powerful experience and can bring home the personal tyranny of such cognition. However, although it can be helpful to see negative aspects of oneself, viewing one's negative self-thoughts as imagery can be overwhelming and some clients will hesitate to produce such imagery or not want to share it. By sensitive education about the process and helping the client to practicing the exercise in session at his or her own pace, the therapist can assist the person in demystifying negative self-thoughts, feelings, and behaviors and help the client to begin to identify and process reactions.

A key to using image making in initial sessions of cognitive-behavioral therapy is to remain directive and structured with the use of images similarly to the way one would with cognitive aids such as charts and worksheets. It is also important to keep directives and materials as simple as possible to increase the likelihood that the client will succeed at the exercise. The worksheets and charts of cognitive work often seem daunting and must be sensitively introduced in order not to overwhelm the client; the same is true with the use of image making in cognitive work. It takes a substantial investment of time and energy to do cognitive-behavioral exercises, and the client must comprehend the reason behind the directive and understand how it works and why it might be helpful.

Image making can also serve as a reinforcement of what is being learned, to help the person reframe or restructure experiences and behaviors (see section below) and to visually develop strategies for positive change. Integrating imagery making into to treatment might take the form of any or all of the following exercises:

• *Make an image of a "stressor."* Identifying stressors which trigger negative feelings are key to understanding and developing strategies of how to cope. The therapist may direct the client to keep an imagery journal of events, situations, or people that initiate negative behaviors or self-talk.

• *Making an image of "how I can prepare for a stressor."* For example, if being in a social setting is stressful, a client may be asked to create an image of "what I can do" or "how would I look if I were successfully meeting this challenge."

• *Make an image of "step-by-step management" of a problem.* For some individuals it is helpful to break down the problem or stressor into steps to a solution. Making an image or series of images that illustrate how the problem can be divided into more manageable parts or components can visually assist some clients in learning how to master difficult situations and any problem behaviors that result from these experiences.

• *Making imagery for stress reduction.* The very act of making images—whether drawing or constructing a collage—can be used as "time out" from negative experiences and may be useful in inducing a relaxation response (DeLue, 1998; Malchiodi, 1999). Meichenbaum's (1985) stress inoculation theory emphasizes techniques such as relaxation training and similar skills that can be used to improve the quality of life. A therapist may also suggest to clients that they collect photo images that they find self-soothing from magazines or other sources and put these into a visual journal or keep them in a prominent place such as the office where they can regularly be seen.

HOMEWORK

In cognitive-behavioral therapy, the client and therapist work together to develop homework assignments that carry treatment beyond the sessions. These assignments may include creating lists of problems, listing beliefs, tracking negative self-talk, and recording internalized self-messages. For example, in REBT, a person may fill out "self-help forms" to encourage them to challenge themselves outside therapy to engage in a risk-taking behavior, such as public speaking, and practice positive self-talk and beliefs.

In a cognitive-behavioral approach to art therapy, a client is also asked to complete homework assignments between sessions. Generally, these assignments involve using images to restructure beliefs and assumptions and to further record, through images, internalized self-messages. For example, the therapist may ask the client to purchase a three-ring binder which will serve an as image journal and workbook for homework purposes. As part of the assigned homework, the client may be asked to visually chart dysfunctional thoughts and feelings (a standard assignment) and also produce at least one image a day that represents the most pervasive thought the client experienced. To make it as easy as possible for the client to accomplish the assignment, the therapist may provide the client with some markers or oil pastels and some collage pictures and encourage the client to supplement these with additional materials. While markers are simple to use, for some clients collage is often the easiest method to record thoughts with imagery. It produces compelling results and helps some people to circumvent the anxiety of having to produce recognizable forms or pictures.

RESTRUCTURING NEGATIVE IMAGERY

Once clients have spent some time identifying and recording negative thoughts, either in session or through homework assignments, they can then start to distance from these cognitions and begin to recognize specific schema that control their perceptions and assumptions. Once these are recognized, the process of cognitive restructuring can begin. This process usually involves analysis of faulty logic, hypothesis testing, generating alternative interpretations, enlarging perspective, and decatastrophizing (Ellis, 1993; Emery, 1989). Once the therapist has led a client through the process of analyzing thoughts and schema, the client may develop more positive assumptions by experimenting with physically altering a negative image through art expression.

CASE ILLUSTRATION

The following case illustrates the use of imagery within a framework of cognitive-behavioral therapy. The client, a women in her early 40s, presented with persistent feelings of low self-worth and depression which were affecting her daily life. The woman felt that "she really had no excuse or reason to feel this way" because she had a supportive husband, had planned her two pregnancies, and had ample financial resources to obtain extra help at home. However, having two young children had made a serious impact on the time she spent making music, but she explained, "I knew this would be the case. I was prepared." The client also described herself as "ruthlessly positive" and "unflappable," so finding herself in her current state represented a failure to her. She was feeling depressed and also upset that she had encountered a situation she "couldn't tackle."

The client was asked to make an initial record of her negative thoughts (List A) followed by an image of what she felt was a problem contributing to her depression. See Figure 6.1.

List A: Initial Record of Negative Thoughts

"I'm overwhelmed."

"I want someone else to take care of me for a change."

"I want to get sick so I can stay in bed and let others handle things."

"I am a hack."

"I have no talent and am wasting my time."

"I'm pretending to have a career to feel worthwhile."

"My songs are rubbish and I might as well be putting recipes and dress patterns in with my CDs because I'm like the Betty Crocker of musicians!"

"I should be using my time to do something valuable, like being a full-time mom."

Figure 6.1 is the image made in response to the thought record and one that the client felt represented a problem contributing to her depression. The primary figure of the desexualized yet perfect homemaker has dwarfed the image of the piano which represents the client's identity as an artist. Not only is the piano in the background,

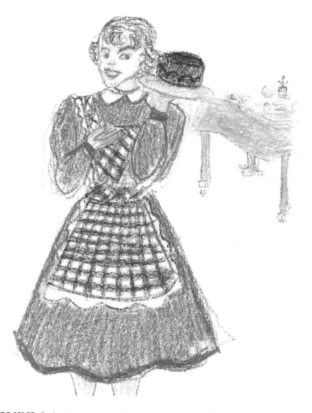

FIGURE 6.1. Drawing of a problem contributing to depression.

but its surface is cluttered with the paraphernalia of homemaking which poses a threat to the condition of the instrument. The imagery depicted a less-than-flattering view of motherhood and one that threatened her core identity as an artist. The client returned to this image several times over the course of therapy because it so accurately reflected her issues. In subsequent sessions, she worked steadily to bring the piano to the foreground as well as coming to terms with her new role as a mother. The therapist worked with the client to define core issues and identify the negative assumptions that were causing her to feel depressed. She was eventually able to challenge the notion that mothering made her less of an artist and she was able to take a more realistic approach to time management. The use of the imagery kept the client focused on the work and kept the definition of her conflicts clear.

The client also wanted to work on her poor self-image which was contributing to her depression and affecting her happiness in her sexual relationship with her spouse. To address this issue, the therapist requested that she again make a record of her negative self-talk concerning her body (List B).

List B: Second Record of Negative Thoughts

"Whatever I try, it never works."
"I just can't make it work."
"I will always feel this way."
"I hate my breasts."
"I am overweight and will never again be fit."
"I have no control over my body."
"My body is trashed and I am no longer attractive."

She was again asked to make an image reflecting her negative self-talk. The drawing (Figure 6.2) was created in two stages: a female figure alone and then adding a male figure. The initial image made by the woman was the female figure alone, representing her overwhelming feelings of self-loathing concerning her physical appearance. She felt the issue was not the weight itself but that she was not losing the weight due to having recently given birth; this feeling triggered a schema about accomplishing goals. Questioning about this image by the therapist along with the negative thought record indicated that it was her lack of progress that made her feel undesirable and unattractive. It also illuminated a schema which insisted that she be energetic, athletic, strong, and unconcerned with her weight.

Working on her own, the client picked one of the negative thoughts—"my body is trashed and I am no longer attractive"—and restructured the image. She chose to add the figure of her spouse, holding her in a protective and desirable way. Her spouse, in fact, did not share her feelings about her appearance and continued to approach her sexually and his behavior actually disproved her belief that she was sexually unattractive. Adding his image to the picture forced her to confront her dysfunctional cognitive schema, as well as providing her with some self-confidence.

The client frequently returned to this image as a way to counter her powerful convictions that she was unattractive. Despite clear evidence to the contrary (her hus-

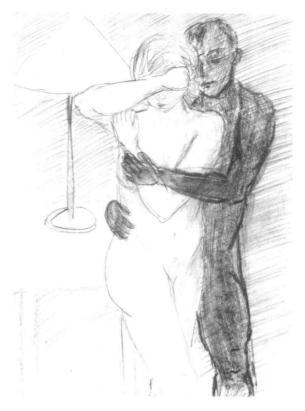

FIGURE 6.2. Drawing reflecting negative self-talk.

band's supportive statements and physical attentions), her dysfunctional rules about her attractiveness continued to fuel persistent negative self-talk and depressed mood. She was able to use her positive statements along with the images she created and she was able to use this final image (Figure 6.2) to reduce negative thoughts, reporting that the image became her "corrective mantra."

CONCLUSION

Combining cognitive-behavioral therapy with image making interweaves linguistic and imaging techniques to help clients reduce or eliminate negative cognitions and self-talk. While cognitive-behavioral therapy has traditionally used verbal modalities as agents for change, image making actually complements cognitive-behavioral approaches, providing therapists with an opportunity to capitalize on visual communication to enhance therapy. The infusion of image making within treatment offers the client an opportunity to collaborate with the therapist on developing creative visual strategies to achieve change. The benefits of therapy continue after the session in the form of imagery-related homework and encourage the client to be an active participant in the process of recovery through hands-on strategies. In summary, a cognitive-behavioral approach to art therapy offers a viable way to reframe dysfunctional patterns of behavior and provides a unique supplement to cognitive techniques that restructure negative patterns and support a positive sense of self.

REFERENCES

Beck, A. (1976). *Cognitive therapy and emotional disorders*. New York: International Universities Press.

Beck, A. (1987). Cognitive therapy. In J. Zeig (Ed.), *The evolution of psychotherapy* (pp. 149–178). New York: Brunner/Mazel.

Beck, A., & Emery, G. (1985). *Anxiety disorders and phobias: A cognitive perspective*. New York: Basic Books.

Camic, P. (1999). Expanding treatment possibilities for chronic pain through the expressive arts. In C. A. Malchiodi (Ed.), *Medical art therapy with adults* (pp. 43–61). London: Jessica Kingsley.

Clark, A. (1989). *Microcognition, philosophy, cognitive science and parallel distributed processing*. Cambridge, MA: MIT Press.

DeLue, C. (1998). Physiological effects of creating mandalas. In C. A. Malchiodi (Ed.), *Medical art therapy with children* (pp. 33–49). London: Jessica Kingsley.

Ellis, A. (1993). Fundamentals of rational-emotive therapy. In W. Dryden & L. Hill (Eds.), *Innovations in rational-emotive therapy* (pp. 1–32). Newbury Park, CA: Sage.

Ellis, A., & Grieger, R. (Eds.). (1996). *Handbook of rational-emotive therapy* (Vols. 1–2). New York: Springer.

Emery, G. (1989). *Own your own life*. New York: Signet.

Hawton, K., Salkovskis, P. M., Kirk, J., & Clark, D. M. (Eds.). (1989). *Cognitive behaviour therapy for psychiatric problems*. New York: Oxford University Press.

Malchiodi, C.A. (1999). *Medical art therapy with adults*. London: Jessica Kingsley.

Malchiodi, C.A. (2001). Using drawing as intervention with traumatized children. *Trauma and Loss: Research and Intervention, 1*(1), 21–28.

Maultsby, M. (1984). *Rational behavior therapy*. Englewood Cliffs, NJ: Prentice-Hall.

McMullin, R. (2000). *Handbook of cognitive therapy techniques*. New York: Norton.

Meichenbaum, D. (1977). *Cognitive behavior modification: An integrative approach*. New York: Plenum Press.

Meichenbaum, D. (1985). *Stress inoculation training*. New York: Pergamon Press.

Rosal, M. (1992). Approaches to art therapy with children. In F. E. Anderson (Ed.), *Art for all the children* (pp. 142–183). Springfield, IL: Charles C Thomas.

Rosal, M. (1993). Comparative group art therapy research to evaluate changes in locus of control in behavior disordered children. *The Arts in Psychotherapy, 20,* 231–241.

Rosal, M. (2001). Cognitive-behavioral art therapy. In J. Rubin (Ed.), *Approaches to art therapy* (pp. 210–225). New York: Brunner-Routledge.

Steele, W., & Raider, M. (2001). Structured sensory intervention with children, adolescents, and parents. *Trauma and Loss: Research and Interventions, 1*(1), 8–20.

Turk, D., Meichenbaum, D., & Genest, M. (1983). *Pain and behavioral medicine: A cognitive-behavioral perspective*. New York: Guilford Press.

CHAPTER 7

Solution-Focused and Narrative Approaches

Shirley Riley
Cathy A. Malchiodi

This chapter offers an overview of the most compelling features of solution-focused and narrative therapies and proposes how art therapy is compatible with these approaches to treatment. To implement these approaches the therapist must put aside the traditional long-term, pathology-oriented theories and accept the client as the expert in an equal position of collaboration with the therapist. This stance establishes that treatment is collaborative and judged by the client's standards, not the therapist's.

Art therapy has been noted for its ability to bring about a more rapid resolution of the presenting difficulties than verbal means alone. It is recognized that two languages, one verbal and one visual, stimulates processes that help the client find solutions to problems in a timely manner (Riley & Malchiodi, 1994). By combining art activities along with solution-focused and narrative approaches, therapeutic change is expedited through both specific interventions and creative expression.

SOLUTION-FOCUSED THERAPY

de Shazer (1980, 1982, 1985, 1991) is the person most frequently associated with solution-focused therapy. de Shazer insists that individuals, couples, and families join with the therapist in therapeutic conversation to describe their life experiences and problems. The therapist leads, directed by the clients' goals, in the construction of possible solutions to reach those objectives. Instead of "problem talk"—a search for explanations to why the problem occurred—the therapist urges "solution talk"—solutions that therapist and client want to work on together. For example, a solution-focused therapist would ask, "How can we work together to help you solve your problem?" This type of question sets the stage for an expectation of change and participation of the client in treatment.

de Shazer believes, like strategic therapists, that problems essentially begin from faulty attempts at problem solution; the client or family has simply run out of ways of dealing with the problem. They may also believe that options for change are extremely limited or nonexistent. Why a particular problem initially arose is less important than helping the client to discover creative ways of solving the problem. de Shazer observes that everyone has the "keys" to unlock the doors that will stimulate positive change; the therapist's task is to help the client find the right keys, rather than understand why the lock won't open.

Solution-focused therapy is also referred to as solution-focused brief therapy (SFBT; Cade & O'Hanlon, 1993); that is, it is conducted in approximately 5 to 10 sessions. By limiting the number of sessions, the therapist also supports the belief that change can occur relatively quickly. Art therapy is compatible with brief approaches such as solution-focused therapy because the process of creating images tends to accelerate the emergence of thoughts and recall of memories and details.

SOLUTION-FOCUSED APPROACHES TO ART THERAPY

Selekman (1997) observes that art activities support a solution-focused approach to treatment because they are less threatening and support the partnership between therapist and client as co-creators of solutions. Although there are many techniques used in solution-focused therapy, several are central to art therapy from a solution-focused approach. These include the role of resistance, exception questions, the miracle question, and facilitating change.

Neutralizing Resistance

Selekman (1993) observes that solution-focused therapy assumes that "resistance is not a useful concept" (p. 141). de Shazer (1994) concurs, noting that the notion of resistance handicaps therapists because it implies that clients do not want to change. If the therapist starts a therapeutic relationship looking for a negative reaction from the client (resistance), chances are that it will be discovered and reinforced.

In solution-focused art therapy, the therapeutic relationship starts with mutual goal setting and a cooperative attitude, with the target of neutralizing resistance. In the initial session, the client may be asked to set some goals through a collage or a simple drawing. A value of art expression in the early phase of treatment is that it allows the client to express the problem in a tangible form and it informs the therapist about the presenting issues through images. When the therapist respectfully explores the art product and listens to how the client perceives it and its meaning, the client feels heard.

In a family session, every member might be asked to draw his or her own view of the major difficulty or the "most pressing problem" that each sees in the family system. The images open the way for subsequent discussion and demystification of the presenting problems. In the case of families, recognition of differing opinions about goals for therapy follow and consensus on the most urgent goal forces some compromise and agreement.

The following brief case may help to illustrate this point. When asked to draw the most pressing problem, a parent may depict her child with undesirable friends who she feels have led her son or daughter astray. The child might draw the "terrible" teacher that has singled him out for unjust punishment. The therapist has the opportunity to take this one step further by asking parent and child to fold or cut away the persons outside the family represented in their drawings and place their images of parent and child close together so that they touch. They are then asked to draw a solution together on a single sheet of paper to combat these external forces. For the parent and child to draw on the same page is an introduction to the notion that they must work together to problem solve. Proceeding sessions could focus on dual drawings that invite multiple ways to cooperate (e.g., mother depicts visiting school and child could illustrate bringing a few friends over to the home).

Exception-Finding Questions

A therapeutic truth that sometimes is forgotten is that change is inevitable (Selekman, 1993). Everyone and every family progresses through life changes. de Shazer (1985) and Berg and Miller (1992) offer a solution-focused intervention to stimulate change that de Shazer calls the "exception-finding question." This type of question helps to deconstruct a problem by focusing on exceptions to the structure. For example, "When you experienced a moment when you were not depressed, how did you accomplish that?" With every client problem, there is usually some sort of exception when the problem does not occur. A common problem often heard in therapy is: "She (or he) always yells at me." A solution-focused therapist will ask, "Can you think of one time when she was not hollering?" Because there is a high chance that an exception can be found, staying closely focused on that one exception and the associated circumstances may be helpful in stimulating problem solving and change.

Over some sessions these questions can be translated into suggestions for an art expression. A change in attitude or behavior becomes more real when it is made concrete. For example, of an adolescent with behavior problems, the therapist might request, "Can you illustrate what change you would experience if you were cooperative with your teachers and other students at school?" With a family, one might ask, "What would dinnertime look like if it did not end in a big fight or a free-for-all?" These types of questions ask clients to imagine what it would be like if the problem were not present in their lives. The physical action of the art activity also reinforces investment in the decision-making process and stimulates thinking through possible solutions.

The Miracle Question

de Shazer (1991) is credited with inventing "the miracle question," which is a technique that asks clients to imagine how their lives would be if they awaken the next day and they were symptom-free (Figure 7.1). He states: "Suppose that one night there is a miracle and while you were sleeping the problem that brought you to therapy is solved: How would you know? What would be different? What would you notice the next morning that will tell you that there has been a miracle?" (p. 113).

The miracle question was designed to envision a hypothetical solution and to encourage the client to speculate on what life would be like when the problem brought to therapy is actually solved. The client is also encouraged to explore other dimensions of the question, including the following questions: "Who would notice?" "Who would care?" "How would you be running your life?" Any number of questions can be created around the notion of positive change and reaching the goal of problem solving.

For example, a 48-year-old woman, socially and professionally successful, was in therapy to explore her marriage and make some changes. The marriage had not been easy and over the last 10 years had deteriorated. Her husband had had several

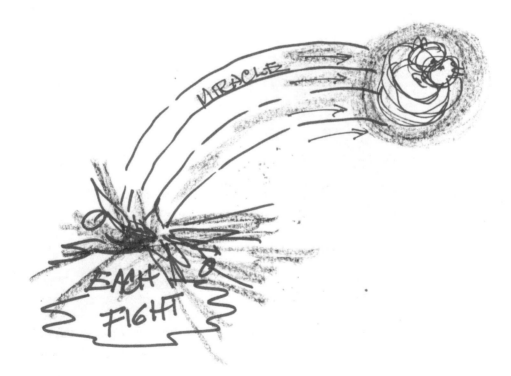

FIGURE 7.1. Author's example of a drawing in response to the "miracle question."

extramarital affairs and blamed them on his wife, whom he accused of getting old and unattractive. He also was showing signs of early dementia, which he refused to acknowledge, and needed a caretaker to watch him, particularly his inappropriate sexual advances to strangers. The wife stayed in the marriage "for the children," who were now grown and independent.

The woman seemed to see herself as a victim but recognized her passive position and was considering how she could leave home and her husband. In art therapy she made many images of living in a miserable small apartment, living in loneliness, and being without the comforts she had in her own home. After several weeks of repetition of these same depressing outcomes of moving out of the home, the therapist asked her to "imagine that she had fallen asleep last evening and when she awakened in the morning, life would be ordered in a way that would be more satisfactory." She closed her eyes spontaneously and remained quiet for quite some time. She then rose from her chair and said in an animated and energetic voice, "Why should I have to move? He is the [expletive] who failed every vow and promise of my marriage. He will go! I will stay. That is what would make me happy and it is just!"

The therapist encouraged her to make some symbols to anchor her decisions in imagery to fortify and reward her beliefs. Within weeks she rented a nice apartment for her husband, moved him out with his caretaker, and became the "owner" of her home. The move was approved by her children and, surprisingly, by her husband.

The task of portraying the miracle question via an art piece, such as a collage, "What will you be doing in the future when this problem no longer exists?" or, "How will you be making decisions differently when the problem has lost its hold on you?" brings a sense of immediacy to this question. In addition to providing a vision of a positive future, the discussion employs language that fits the client's dominant problem-solving approach.

Facilitating Change

O'Hanlon and Weiner-Davis (1989) believe a therapist using a solution-focused approach is trying to achieve three things: "1) change the 'doing' of the situation that is perceived as problematic; 2) change the 'viewing' of the situation that is perceived as problematic; and 3) evoke resources, solutions, and strengths to bring to the situation that is problematic" (pp. 126–127).

For example, a harassed single mother who works day and night to keep her family together can be validated through a simple clarification of the burdens she bears daily by creating an art piece, with the children's help, of all the duties she attempts to do every day. The parent often is surprised to see the number of tasks and the children can come to a new appreciation of the energy it takes to provide their home life. In this situation, the therapist offers encouragement to the client by observing times she has done something extra. The therapist might ask, "How did you ever find time to do that?"

In single-parent families, communication often turns into shouting when the parent is pushed over the edge. To change the "viewing" of the situation, the therapist can identify exceptions and focus on a time (no matter how brief) when messages were sent without negativity. For example, the therapist might ask the mother to illustrate "how you mustered the inner strength that stopped you from screaming at Johnny." "Can you illustrate how Johnny acted differently, even for a short time, after you explained the reason you were upset?" "Johnny, make a picture for Mom that shows her how you will help each other not to yell." A solution-focused therapist joins with the client to solve the immediate stressor and to change both "doing" and "viewing" of a problem situation.

Problems are exacerbated by repetitive failed attempts to problem solve; this is the time when identification of resources and strengths becomes important for change. Clients often experience guilt because they are ashamed of their lack of success, but they are relieved when they can let go of the guilt that accompanies failure by joining the therapist in creating alternate approaches to problem solving. A task that leads to discussion of success and failure follows: The family makes an image of the "problem" in the center of the paper in the form of an "insurmountable" mountain. They are challenged to find a way to "move the mountain." This is a common metaphor which most adults can relate to easily and calls on them to use their resources to change the picture. Mountains may be blown up, tunneled through, gone around, scaled, and cut out (Figure 7.2). It is immaterial how the mountain was top-

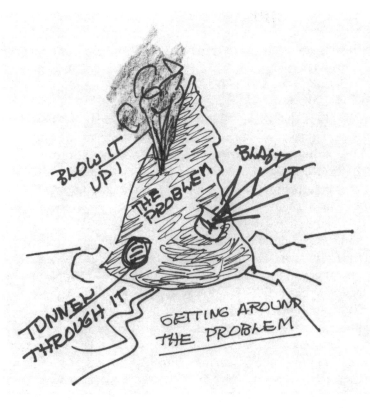

FIGURE 7.2. Author's example of a "moving the mountain," an example of helping clients to envision getting around a problem.

pled, but it is important how the family used their resources to make a change. The problem can be destroyed in one way or many ways and can become the family metaphor for solving the problem in a new manner.

At some point, the therapist can reinforce change by using additional solution-focused strategies. For example, it may be helpful to ask the client to illustrate any of the following: "How often do you plan to repeat this positive action this coming week?" "Which part of these exceptions (pointing to the images) do you think will happen first?" "Would you like to take that piece of the artwork home and check the frequency that this transformed behavior is recognized?" "How will I know when you have satisfactorily reached the goal you desired? Illustrate those circumstances."

NARRATIVE THERAPY

Narrative therapy (White & Epston, 1990) is considered a relatively new direction in family therapy and is similar to solution-focused approaches to treatment. The term "narrative" has been used to refer to the telling or retelling of stories as part of therapy. While narrative therapy involves a highly focused set of intervention techniques, its basic principles complement those of art therapy, and for this reason, it is a useful approach in work with children, adults, and families.

The primary goal of narrative therapy is to help people externalize their problems (White 1989; White & Epston, 1990) to separate the individual from the problem. In fact, the maxim of narrative therapy is "the problem is the problem, the person is not the problem." When a person believes the problem is part of his or her character, it is difficult to make changes and to call on inner resources to make those changes. Separating the problem from the person relieves the pressure of blame and responsibility and frees the therapist and client to focus on how to solve the problem.

Narrative therapy uses primarily verbal means—storytelling and therapeutic letters—to help people externalize their problems. In taking a narrative approach to art therapy, the art expression also becomes a form of externalization with added benefits to the therapeutic process. For example, a drawing, painting, or collage of the presenting problem is a natural way of separating the person from the problem because through art, the problem becomes visible. It allows the person to literally see the problem and think about it as something outside him- or herself. Visual modes of externalization are particularly helpful with children who do not have the verbal capacity to communicate details. It also is a viable therapeutic option when solution-focused strategies are not helping to alter responses or beliefs. Creative expression in the form of art is especially helpful if an adult or family is wedded to a label, habit, behavior, or lifestyle that is difficult to successfully externalize through words alone. It also can evoke a physical sense of how the problem feels and provides the opportunity to make meaning and rework images into new stories.

Freeman, Epston, and Lobovits (1997) see expressive activities as an integral part of the narrative therapy approach, particularly with children and their families. They note that "an externalizing conversation is easily enhanced with other forms of expression favored by children, such as play and expressive arts therapy" (p. 11).

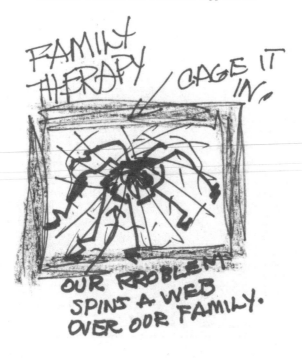

FIGURE 7.3. Author's example of a depiction of the family's problem.

Children and their families can more effectively participate in the narrative process using drawing, painting, cartoons, sculpture, dramatic play with puppets, dress-ups, and mask making. Child clients are already "experts" at art and naturally enjoy using expressive modalities to create stories and retell them to others.

Riley (1997) observes that a narrative approach to art therapy allows for multiple perspectives to emerge, particularly in work with families. In most families, a myth persists that everyone is in agreement about "how they understand the problem" and, moreover, what to do about it. However, it is not likely for the family to have an agreement or a consensus concerning problem solving. Art expression can address multiple perspectives, helping the family to see how each other defines the problem and its solution. For example, the members of a family can be asked to individually depict the dominant "problem" that concerns them (Figure 7.3). Multiple images of the same problem can be expressed and all can be witnessed by the family and therapist.

Riley and Malchiodi (1994) also note that "When the family begins telling their stories, imaging a new ending, finding new truths, they are becoming creative. Being aware of these variants should improve the chances for a good outcome to therapy. The block to success is that of language. It takes many years for newlyweds, for example, to understand what their spouse really means. How can therapists, newly wed to the client family, learn a foreign language and exotic legends of their clients rapidly enough to be effective?" (p. 21). This observation underscores the possibilities for art expression to assist both therapist and client in understanding the client's narrative and using images to supplement communication and problem resolution.

NARRATIVE STRATEGIES AND ART THERAPY

Much of narrative therapy is predicated on how the therapist uses questions to help people understand and separate from the "problem-saturated story" about themselves. In a narrative approach to art therapy, these questions might include the following:

- How long has the problem (attitude, behavior, emotional difficulty, habit, illness) been pushing you around? What does it make you do that you don't want to do? Can you show me through a drawing what it looks like when it is pushing you around?
- Are there times when you didn't allow the problem to get you into trouble? Can you draw or imagine a time lately when the problem was present but you didn't allow it to get the better of you?
- Are there times when you feel you can push the problem around? Can you show me through a drawing what it looks like when you are pushing the problem around?

The following brief case example illustrates how a therapist using a narrative approach employs art expression to help an individual separate from the problem. A young woman came to therapy to explore her struggles with her family's expectations for her after her graduation from college. She was the first person in her family to obtain a college degree and the first young woman to move out of the family home before marriage. Her parents had immigrated and had lived in the United States since their early 20s; the woman's mother had not mastered English and was still very much involved in the customs and belief systems of her country. In her parent's culture a woman had a lesser stature than a man and was expected to behave according to old world rules of feminine behavior. The young woman wanted to choose her male relationships independently, but her family's influence created deeply ambivalent feelings in her.

The therapist asked her to create a collage image of the demands of her culture to externalize the "problem-saturated story" and ascribe to this image all the positive and negative demands that had taken control of her life. The therapist then asked her to cut out from the image those traits that she wanted to keep and those she wished to discard. With the preferred traits, the woman made a collage that illustrated both her attachment to her family's culture and the freedom to decide how she wanted to live. By visually separating the problem from her family and herself she was able to create an alternate definition of her life choices.

By helping this young woman express in tangible form a "unique outcome" (Epston, White, & Murray, 1993)—exceptional events, actions, or thoughts that contradict the problem-saturated story where the problem did not win out—it becomes possible to deconstruct fixed beliefs about the problem. In this case, it helped the woman to see that she was empowered to do something to change the dominant story. Unique outcomes provide a way to explore and experiment with alternative stories. This is somewhat similar to de Shazer's "miracle question," which is employed to help individuals imagine other scenarios that move from problem-focused to solution-focused.

Riley (1997), in work with women and families, suggests the following art therapy strategies that complement a narrative approach:

- Trace back in your life to when messages or events emerged that established your expectations for relationships and sexuality. Illustrate those stories and then explore through additional illustrations new images that reauthor the original script.
- Create visual illustrations introducing a "new self" to your family.
- Try out new roles through art expression before trying them in the real world.

These directives are similar to the "unique outcome" and offer the client the opportunity not only to reflect on alternative stories but to actually see them through images.

CONCLUSION

According to Alter-Muri (1998), "Art therapists embracing a post-modernist approach become co-creators with their clients in a life of meaningfulness rather than continuing to act as mere interpreters of signs and symbols of pathology or the continuum of health in their client's products" (p. 250). Solution-focused and narrative approaches support the idea of therapist and client as partners and collaborators in problem solving. Art expression complements the approaches addressed in this chapter because imagery assists both therapist and client in finding alternative solutions to problem-saturated stories. There is no other form of therapy where internal processes can actually be made visible and tangible. It adds another dimension to these approaches by providing creative ways to externalize, reframe, and "restory" the problem.

REFERENCES

Alter-Muri, S. (1998). Texture in the melting pot: Post modernist art and art therapy. *Art Therapy: Journal of the American Art Therapy Association, 15*(4), 245–251.

Berg, I. K., & Miller, S. (1992). *Working with the problem drinker: A solution-focused approach.* New York: Norton.

Cade, B., & O'Hanlon, W. H. (1993). *A brief guide to brief therapy.* New York: Norton

de Shazer, S. (1980). Brief family therapy: A metaphorical task. *Journal of Marital and Family Therapy, 6,* 471–476.

de Shazer, S. (1982). *Patterns of brief family therapy: An ecosystemic approach.* New York: Guilford Press.

de Shazer, S. (1985). *Keys to solution in brief therapy*. New York: Norton.

de Shazer, S. (1991). *Putting differences to work*. New York: Norton.

de Shazer, S. (1994). *Words were originally magic*. New York: Norton.

Epston, D., White, M., & Murray, K. (1993). A proposal for re-authoring therapy. In S. McNamee & K. Gergen (Eds.), *Therapy as social construction*. Newbury Park, CA: Sage.

Freeman, J., Epston, D., & Lobovits, D. (1997). *Playful approaches to serious problems*. New York: Norton.

O'Hanlon, W., & Weiner-Davis, M. (1989). *In search of solutions: A new direction in psychotherapy*. New York: Norton.

Riley, S. (1997). Conflicts in treatment, issues of liberation, connection, and culture: Art therapy for women and their families. *Art Therapy: Journal of the American Art Therapy Association, 14*(2), 102–108.

Riley, S., & Malchiodi, C. (1994). *Integrative approaches to family art therapy*. Chicago: Magnolia Street.

Selekman, M. D. (1993). *Pathways to change: Brief therapy solutions with difficult adolescents*. New York: Guilford Press.

Selekman, M. D. (1997). *Solution-focused therapy with children: Harnessing family strengths for systemic change*. New York: Guilford Press.

White, M. (1989). *Selected papers*. Adelaide, Australia: Dulwich Centre.

White, M., & Epston, D. (1990). *Narrative means to therapeutic ends*. New York: Norton.

CHAPTER 8

Developmental Art Therapy

Cathy A. Malchiodi
Dong-Yeun Kim
Wae Soon Choi

Many therapists who use art therapy integrate a variety of developmental frameworks into their work, including psychosexual (Freud, 1905/1962) and psychosocial (Erikson, 1963) approaches and object relations (Mahler, Pine, & Bergman, 1975). Clinicians may use one or more developmental frameworks to guide therapy, but art therapy is most often informed by the stages of normal artistic development presented by Lowenfeld (1957), Gardner (1980), Kellogg (1970), and Golomb (1990) and the general principles of cognitive development proposed by Piaget (Piaget, 1959; Piaget & Inhelder, 1971). Developmental art therapy is most often used in work with children, but it may be applied to individuals of any age, especially those with physical handicaps, cognitive impairments, or developmental delays. It may also be valuable in therapy with adults who have experienced emotional stress or trauma, because art making evokes early sensory experiences and taps symbolic expression that is found throughout the developmental continuum (Malchiodi, 1993, 2002).

This chapter presents an overview of developmental art therapy, including a summary of the stages of normal artistic expression in children and goals in treatment. We offer a brief case presentation to demonstrate a developmental approach to art therapy in a rehabilitation setting and to underscore the major goals in this approach to treatment.

THEORIES OF DEVELOPMENTAL ART THERAPY

A developmental approach to art therapy uses normative creative and mental growth as a guide to understanding the individual. The work of Victor Lowenfeld (1957), an educator who believed that the art process contributed to many aspects of children's creative and mental growth, is undoubtedly one of the most important influences on the practice of developmental art therapy. Lowenfeld believed that art making not only was a source of self-expression but also had the potential to enhance emotional well-being. He coined the term "art education therapy" to describe a therapeutic and educational use of art activities with children with handicaps. Lowenfeld was somewhat influenced by the psychoanalytic concepts of his time and, as a result, became interested in how handicapping conditions influenced children's self-concept and how the art process might be used to support children's development.

Many of Lowenfeld's concepts are echoed in the work of art therapists who have applied developmental principles to their work with children and adults. Kramer (1971), who worked with culturally disadvantaged and emotionally handicapped children, recognized the power of art to developmentally enrich the lives of children. Uhlin (1972) published studies of neurologically handicapped children and provided a theory for developmental art therapy informed by normal artistic development and psychoanalytic and analytic principles. Williams and Woods (1977) actually coined the phrase "developmental art therapy" and focused their work with children on acquisition of cognitive and motor skills. Silver (1978, 2000) has contributed several decades of research on how art expression can be used to recognize and understand cognitive and developmental abilities in children and adults (see Appendix I, this volume, for a description of the Silver Drawing Test).

Henley (1992) synthesized the theories of Lowenfeld and Kramer to create an approach to treating children with physical and emotional disabilities; his work provides an excellent framework for application of the principles of art therapy and art education to children in both therapy and the classroom. Aach-Feldman and Kunkle-Miller (Aach-Feldman, 1981; Aach-Feldman & Kunkle-Miller, 1987) and Rubin (1978) used not only developmental theories of art expression but also concepts of psychosexual, psychosocial, and motor development in work with children with various disabilities and emotional disorders. More recently, the impact of neuroscience as it relates to the brain's capacity to create images, both mentally and through image-making activities, is influencing how we look at human development, particularly the function of art expression in early childhood and throughout the lifespan (Malchiodi, Riley, & Hass-Cohen, 2001).

STAGES OF NORMAL ARTISTIC DEVELOPMENT

The therapist who uses a developmental approach generally uses the normal developmental stages of artistic expression, as well as normal play, motor skills, and social interactions, as a basis for evaluation and subsequent interventions. Most art therapists and developmental psychologists are familiar with the stages and characteristics of normal artistic development in children; however, for therapists who are not acquainted with these concepts, we provide the following brief section. Because an in-depth coverage of the developmental characteristics of children's art expressions cannot be fully addressed within the scope of this chapter, readers are referred to the work of Gardner (1980), Winner (1982), Golumb (1990), Kellogg (1970), and Lowenfeld and Brittain (1987) for more information. Malchiodi (1998) and Henley (1992) also provide frameworks for therapists who work with children with handicaps or developmental disabilities. Currently, art therapists are collecting data to reevaluate the established developmental norms, examine children's drawings from a cross-cultural perspective, and create an archive of normal children's art to assist researchers in future studies (Deaver, Bernier, Sanderson, & Stovall, 2000).

Throughout childhood, all children follow expected, progressive changes in their art expression, changes that are characteristic of each age group. Table 8.1 provides an overview of the basic characteristics and graphic elements of these stages and approximate age ranges for each stage (Note: Most of the current research has been on how children draw, while less attention has been paid to other art modalities such as paint and clay.) These stages of artistic development appear to be universal to children throughout the world and are commonalties of image making that are part of every normal child's ability to communicate through art. Some children may remain in one developmental stage for years; in other cases, the child may possess the ability to move forward but may need prompting or support from a skilled therapist to do so.

It is important to have a solid understanding of the normal stages of artistic development, not only in using a developmental approach but in using any approach to art therapy. By understanding these stages and their graphic characteristics, one will be able to judge what qualities in art expressions are unusual for a child of a particular age and spot deviations in content and form. As with developmental skills and cognitive abilities, artistic expression is a sequential process. However, like motor development and cognition, there may be some overlap in age range and drawing skills and most children fluctuate between stages. For example, a child may draw human figures one day (Stage III) and makes less complex forms (Stage II) a day later. It is also important to remember that although there are many universal commonalities in how children draw at each developmental stage, children also may have a "personal visual logic" (Winner, 1982) that influences how they place objects on the page, use color and line, or develop individual symbols for people and objects in their environments; this is considered to be a normal aspect of developing artistic expression.

In a developmental art therapy approach, assessment is based less on the symbolic content of the art expression but relies more on the stages of normal artistic development as a basis for comparison and evaluation. A developmental art assessment might determine if the individual could benefit from art as self-expression. In an art therapy session with an 8-year-old girl with emotional trauma, does the child create human figures appropriate for her age or are they more characteristic of those of a 4- or 5-year-old? Children with developmental disorders are likely to have some sort of delay in artistic expression. For example, is an 11-year-old boy with mental retardation still making scribbles like a 3-year-old? For children with varying degrees of mental retardation, a therapist generally sees some sort of developmental delays in artistic expression. These are only a few of the issues that may arise in evaluating the drawings or paintings of a particular child.

The therapist may also use the stages of artistic development to evaluate motor,

TABLE 8.1. Stages of Artistic Expression

Stage	Age	Description
Stage I: Scribbling	18 months–3 years	During this stage the very first marks are made by a child on paper. At first there is little control of the motions that used to make the scribble; accidental results occur and the line quality of these early drawings varies greatly.
		As motor skills improve scribbles include repeated motions, making horizontal or longitudinal lines, circular shapes, and assorted dots, marks, and other forms. At this stage there is also not much conscious use of color (i.e., the color is used for enjoyment without specific intentions) and drawing is enjoyed for the kinesthetic experience it provides. Limited attention span and not much narrative about the art product.
Stage II: Basic forms	3–4 years	Children may still make scribbles at this age, but they also become more involved in naming and inventing stories about them. The connection of one's marks on paper to the world around him or her occurs. Children want to talk about their drawings, even if they appear to adults as unidentifiable scribbles. Attention span is still limited and concentration is restricted. Meanings for images change; a child may start a scribble drawing by saying "this is my mommy," only to quickly label it as something else soon after.
		Other configurations emerge at this time, including the mandala, a circular shape, design, or pattern and combinations of basic forms and shapes such as triangles, circles, crosses, squares and rectangle. These are the forms that are the precursors of human figures and other objects, the milestone in the next stage.
Stage III: Human forms and beginning schema	4–6 years	The major milestone of this stage is the emergence of rudimentary human figures, often called tadpoles, cephlapods, and prototypes. These human figures are often primitive and sometimes quite charming.
		There is still a subjective use of color at this stage, although some children may begin to associate color in their drawings with what they perceive to be in the environment (e.g., leaves are green). Children of this age are more interested in drawing the figure or object than the color of it. Also, there is no conscious approach to composition or design, and children may place objects throughout a page without concern for a groundline or relationships to size. A figure may float freely across the page, at the top or sides, and some things may be appear upside down because children are not concerned with direction or relationship of objects.

Stage IV: Development of a visual schema   6–9 years

Children rapidly progress in their artistic abilities during this stage. The first and foremost is the development of visual symbols or schema for human figures, animals, houses, trees, and other objects in the environment. Many of these symbols are fairly standard, such as a particular way to depict a head with a circle, hairstyles, arms and legs, a tree with a brown trunk and green top; a yellow sun in the upper corner of the page; and a house with a triangular, pitched roof. Color is used objectively and sometimes rigidly (e.g., all leaves must be the same color green). There is the development of a baseline (a groundline upon which objects sit) and often a skyline (a blue line across the top the drawing to indicate the sky). During these years children also draw see-through or x-ray pictures (such as cut-away images of a house, where one can see everything inside) and attempt beginning perspective by placing more distant objects higher on the drawing page.

It is normal at this age to use variations in size to emphasize importance; for example, children may depict themselves as bigger than the house or tree in the same drawing, if they wish to emphasize the figure. Or a child depicting a person throwing a ball may draw a much longer arm than usual.

Stage V: Realism   9–12 years

At this stage, children become interested in depicting what they perceive to be realistic elements in their drawings. This includes the first attempts at perspective; children no longer draw a simple baseline but instead draw the ground meeting the sky to create depth. There is a more accurate depiction of color in nature (e.g., leaves can be many different colors rather than just one shade of green), and the human figure is more detailed and differentiated in gender characteristics (e.g., more details in hair, clothing, and build).

At this stage, children begin to become more conventional in their art expressions and are more literal because they want to achieve a "photographic effect" in their renditions. They may also make drawings of cartoon or comic strip characters in order to imitate an adult-like quality in their pictures. In this stage children have increasing technical abilities and enjoy exploring new materials and can work on more detailed, complicated art expressions.

Stage VI: Adolescence   12 years and onward

Many children (and adults) never reach this stage of artistic development because they may discontinue drawing or making art at around the age of 10 or 11 due to other interests. However, by the age of 13, children who have continued to make art or have art training will be able to use perspective more accurately and effectively in their drawings, will include greater detail in their work, will have increasing mastery of materials, will be more attentive to color and design, and will be able to create abstract images.

Note. Based on the work of Lowenfeld and Brittain (1987), Gardner (1980), Kellogg (1969), and Winner (1982). Adapted from Malchiodi (1998). Copyright 1998 by Cathy A. Malchiodi. Adapted by permission.

cognitive, or social skills. For example, does a child who is sensory impaired, such as a blind or autistic child, have an age-appropriate ability to grasp or make marks and other fine motor skills? Has an adolescent with developmental delays reached the stage of concrete operations? Does a child with disabilities make appropriate eye contact with the therapist and respond to modeling or directions during art activities? Both the art product and the process of art making are used to evaluate these and related skill areas.

TREATMENT GOALS

There are many areas that a developmental approach to art therapy may address, but several are particularly important:

- *Sensory stimulation.* Sensory stimulation refers to the use of art and play materials to enhance sensory, visual, motor, and even interactive skills with the therapist and other children. The therapist may introduce a water play table where, for example, a child can touch or splash and eventually perhaps learn to use cups or other toys. This activity might serve as a prelude to learning to use a brush in water, followed by learning to use a simple set of paints or watercolors. Other sensory-related developmental tasks might include using a sandtray, interacting with a puppet, or touching different textures of fabric, oatmeal, pudding, or other tactile materials.
- *Skill acquisition.* Skill acquisition refers to learning a particular activity through a series of sequential steps for the purpose of assimilating increasing complex motor skills. For example, the therapist may break a task down into the following steps with an individual: (1) learning to sit a the work table; (2) making eye contact with the therapist; (3) learning to hold a brush; (4) learning to dip the brush into the water, then into paint; and (5) learning to use a brush, water, and paint on paper. For some individuals, this process may take several sessions, whereas for others, learning these skills may take weeks, months, or longer.
- *Adaptation.* For some individuals, adaptations of art materials and tools are a necessary prelude to art making. For example, an older woman who has suffered a stroke may not be able to hold a pencil or pen any longer; the therapist might adapt the activity by providing an ink pad or paint roller as alternatives, or provide a splint so that the person can hold the drawing instrument. A therapist working with a child with hyperactivity disorder may remove extraneous materials from the art therapy room or set up a partition to decrease overstimulation. Creating a consistent environment in which shelves and containers hold similar items is another example of an adaptation that encourages self-confidence and self-reliance (Henley, 1992; Malchiodi, 1997).

In a developmental approach, the therapist takes an active role in facilitating the aforementioned goals. Kramer (1986) explained a concept which she refers to as the "third hand" to describe the therapist's use of suggestion, metaphors, or other techniques to enhance the child's progress in therapy. The therapist is the third hand in strategically helping the individual to have successful experiences with the creative process. Henley (1992) provides an good example through his work with Peter, a boy with a hearing impairment. After being reprimanded for fighting in school, Peter drew a figure with distorted hands to which Henley responded by encouraging him to continue drawing hands, as opposed to not giving the boy any suggestion of theme. He also stimulated his interest with drawings of hands by famous artists and demonstrated artistic skills to the boy, such as shading to convey depth and contour drawing as a way to create lines and forms. Eventually, Peter, who was initially angry, anxious, and frustrated, began to become deeply engaged in the process of drawing, experiencing a great satisfaction and appreciation of his growing skills and development of his own drawing style. Henley believes that through third-hand interventions such as this one a therapist can encourage a child to reflect on his or her feelings while supporting artistic exploration as well as creative and mental growth.

DEVELOPMENTAL ART THERAPY IN PRACTICE

The following case illustration demonstrates a developmental approach to art therapy in practice. Therapy was conducted for 11 months in 49 separate sessions of 40 minutes. The therapist initially considered the child's developmental and cognitive capacity through art tasks and psychological testing. In taking a developmental approach, many of the tasks were repeated to increase the child's familiarity with the activities, self-confidence, and personal satisfaction with her work. Once a level of competence was reached, the therapist allowed the child to eventually make her own choice of art activity and encouraged her engagement in the tasks.

CASE EXAMPLE

Nari, a 5-year-old female with physical and mental developmental delays and speech problems, was enrolled in a special program for children and a speech pathology clinic. She lived in a family including grandparents, parents, and one elder sister, all of whom were generous and accepting of Nari despite her problems. The speech pathologist's evaluation indicated that Nari's lips and tongue did not work properly, causing problems with the development of normal speech. Her mother reported that Nari's physical development was delayed as a baby and toddler. She could not use a spoon properly, had difficulty putting on clothing, and could not take care of simple needs by herself.

In the first session, Nari did not make eye contact with the therapist. Her mother asked her to greet the therapist, but Nari's speech was fast and inarticulate. She seemed curious and happy about the variety of art and play materials available in the room. To determine the level of Nari's physical skills, the therapist engaged her in basic art activities such as paper folding, clay work, and line drawing. The therapist demonstrated working with clay and Nari cautiously, but with a shy smile, imitated the therapist. However, her muscles were very weak and she could not continue for very long. In a paper-folding activity Nari displayed a lack of coordination between her eyes and hands. Her paper-cutting work along the line was also poor and she could not grasp a pencil, revealing weak muscle control. In general, Nari was developmentally delayed and appeared slightly delayed in her abilities.

In a subsequent session, the therapist asked Nari to draw a house, tree, and person, a standard projective drawing task (Kim & Kong, 2000). Nari drew a circle in the middle of the paper and added another circle, triangle, and squares (Figure 8.1); when asked what she had drawn, Nari replied with inaudible speech. Her drawing suggests that Nari is developmentally behind in symbolic representational ability. In her person drawing, Nari showed more developmentally appropriate expression by drawing head and legs on a circle (Figure 8.2). However, in her tree drawing Nari was not yet able to produce a formed idea of a tree. According to Kellogg (1970), a child of 4 to 5 years of age begins to link simple figures as triangles and squares with her object face or tree. In this light, Nari was in the stage of naming of scribbling, at a chronological age (CA) of about 2 to 3 years.

To analyze and assess Nari's current level of ability in areas of cognitive and developmental function, the therapist also conducted a standardized Psycho-Educational Profile (Kim, 1989) test before and after the treatment. Nari's level was assessed to be in the 2 years, 10 months stage, not up to her normal chronological age. Her small muscles were not fully developed; she displayed distracted attention, had difficulties in relating to others, was delayed in cognitive abilities, and had a poor command of language. Nari's developmental delays were mainly attributed to difficulty in birth and malnutrition of her mother. Her mother's inconsistent attitude toward her and Nari's linguistic defect also were assumed to be additional factors in her developmental problems. The therapist considered all these factors during the process of treatment.

The long-terms goals of art therapy were (1) to enhance Nari's communication

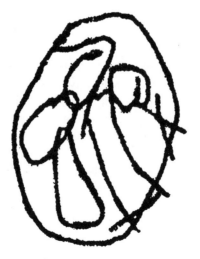

FIGURE 8.1. Nari's initial house drawing.

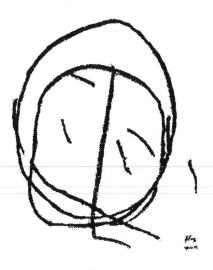

FIGURE 8.2. Nari's initial person drawing.

ability through various art activities, (2) to build her self-confidence and sense of achievement in her work, (3) to increase her sense of independence through voluntary participation in the work and free choice of art materials, and (4) to help her improve interpersonal relationships. In subsequent sessions, Nari engaged in drawing, coloring, clay work, and making things of her own choosing, using various art materials. These experiences were designed to encourage her coordination skills and perception and to expand her field of experiences. In the fourth session Nari positively accepted the therapist's suggestion to color a fish image that the therapist drew. Given the therapist's fish she began to color and cut it along one of the lines. Coordination between her hands and eyes was poor her and her coloring went over the lines. Disappointed with her poor work, Nari cut the fish at random as if frustrated with her abilities.

In the eighth session, Nari was to make a house with colored sand with glue on paper. Therapist first let her feel the sand and glue on the outline of the house and then demonstrated how to place the sand on the paper. Nari began to spread the sand on the paper and was so interested in her artistic work that she insisted on extending the activity even after the session had ended. She seemed very satisfied with the task and stayed at the table for the entire session, which was an achievement for Nari.

In sessions 9–29, Nari was to have puzzles, clay, chalk pastels, marbles, and a variety of play things at her disposal. The therapist allowed Nari to express her choices of materials and an exhibition of her works was encouraged to promote her sense of achievement and awareness of self. During the 9th through 29th sessions the therapist conducted various experiments to have a clearer understanding of Nari's inner world and to enhance Nari's self-expression. Nari now felt comfortable with the therapist and began to open up. There was another turning point, too; before the 18th session Nari would only draw what the therapist asked her to draw. From the 18th session onward, Nari felt comfortable and confident enough to engage in spontaneous expression beyond the therapist's requests or suggestions.

At the end of the 25th session, Nari went to the hospital with a bad case of meningitis. Meeting the therapist in hospital, she was overjoyed with the encounter. After a month she reappeared in the clinic with bright smile. When asked what she wanted to draw, she instantly engaged herself in creating a crocodile. On an oval shape drawn by the therapist she drew the head of the crocodile in yellow-green pastel. Nari then added four legs to the crocodile and jumped with joy and clapped.

By this time in therapy Nari could remove her shoes and jacket all by herself. She showed energy and motivation in her work and increased curiosity and questions. The therapist decided to provide clay as a medium for creative expression to encourage Nari's growing creativity and confidence but also to help her with developing motor skills.

Sessions 30–49 were used to enhance Nari's independence and creativity through more diverse art activities. Taking into consideration her abilities, Nari was offered a full range of tasks in drawing, coloring, clay work, and play to help her to continue to develop skills and to express herself. During this time, the therapist became decreasingly involved in stimulating Nari's creative expression, allowing Nari to develop more self-confidence, increase self-esteem, and improve her interpersonal relations with others. Figure 8.3 is Nari's drawing of a house. Unlike the mere maze of lines in earlier sessions, it was more in accordance with a recognizable house with roof windows and doors. The therapist felt that this artwork was significant evidence that Nari had acquired the ability to create a house drawing appropriate for her age. Figure 8.4 is a face drawing of Nari. In contrast with the earlier ones, this drawing has two eyes, nose, mouth, and two ears in the right places.

Posttherapy, Nari's level of development was assessed to be 3 years, 11 months chronological age. Compared to the earlier test, it reveals that her imitation, perception, muscle control, and coordination had made striking improvements. Since her

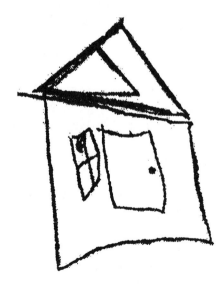

FIGURE 8.3. Nari's house drawing, postintervention.

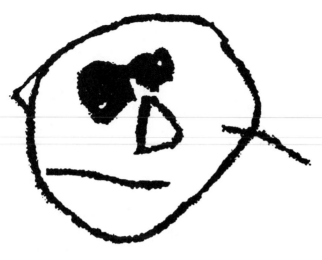

FIGURE 8.4. Nari's person drawing, postintervention.

self-expression still was delayed for her social age, an extended treatment was recommended.

The treatment described in this case example is based a developmental approach to art therapy and focused on cultivating Nari's sense of achievement, self-confidence, independence, and relationships with others. Expressive tasks such as games and play activities and art tasks such as drawing, paper folding, and clay sculpting were used to improve and increase developmental skills appropriate for Nari's age. As a result of developmental art therapy for approximately 1 year, Nari became less negative and more socially interactive with her peers. She also was more capable of self-care, such as washing her hands; brushing her teeth; and using a knife, fork, and spoon with little or no difficulties.

In the early stages, Nari tended to engage herself in only simple and repetitive muscle exercise games. But in later sessions her work became more creative and self-confident, and Nari showed development in social and intellectual faculties. She also showed improvement in emotional areas. In the early sessions, Nari felt uneasy in the company of the therapist. By the end of treatment, she was more interactive with the therapist and expressed herself more freely in art and play activities, displayed enthusiasm about her artistic creations, and appeared happier and more self-assured in the company of other children.

COGNITIVE DEVELOPMENT

In addition to the strategies used in the preceding case example, many therapists see art expression as a way of evaluating cognitive development. Components of the Silver Drawing Test (Silver, 2001, 2002) (also described in Appendix I, this volume) are useful to understand the individual based on constructs of cognitive development set forth by Piaget and Inhelder (1971). The following tasks designed by Silver are useful in cognitive assessment and skill acquisition:

- Predictive drawing—assesses the ability to sequence.
- Drawing from observation—assesses the ability to represent spatial relationships of height, width, and depth.
- Drawing from imagination—assesses the ability to deal with abstract concepts, use personal creativity, and project feelings.

Postassessment, Silver (2001) suggests specific interventions involving paint, drawing, and clay to help the individual make cognitive and creative gains. Although widely used with children, Silver's assessment and methods have been also used with adolescents, adults, and the elderly, establishing that artistic and cognitive development are an effective basis for evaluation and intervention.

CONCLUSION

Developmental art therapy is reflected in several chapters of this text, including that of Safran, who applies art therapy to children with attention-deficit/hyperactivity disorder (see Chapter 14); Gabriels, who describes interventions with children with autism (Chapter 15); and Riley, in working with adolescents (see Chapter 17). As this chapter illustrates, it is a particularly popular approach among therapists who work with individuals with developmental delays; cognitive, visual, or auditory impairments; and physical handicaps. Although it is applicable to specific populations, developmental approaches can serve as a basis for all art therapy approaches with children and adults. It provides therapists not only a method of evaluating development but also norms for establishing goals for treatment based on the rich foundation of artistic development.

REFERENCES

Aach-Feldman, S. (1981). Art and the IEP. In L. Kearns, M. Ditson, & B. Roehner (Eds.), *Readings: Developing arts programs for handicapped students.* Harrisburg, PA: Arts in Special Education Project of Pennsylvania.

Aach-Feldman, S., & Kunkle-Miller, C. (1987). A developmental approach to art therapy. In J. Rubin (Ed.), *Approaches to art therapy* (pp. 251–274). New York: Brunner/Mazel.

Deaver, S., Bernier, M., Sanderson, T., & Stovall, K. (2000). *A collection of children's drawings.* Unpublished research presented at Research Roundtable, Annual Conference of the American Art Therapy Association, St. Louis, MO.

Erikson, E. H. (1963). *Childhood and society.* New York: Norton.

Freud, S. (1905/1962). Three essays on the theory of sexuality. In *The standard edition of the complete psychological works of Sigmund Freud* (Vol. 7). London: Hogarth Press.

Gardner, H. (1980). *Artful scribbles.* New York: Basic Books.

Golomb, C. (1990). *The child's creation of the pictorial world.* Berkeley: University of California Press.

Henley, D. (1992). *Exceptional children, exceptional art.* Springfield, MA: Davis.

Kellogg, R. (1970). *Analyzing children's art.* Palo Alto, CA: Mayfield.

Kim, D. Y., & Kong, M. (2000). *Korean DAP & HTP.* Taegu, Korea: Korean Art Therapy Association.

Kim, J. K. (1989). *Korean Psycho-Educational Profile.* Taegu, Korea: Taegu University Press.

Kramer, E. (1971). *Art as therapy with children.* New York: Schocken.

Kramer, E. (1986). The art therapist's third hand: Reflections on art, art therapy, and society at large. *American Journal of Art Therapy, 24*(3), 71–86.

Lowenfeld, V. (1957). *Creative and mental growth* (3rd ed.). New York: Macmillan.

Lowenfeld, V., & Brittain, W. (1987). *Creative and mental growth* (7th ed.). New York: Macmillan.

Mahler, M., Pine, F., & Bergman, A. (1975). *The psychological birth of the human infant: Symbiosis and individuation.* New York: Basic Books.

Malchiodi, C. A. (1993). *Developmental stages and art therapy techniques.* Unpublished graduate-level syllabus, University of California, Sacramento.

Malchiodi, C. A. (1997). *Breaking the silence: Art therapy with children from violent homes.* Philadelphia: Brunner/Mazel.

Malchiodi, C. A. (1998). *Understanding children's drawings.* New York: Guilford Press.

Malchiodi, C. A. (2002). Using drawing in short-term assessment and intervention of child maltreatment and trauma. In A. Giardino (Ed.), *Child maltreatment* (3rd ed., pp. 201–220). St. Louis, MO: GW Medical Press.

Malchiodi, C. A., Riley, S., & Hass-Cohen, N. (2001). *Art therapy mind-body landscapes* (Audiotape presentation #108-1525). Denver, CO: National Audio Video.

Piaget, J. (1959). *Judgment and reasoning in the child.* Patterson, NJ: Littlefield Adams.

Piaget, J., & Inhelder, B. (1971). *Mental imagery in the child.* New York: Basic Books.

Rubin, J. (1978). *Child art therapy.* New York: Van Nostrand Reinhold.

Silver, R. (1978). *Developing cognitive and creative skills through art.* Baltimore, MD: University Park Press.

Silver, R. (2001). *Art as language.* Philadelphia: Brunner-Routledge.

Silver, R. (2002). *The Silver Drawing Test.* New York: Brunner-Routledge.

Uhlin, D. (1972). *Art for exceptional children.* Dubuque, IA: William Brown.

Williams, G., & Wood, M. (1977). *Developmental art therapy.* Baltimore, MD: University Park Press.

Winner, E. (1982). *Invented worlds: The psychology of the arts.* Cambridge, MA: Harvard University.

CHAPTER 9

Expressive Arts Therapy and Multimodal Approaches

Cathy A. Malchiodi

Art therapy is a distinct field with many approaches, as described in this volume and throughout the art therapy literature (Malchiodi, 1998; Rubin, 1998). However, some practitioners see art therapy as part of a larger discipline referred to as expressive arts therapy (the therapeutic use of art, music, dance/movement, drama, and poetry/writing) and intermodal or multimodal (moving from one art form to another) approaches. This chapter provides a brief history of expressive arts therapy and multimodal approaches, theoretical foundations, and expressive arts therapy assessment and evaluation and demonstrates the integration of art therapy, expressive arts therapy, and intermodal approaches in treatment through case examples.

WHAT IS EXPRESSIVE ARTS THERAPY?

Expressive arts therapy has been linked to the traditions and cultural precedents of world healing practices because they frequently involve the integration of all the arts (McNiff, 1981). Ceremonies in which a indigenous healer or shaman might sing, dance, make images, or tell stories recall the early roots of psychology and psychiatry. For example, in ancient Greece, dramatic enactments including dance, music and storytelling brought people together to experience cathartic release. The Navaho people in the Southwestern United States still employ the arts, including sand paintings, songs, dance, and chanting, to heal ill members of their communities.

Although the idea of expressive arts therapy is a development of the last half of the 20th century, it is still growing in scope and definition (Malchiodi, in press). Some characterize expressive arts therapy as the inclusion of any of the arts therapies—art, music, dance/movement, drama, and poetry/writing. Thus, using one or more of these therapies in work with individuals or groups is defined as expressive arts therapy. To make matters more confusing, the term "expressive therapy" is sometimes used interchangeably with expressive arts therapy. Expressive therapy has been defined as using the arts and their products to foster awareness, encourage emotional growth, and enhance relationships with others through access to imagination; including arts as therapy, arts psychotherapy, and the use of arts for traditional healing; and emphasizing the interrelatedness of the arts in therapy (Lesley College, 1995).

Some characterize expressive arts therapy as using one or two disciplines within treatment (Levine & Levine, 1999), whereas others take a more interdisciplinary view of these modalities (Knill, 1978; Knill, Barba, & Fuchs, 1995; McNiff, 1978, 1992). Rogers (1993) defines expressive arts therapy as using "various arts—movement, drawing, painting, sculpting, music, writing, sound, and improvisation—in a supportive setting to experience and express feelings" (p. 115). As in art therapy, the aesthetics of the art work are not primary, and the arts are used to self-express and to gain insight.

Some practitioners believe that expressive art therapies should be strictly delineated as the "intermodal" or "multimodal" use of various arts therapies. The idea of "multimodal expressive arts therapy" has also been proposed and is defined as integrating various art forms into a therapeutic relationship and by working within more than one medium (Spaniol, Spieser, & Cattaneo, 1999). That is, any of the arts therapies may be used in therapeutic work as the therapist deems appropriate to meet the needs of the client, and in a given session, more than one art form is used to enhance therapy.

THEORETICAL FOUNDATIONS

Therapists working from an expressive arts therapy or intermodal approach have a variety of theoretical stances. Just as those practicing art therapy, practitioners of expressive arts therapy might have a Jungian, object relations, or other theoretical orientation that guides their understanding and frames the process of therapy. An underlying belief common to many approaches is the principle of unconscious expression that echoes the psychoanalytic principles discussed in Chapter 4 (this volume). The basic premise is that the expressive arts experiences—visual art, music, dance, and drama—allow people to explore unknown facets of themselves, communicate nonverbally, and achieve insight.

Natalie Rogers, the daughter of psychologist Carl Rogers, has proposed one of the more accepted theories of expressive arts therapy and intermodal work and integrates a "person-centered" approach in her work. As previously discussed in Chapter 5 (this volume), "person-centered" or "client-centered" approaches were developed by Carl Rogers and emphasize the therapist's role as a sensitive, reflective, and

empathetic individual. Person-centered expressive arts therapy embraces similar tenets, including the premise that each person has the capacity for self-direction and has
an impulse toward personal growth and full potential.

Rogers (1993) also coined a term for encouraging and enhancing the interplay
between the arts in therapy: the creative connection. She believes that one art form
naturally stimulates another; for example, creative movement can affect what we
express through drawing, and drawing may activate what we feel or think. This creative connection can involve a variety of different sequential experiences of the arts
for therapy; however, the individual is central to the process and determines, with
guidance and facilitation of the therapist, the direction the process takes and the art
forms used.

Other humanistic approaches to psychotherapy often use expressive arts therapy
and multimodal techniques within treatment. For example, some practitioners of
Gestalt therapy use what could be considered multimodal approaches, combining
art, movement, and other modalities (Rhyne, 1973/1995). Therapists with a transpersonal approach may combine some form of imagery, music, movement, and creative writing in their work with clients (Farelly, 2001).

Some believe that expressive arts therapy and intermodal approaches are based
on the interrelationship of the arts and theories of creativity and imagination, rather
than integration with psychological principles. Knill (1978; Knill et al., 1995) proposes that the connection between self-expression through the arts taps the healing
power of imagination and is a fundamental phenomenon of human existence, as opposed to a theory of psychotherapy. McNiff (1992) also proposes a similar philosophy, seeing the arts as medicine for the soul, grounded in traditional uses of art
throughout history to heal and transform human suffering.

The introduction of action into psychotherapy is the basis for expressive arts
therapy, no matter what theoretical stance is used. According to McNiff (1981),
action within therapy is rarely limited to a single mode of expression, one form of
expression tends to flow from another, and art forms complement each other in
therapy. The approach also honors that each person has a different expressive
style. For example, one person will be more verbal, another more visual, and a
third more kinesthetic or tactile. Each art form (visual art, dance, music, drama,
and poetry/writing) helps people to make sense and meaning in a specific way—visual arts through image, dance through movement, music through sound and
rhythm, drama through action, and poetry/writing through words (Knill et al.,
1995). By opening the therapeutic experience beyond visual art alone, the therapy
is enhanced in clinical depth and facilitates expression in a manner most appropriate to the particular client.

Although there are various theories and orientations in expressive arts therapy
and intermodal work, all theorists who agree to employ them in treatment must possess a practical knowledge of how each of the art forms functions, how people respond to each art form, and how to guide the client from one art form to another.
Some therapists comfortably use all arts in treatment, but, in reality, most rely on
two or three that they feel qualified to use.

ASSESSMENT AND EVALUATION IN EXPRESSIVE ARTS THERAPY AND INTERMODAL WORK

There are no formalized assessments that use expressive arts therapy as a foundation. The lack of a formal, standardized assessment is, in part, the result of a lack of quantifiable research on the intermodal use of arts as therapy. Therapists using an expressive arts therapy or intermodal approach generally make clinical observations, based on their own training, experience, and orientation, to evaluate how to proceed with treatment. However, there are a few models for understanding and evaluating clients' uses of arts media in therapy which are used by some practitioners to guide the therapeutic process and establish goals for future treatment. These models include the expressive therapies continuum (Kagin & Lusebrink, 1978; Lusebrink, 1990), the mode of representation model (Johnson, 1999), and the creative axis model (Goren-Bar, 1997).

Expressive Therapies Continuum

Kagin and Lusebrink (1978) first proposed the expressive therapies continuum (ETC), a model for understanding expressive arts therapy. Initially, the ETC was designed to focus on art therapy, but in later work, the model has been extended to all art forms used in therapy (Lusebrink, 1990, 1991). The ETC integrates information from neurological research on how the brain processes imagery with theories of sensory–motor development, cognition, psychosocial behavior, and self-psychology (Lusebrink, 1990). It demonstrates the commonalities between the various art forms, defines the properties of each medium, and provides a common language for those using expressive arts therapy in assessment and treatment. The ETC is based on a developmental model reflecting the ideas of Piaget (1951) and Bruner (1964), and it proposes four levels of experience: kinesthetic/sensory (action), perceptual/affective (form), cognitive/symbolic (schema), and creative. Each level is distinguished by a greater complexity and reflective distance than the one previous.

On the kinesthetic/sensory level, a person is generally interacting with an art form in an exploratory way. Kinesthetic aspects are characterized by movement and motor activity, while sensory aspects imply the use of tactile or other senses to explore media. Free movement or scribble drawings could be seen as kinesthetic; a hands-on experience with clay is an example of the sensory level. The details of what is created are not important, only the bodily expression of movement through the art form.

On the perceptual/affective level, an individual engages with an art form to develop form for ideas and to communicate emotions. This level reflects the person's ability to explore the structural properties of an art form and to imbue the form with feeling. For example, using lines and colors to create form through a painting is an expression at the perceptual level; creating a piece of music to convey an emotion is an example of the affective level. At this level, the individual is able to develop some reflective distance and to self-observe his or her process with the art form.

On the cognitive/symbolic level, a person uses an art form for problem solving and, in some cases, meaning seeking. Cohen and Mills (1993) note at the cognitive level there is structuring, sequencing, and naming, in addition to problem solving through media. A person operating on this level is able to use analytic, logical, and sequential skills while engaging in the art process. This experience may lead to the symbolic level in which personal meaning can be explored. Clients working at the cognitive/symbolic level of the ETC may demonstrate the use of rational thought and intellect in the art process and may naturally look for meaning in their images and arts experiences.

The creative level requires the integration of all other levels of the ETC into the expressive arts therapy process and all previous levels (kinesthetic/sensory, perceptual/affective, and cognitive/symbolic) are apparent in an art form. Not all individuals or art forms necessarily reach this level, but a form of creativity can be experienced at each of the three levels of the ETC. For example, someone could experience creativity through spontaneous movement, although the experience would be defined as kinesthetic on the continuum.

The ETC is a model for helping therapists understand how expressive arts therapy can be used in therapeutic work with clients. A therapist might use the ETC to evaluate the art work of an individual and determine whether another art form (such as dance or creative writing) can enhance therapy. If using a multimodal expressive arts therapy approach, the therapist might use the ETC as a guideline for understanding client expression in a variety of media and may use the model to choose additional modes of expression for therapeutic purposes. For example, an individual who is in need of expressing emotion might be guided by the therapist to use music or painting to communicate affect while a child who responds to sensory modes of communication may be encouraged to explore the tactile qualities of clay.

Some therapists have used the ETC to evaluate, understand, and treat specific populations with an expressive arts therapy approach in mind. Cohen and Mills (1993) describe their use of the ETC to understand and assess people with dissociative identity disorder who have also experienced trauma such as abuse. They note that the ETC helps clinicians learn how to pace, contain, and sequence therapy. Johnson (1999) observes that developmental models such as the ETC are useful not only in evaluating clients in art therapy but also in integrating various arts media into therapy. (For in-depth information on the ETC, consult the work of Lusebrink, 1990, 1991).

Mode of Representation Model

Johnson and Sandel (cited in Johnson, 1999) delineate a developmental model for the arts therapies based on what they refer to as the "mode of representation." They base their model on the stance that cognitive development proceeds from kinesthetic and movement-oriented expression to expression through gesture and image and finally to linguistic forms of expression. Developmental theorists such as Piaget and Bruner have referred to these stages as kinesthetic, enactive, imagistic, iconic, symbolic, and lexical. This sequence can be used to understand a client's progress through various art forms (e.g., from the kinesthetic experience of scribbling on paper to creating a dance with symbolic meaning). It also can be used to characterize the therapeutic process within each art form (the kinesthetic experience of pounding clay to making a clay object to creating a series of sculptures that are used to tell a story and thus have lexical meaning).

Within this model, Johnson and Sandel have explored the impact of different media and arts interventions on therapeutic process and outcome. For example, they found that people with severe schizophrenia were able to more fully participate in music and movement rather than drama and poetry (Sandel & Johnson, 1974). They do note that relatively few studies have been done with this developmental model and more research is needed to understand implications for evaluating expressive arts therapy and intermodal expression. However, it still provides a useful framework for clinical observations when using multiple art forms in treatment.

Creative Axis Model

Some practitioners have explored ways of understanding the process of expressive arts therapy within a single session or a series of sessions to help evaluate the individual's use of various art forms. Goren-Bar (1997) offers a "creative axis model," another stage model that can be used a guide to expressive arts therapy treatment. These stages can be summarized as follows:

1. *Stage 1: Contact.* This is the initial period in which a client makes contact with the art form (handling art materials, experimenting with musical instruments, etc.).
2. *Stage 2: Organization.* After choosing the art form, the client organizes the various elements (preparation of materials to create a drawing, playing notes or scales on a musical instrument, etc.).
3. *Stage 3: Improvisation.* A continuation of the organization stage, the client uses trial and error to explore materials and characteristics of the medium (such as exploring the relationship of lines on paper, or changing the range or chord of musical notes).
4. *Stage 4: Central theme.* This is the time during the session when a theme becomes clear and the person invests more attention and effort in that particular aspect of the artwork (such as creating an image from lines in a drawing, or repeating a rhythm or melody).
5. *Stage 5: Elaboration (Variation).* This is the time following the formation of a central theme when the person is preoccupied with the modification, development, or improvement of the artwork.
6. *Stage 6: Preservation.* This is the ending of the experience, which may include distancing, preserving the work, putting it away, or presenting it (displaying or storing an art piece or performing a musical piece) (adapted from Goren-Bar, 1997, pp. 413–414).

This sequence can be used to consider how a person progresses through the various stages, how the person transitions from one stage to another, or how an individual struggles with particular stages or regresses to earlier stages. Goren-Bar hypothesizes that there are possible emotional reactions to each stage and that certain populations may experience difficulties at various stages in the sequence. For example, children and adults with learning difficulties may have difficulties at stages 1, 2, and 3, and prefer to go immediately to stage 4 (central theme). A child with a learning disability might enter a session and, instead of experimenting with materials, quickly execute repetitive drawings of an airplane. Individuals with behavioral difficulties or personality disorders may stay in stage 3, improvisation, because it is hard to move to and remain with a central theme. Although Goren-Bar's hypotheses are the result of clinical observations and not systematic research, this model underscores the importance of noting points of reference during an expressive arts therapy session with regard to how a person engages in the creative process and how he or she uses an art form.

TREATMENT ISSUES

Expressive arts therapy is tailored to the individual. There is no set way to begin a session, although, depending on the practitioner, any art form could be used as a starting point for further art expression. For one person the art form may start from drawing, for another a piece of creative writing or poetry, and for others, improvised movements or dance. The following vignette provides an example of an expressive arts therapy session.

A expressive arts therapy group session in an inpatient unit of a psychiatric hospital begins with a warm-up activity and the therapist leads the participants in a brief series of movements and simple stretches from a seated position. After several minutes of movement the participants are then asked to make an oil pastel drawing using lines, shapes, and colors, showing a movement or stretch experienced in the warm-up (Figure 9.1). After completing these drawings, the therapist instructs the group members to select a musical instrument (drum, bells, maracas, keyboard) and make a sound to depict the rhythms of their drawings. From there the therapist may facilitate the group in working together with the musical instruments to create a group musical piece. At the close of the group, the participants return to their seats in the circle and discuss their experiences with movement, drawing, and music.

Spaniol et al. (1999) offer another example of a multimodal session:

A multimodal expressive arts therapy session might begin by having participants stand in a circle and take turns making a movement that expresses their immediate feelings. In the second phase of the session, they might use oil crayons, pastels, or a felt-tipped pen first to transfer that movement onto a large piece of drawing paper, then elaborate the graphic mark into a picture. . . . The therapists might suggest that the participants look at one an-

FIGURE 9.1. Drawing using lines, shapes, and colors to show body movement.

other's pictures and leave a written response on a nearby piece of paper. Each participant then uses the words and phrases to compose a poem that she or he recites to the group. The sequential unfolding of expression, from physical gesture to recited poem, becomes the basis for a concluding discussion that might consider the interplay of emotion, bodily movement, and verbal expression or the insights gained through group interaction. (pp. 364–365)

A typical session with an individual might begin with a warm-up activity, such as spontaneous movement or drawing, similar to what was described in the vignette. The therapist may also choose to engage the client in a modality that the person finds most comfortable and nonthreatening. In some situations, a person may naturally be attracted to one art form over another and begin to express through that modality without any suggestion from the therapist. As the level of comfort with a modality increases and expression becomes more spontaneous, the therapist may encourage "transition" to another mode of expression (Knill, 1978). Children, in nondirective play, naturally move from one activity to another (e.g., finger painting to dramatic enactment to puppets); transition to another modality is a natural occurrence. Adults may also express themselves in several modes, but it is more likely that the therapist will need to direct and support movement from one form of expression to another. The purpose of facilitating transition is to encourage spontaneous expression, stimulate creativity, and enhance the experience feelings, allowing for deeper understanding. In the final part of the session, the individual may reflect on the images, words, sounds, or movements that were created and discuss the process of making them with the therapist.

ART THERAPY AND MULTIMODAL TECHNIQUES

As mentioned, therapists using an expressive arts therapy or multimodal approach to art therapy may use other art forms along with visual expression to facilitate an individual's or group's self-expression. Because this chapter is part of a text on clinical art therapy theory and applications, some of the more common techniques in multimodal work using art expression as central to expressive arts therapy are briefly discussed in the following sections: creative writing and art expression, movement and art expression, and an intermodal experiential starting with art and including a number of different art forms.

Creative Writing and Art

Many therapists using an intermodal approach believe writing about art images is helpful and necessary to enhance the individual's understanding of images. Writing may involve simply listing words that spontaneously come to mind when looking at the image (like the process of free association), creating a story, or simply giving the piece a title. Some therapists use specific techniques based on psychological theories; for example, a Gestalt approach might be used and the person might be asked to write three statements starting with "I am," "I feel," or "I think" about the imagery. Letting the image also have a voice and writing a dialogue between oneself and the image is another common technique. A therapist might encourage the person to disagree, argue, or debate with the image or let the dialogue take the person wherever it will.

There is evidence that writing has a profound effect on both physical and psychological health. For example, Pennebaker (1997) notes that writing about trauma, in contrast to writing about trivia or daily routine, has a significant effect on the immune system. He observes that people who write about traumatic events are healthier during the subsequent year than those who do not engage in self-expression of unpleasant experiences. Studies also point to positive effects of writing on chronic illnesses such as arthritis and it has been suggested that regular writing about one's illness can have beneficial outcome on symptoms and perception of pain. Although there have not been specific studies on the impact of art expression and writing, the inclusion of some form writing as part of the art therapy experience may be beneficial to some individuals, particularly those who have experienced trauma or have chronic physical illness.

Movement and Art

As described by Lusebrink (1991) in the ETC and Johnson and Sandel (cited in Johnson, 1999), the kinesthetic quality of rhythm or movement is present in all art forms. An intermodal activity involving art and movement that I have employed for many years with groups involves using simple movements as an inspiration for drawing. Participants are asked to create a movement describing "how they feel today," using any part or all parts of their bodies. Group members practice the movement for several minutes, mentally noting how it feels to make that movement and what lines, shapes, and colors come to mind while repeating it. Next, each person is given a large piece of paper and a set of oil pastels with which to depict the lines, shapes, and colors of their movements.

When the drawings are completed I ask the participants to walk around the room and look at the drawings the others in the group have created. At this point I may ask each group member to choose another person's drawing that he or she likes or feels attracted to because of the lines, shapes, or colors in it. Next, if the participants are willing, I ask each person to imagine what the drawing is conveying in terms of movement and feeling and, if possible, to show the group the movement that he or she thinks is depicted in the drawing. If time permits, I may also ask the drawing's creator to show the group what movement was described in the artwork and to have both participants repeat their movements together, creating a simple dance between two people.

Intermodal activities combining art and movement can be particularly helpful in groupwork where interaction is encouraged and dynamics between participants is an important part of the experience. This type of arts therapy process also provides individuals who respond to kinesthetic and sensory experiences the opportunity for more satisfying and personally meaningful self-expression.

Scribble Chase

Based on the work of Lusebrink (1990), called "scribble chase" (an art therapy process also discussed in Chapter 4 in individual treatment) illustrates the various aspects of the ETC and the mode of representation model proposed by Johnson and Sandel (cited in Johnson, 1999). Depending on how the therapist guides the process, this activity can also include multimodal work involving movement, music/sound, or storytelling and creative writing.

The activity begins with a scribble drawings created in dyads; the participants each take turns making a scribble with chalk on paper while the other attempts to follow the lines with another chalk. Because no specific imagery is intended, it usually results in drawings with a maze of chaotic lines similar to those of a child's scribble. This initial experience is often perceived as playful and reminiscent of the kinesthetic/sensory level of the ETC.

Next participants are asked to take their scribble drawings and find images in them. Lusebrink (1991) notes that finding forms in the scribble and then adding additional colors, lines, and details to these forms first involves the perceptual level and may lead to other levels of the ETC, including cognitive, symbolic, and creative levels. To guide participants to experience other cognitive/symbolic levels, the therapist may encourage the individual to describe the images created, "talk with the image," or write a story or poem about the image. This sequence of activities, from movement-oriented scribbling to finding forms to developing a story, also reflects Johnson and Sandel's continuum from kinesthetic to symbolic and lexical expression. Other modalities, in addition to writing, may be used to help the individual explore and expand on the images created through the scribble chase activity. For example, the therapist might ask the individual to make a sound or movement for each image in the picture.

This activity can be adapted to groupwork by facilitating participants to combine their images into a single drawing or mural. At that point the group can be encouraged to create a story about the joint drawing or improvise a short drama or musical piece to express the content of their artwork. Participants might be encouraged to make sounds or movements simultaneously and group dynamics, rather than person insight or expression, would be emphasized as a goal of the experience. Figure 9.2 is an example of this group process; two dyads (four people) completed individual scribble drawings, found images in their scribbles, and finally selected several images from all four of their drawings to use in a group mural. The joint artwork is called "A Whale Out of His Element" and the group gave a short performance using dance, each member using simple movements to describe a detail of the mural. Through this experience the participants were not only able to learn more about how they interact within a small group but also to expand on their understanding of the themes and images contained in their group art piece through storytelling and creative movement.

CONCLUSION

An expressive arts therapy or multimodal approach to art therapy capitalizes on the integration of two or more forms of art expression into treatment. Although many

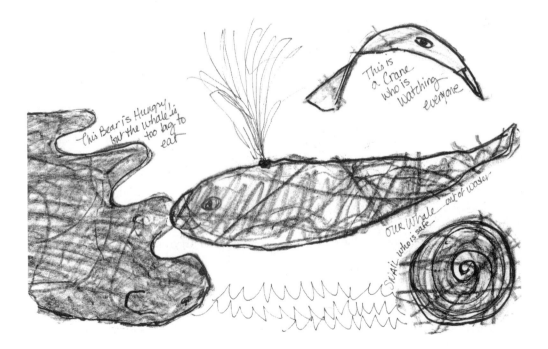

FIGURE 9.2. "A Whale Out of His Element," group mural using scribble images chosen by participants.

theoretical frameworks of psychology are used within this approach, expressive arts therapy and multimodal work are considered to have a unique philosophy separate from that of art therapy. However, although recognized as separate philosophy, expressive arts therapy shares methods of practice that are similar to that of art therapy. A multimodal, art therapy approach to treatment, like other art therapy approaches described throughout this text, offers creative modalities through which individuals can express thoughts and feelings, communicate nonverbally, achieve insight, and experience the curative potential of the creative process.

REFERENCES

Bruner, J. (1964). The course of cognitive growth. *American Psychologist, 19,* 1–6.

Cohen, B., & Mills, A. (1993). *Expressive therapies continuum and the treatment of multiple personality disorder.* Unpublished paper.

Farrelly, M. (2001). *Spirituality and art therapy: Living the connection.* London: Jessica Kingsley.

Goren-Bar, A. (1997). The "creative axis" in expressive therapies. *The Arts in Psychotherapy, 24*(5), 411–418.

Johnson, D. R. (1999). *Essays on the creative arts therapies.* Springfield, IL: Charles C Thomas.

Lesley College. (1995). *Definition of expressive therapy* [On-line]. Available: http://www.lesley.edu/faculty/estrella/intermod.htm.

Levine, S., & Levine, E. (1999). *Foundations of expressive arts therapy.* London: Jessica Kingsley.

Lusebrink, V. (1990). *Imagery and visual expression in therapy.* New York: Plenum Press.

Lusebrink, V. (1991). A systems-oriented approach to the expressive therapies: The Expressive Therapies Continuum. *The Arts in Psychotherapy, 18*(4), 395–404.

Kagin, S., & Lusebrink, V. (1978). The expressive therapies continuum. *Arts in Psychotherapy, 5,* 171–180.

Knill, P. (1978). *Ausdruckstherapie.* Lilienthal, Germany: ERES.

Knill, P., Barba, H., & Fuchs, M. (1995). *Minstrels of the soul: Intermodal expressive therapy.* Toronto: Palmerson Press.

Malchiodi, C. A. (1998). *The art therapy sourcebook.* Columbus, OH: McGraw-Hill.

Malchiodi, C. A. (in press). *The expressive arts therapies handbook.* New York: Guilford Press.

McNiff, S. (1978). From shamanism to art therapy. *Arts in Psychotherapy, 15,* 285–292.

McNiff, S. (1981). *The arts and psychotherapy.* Springfield, IL: Charles C Thomas.

McNiff, S. (1992). *Art as medicine.* Boston: Shambhala.

Pennebaker, J. (1997). *Opening up: The healing power of expressing emotion.* New York: Guilford Press.

Piaget, J. (1951). *Plays, dreams, and imitation in childhood.* New York: Norton.

Rhyne, J. (1973/1995). *The Gestalt art experience.* Monterey, CA: Brooks/Cole/Chicago: Magnolia Street.

Rogers, N. (1993). *The creative connection: Expressive arts as healing.* Palo Alto, CA: Science & Behavior Books.

Rubin, J. (1998). *Art therapy: An introduction.* New York: Brunner-Routledge.

Sandel, S., & Johnson, D. (1974). Indications and contraindications for dance therapy and sociodrama in a long-term psychiatric hospital. *American Dance Therapy Association Monograph, 3,* 47–65.

Spaniol, S., Spieser, P., & Cattaneo, M. (1999). Multimodal expressive arts therapy. In N. Allison (Ed.), *Illustrated encyclopedia of body–mind disciplines* (pp. 363–366). New York: Rosen.

PART III

Clinical Applications with Children and Adolescents

This section introduces the reader to some of the many clinical applications of art therapy with children and adolescents. Art expression has been extensively used in therapy with children for several reasons. It is a natural language for most children and can be a valuable modality in enhancing expression of trauma, distress, or loss (Malchiodi, 1997, 1998, 2001). Also, children do not have the verbal capacity to articulate crisis and for those who have been violated or abused, art is a way to communicate feelings and experiences without words. Gross and Haynes (1998) hypothesized that there may be several reasons why art expressions are helpful adjuncts in child therapy:

- They may reduce anxiety and help children feel more comfortable with the therapist.
- They may increase memory retrieval.
- They may help children organize their narratives.
- They may prompt children to tell more than they would during a solely verbal interview.

When working with children and their art expressions, it is important to avoid imposing adult standards on children's creative work and making assumptions about content and meaning. Because it is difficult to make conclusive interpretations about content and meaning, using a phenomenological approach to understanding children and their art is helpful (Malchiodi, 1998). This means looking at their art expressions with an openness to a variety of meanings, the context in which they were created, and the child's way of viewing the world. The first step in doing this is to see the child as the expert on his or her experiences and to encourage the child to develop narratives for artistic expressions. When therapists use lists of predetermined meanings for content, it is more likely that the child's meanings will not be conveyed, will be misunderstood, or may be disrespected.

Another feature of the phenomenological approach is the opportunity to acknowledge many different aspects of art expressions, including cognitive, emotional, interpersonal, and developmental. A therapist may also consider somatic (physical) and spiritual aspects, depending on one's theoretical framework. Looking for a multiplicity of meaning provides a therapist with information for developing and deepening the therapeutic relationship as well as honoring the uniqueness of the individual (For more detailed information on this approach, see Malchiodi, 1998.)

Many therapists who use art activities with children in therapy wonder: "Is talking necessary?", "If so, when is it appropriate to talk?", and "How much should I talk with the child during an art activity?" The answers to these questions are dependent on the child, the relationship between therapist and client, and the context and course of therapy. Some children become extremely engrossed in art activities and find it disruptive to speak with the therapist while creating. Others, particularly adolescents, may be resistant to speaking about it directly and may require some encouragement and a degree of patience on the part of the therapist. On the other hand, many children enjoy the therapist's taking an interest in their art as they are working on it, especially when a sense of trust has been developed between therapist and child client. For some children, talking during drawing is helpful, especially if there has been trauma; talking can actually help diffuse some of the powerful and overwhelming feelings that arise during the process of drawing a traumatic event (Malchiodi, 2001; Steele & Raider, 2001).

Talking at the end of a session about finished art works is important and encouraging the child to communicate is useful for two reasons: (1) it helps the child to externalize thoughts, feelings, and experiences through both art expression and storytelling; and (2) it helps the therapist to better understand the child and provide the best possible intervention on behalf of the child. With children who are resistant to talking, art expressions can be a way to facilitate conversation through storytelling, pretend, and play activities. In fact, most children do not know what their art expressions mean but can, with the help of the therapist, develop imaginative narratives about the elements of a drawing or painting that reveal a great deal about their feelings, perceptions, and world views.

The authors in this section demonstrate both the basic principles of art therapy with children and adolescents as well as the diversity in application of art therapy with a variety of child and adolescent populations. Tanaka, Kakuyama, and Urhausen (Chapter 10) illustrate how storytelling and art work hand in hand, resulting in effective child therapy. The lead author based his innovative techniques on the seminal work of Donald Winnicott, a pediatrician, who created the "squiggle game," a simple method that involves both therapist and child in drawing and storytelling. Winnicott's work inspired Tanaka to develop the "Egg Drawing" and "Cave Drawing," his own versions of drawing activities with children. Along with coauthors Kakuyama and Urhausen, he explores the value of drawing and personal narratives as both a creative assessment tool and a therapeutic intervention that engages the child's imagination through metaphor and story.

Chapters 11 (Steele) and 12 (Gil) discuss ways that clinicians can use art and play activities to process trauma. Interventions using drawing have been successful in ameliorating posttraumatic stress disorder (PTSD) in children exposed to school shootings, family violence, abuse, and traumatic loss. During the completion of this book, therapists witnessed the value of drawing when terrorist attacks on the World Trade Center and the Pentagon created fear and anxiety in millions. Art interventions proved to be one of few ways to reach children's fears, anxiety, and other sequelae of trauma created by subsequent terrorist alerts and biological threats to safety. Because of the prevalence of televised images of terrorist attacks, most children initially portrayed airplanes crashing into buildings, the Twin Towers of the World Trade Center on fire, and rescue efforts by fire trucks and helicopters (see Figures III.1 and III.2). Content of these images often reflected the more typical responses of children exposed to acute trauma—simple renderings and predominant use of red and black. Children most exposed to the terrorist attacks continued to repeat these images for many months after the incidents of September 11, 2001, a response typical to severe trauma or loss. Trauma interventions such as those described by Steele (Chapter 11) have been successful in ameliorating PTSD in those who have witnessed violence, including school shootings and terrorism.

In addition to intervention, art expression is also used as a tool in forensic investigations of children, particularly those traumatized by physical or sexual abuse. Cohen-Liebman (Chapter 13) explains the concepts of "forensic art evaluation" as a method of evaluating child abuse and discusses how drawings are being used as novel scientific evidence in courts. Because children's drawings may reveal physical or sex-

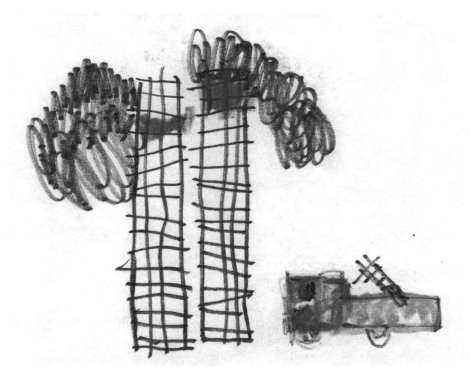

FIGURE III.1. A 5-year-old girl's drawing of the World Trade Center attack.

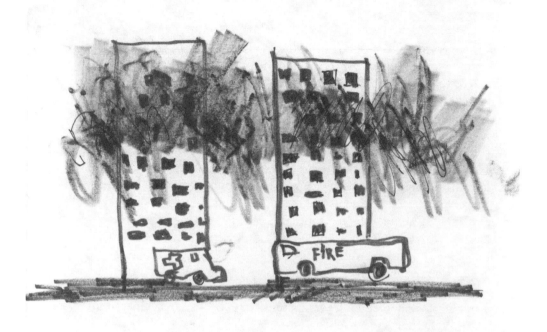

FIGURE III.2. A 9-year-old boy's drawing of "what happened" when the World Trade Center was hit by airplanes.

ual abuse and can supplement verbal interviews of children suspected of abuse, they are an important method for all therapists who work with children subjected to possible violence or molestation. Liebmann addresses how drawings can help the therapist understand children who have been abused and how art expressions are an effective adjunct to verbal forensic interviews.

Art therapy is useful in the treatment of many disorders in children, and attention-deficit/hyperactivity disorder (AD/HD) and autism are two that are particularly suited to creative expression in therapy. In Chapter 14, Safran explains how art therapy is effective with children with AD/HD, outlining its advantages in addressing impulsivity and inattentiveness in this population. Case material on working with individual children and groups gives the reader a more complete understanding of how art therapy can be integrated within all phases of treatment. In Chapter 15, Gabriels offers a comprehensive overview of childhood autism and provides specific methods she has found helpful in intervention for a variety of issues. Both authors include valuable observations on the importance of family art therapy in the treatment of these children, underscoring the need to work with the child in the context of parents and siblings in order to achieve the greatest impact on behavioral change.

Councill (Chapter 16) provides a model with how art therapy is used with pediatric populations, particularly children with cancer. Medical art therapy is a growing area of application and has been used with children with cancer, HIV, asthma, juvenile arthritis, severe burns, and other medical conditions (Malchiodi, 1999). It is used not only to address trauma associated with illness, surgery, medication, and medical interventions but also as a form of psychosocial treatment and stress reduction. Art therapy with pediatric patients may minimize preoperative anxieties and fears, reduce pain, and enhance a sense of self-empowerment in medical treatment. Council brings a wide range of techniques in both art-based assessment and art therapy, vividly illustrating how pediatric patients benefit from creative expression in hospital settings.

The final chapters of this section cover two contemporary issues clinicians face in work with adolescents: depression and violence. Riley (Chapter 17) provides guidelines for how art expression complements the treatment of adolescent depression, underscoring how drawings can reveal unspoken indications of suicidal thoughts and depressed affect. Art for adolescents is one way to reach both those who are withdrawn as well as the resistant teenager; it provides a creative way to communicate without words that most adolescents find preferable to solely verbal interviews. Phillips (Chapter 18) tackles the topic of violent imagery in adolescents and discusses why both normal adolescents as well as teenagers with violent tendencies make violent images. Violence, whether in the form of school shootings and assaults, gang-related violence, or conduct disorders, is a serious concern to most therapists who work with adolescents. Events such as those at Columbine and other high schools have heightened interest in violence among those who work with youth and many therapists are interested in identifying those who have violence tendencies and effectively addressing the appearance of violent imagery in art expressions. Phillips explains ways the therapist can evaluate and work with these images in ways productive to the course of therapy.

All the applications described in this section underscore how therapists who work with children and adolescents can integrate art therapy in their work. Art can provide a window to children's and adolescents' problems, traumatic memories, development, and world views. Its primary purpose is to give these young clients another language with which to share feelings, ideas, perceptions, and observations about themselves, others, and the environment. Art therapy can serve as an important catalyst for increased interaction and exchange between therapist and child or adolescent, thus expanding and deepening the effectiveness of the relationship and its impact on young clients.

REFERENCES

Gross, J., & Haynes, H. (1998). Drawing facilitates children's verbal reports of emotionally laden events. *Journal of Experimental Psychology, 4,* 163–179.

Malchiodi, C. A. (1997). *Breaking the silence: Art therapy with children from violent homes.* Philadelphia: Brunner/Mazel.

Malchiodi, C. A. (1998). *Understanding children's drawings.* New York: Guilford Press.

Malchiodi, C. A. (1999). *Medical art therapy with children.* London: Jessica Kingsley.

Malchiodi, C. A. (2001). Using drawing as intervention with traumatized children. *Trauma and Loss: Research and Interventions, 1*(1), 21–28.

Steele, W., & Raider, M. (2001). Structured sensory intervention for traumatized children, adolescents, and parents. *Trauma and Loss: Research and Interventions, 1*(1), 8–20.

CHAPTER 10

Drawing and Storytelling as Psychotherapy with Children

Masahiro Tanaka
Tomio Kakuyama
Madoka Takada Urhausen

Many Japanese children referred to the Child Guidance Center and Educational Counseling Center display a wide range of emotional problems including social withdrawal, school refusal, anxiety disorder, selective mutism, social phobia, and posttraumatic stress disorder (PTSD) from abuse and neglect. Others seek counseling to cope with depression due to medical conditions. The children entering psychotherapy often have difficulty verbalizing their concerns regarding themselves and any traumatic experiences they have had. It is also common that they do not respond well to direct questions. In particular, if children have been physically or sexual abused, they may feel embarrassed to talk about the incident or feel guilty expressing their feelings. In addition, they may have to grapple with the cultural dilemma that prohibits the sharing of personal or family secrets with others. As a result, these children have an extraordinary amount of internalized shame and low self-esteem.

In verbal therapy, additional clinical challenges are present if these children suffer from speech disorders due to developmental arrest exacerbated by trauma or developmental delay from organic problems. Children's lack of verbalization about the trauma experience puts them at higher risk for the continuation of the trauma as it prevents them from seeking proper help. This phenomenon often leads to victimized children's increased sense of helplessness and isolation which in turn contributes to the vicious cycle of self-victimization.

One of the effective interventions known to assist children in verbalizing their feelings safely is storytelling, a technique that includes various expressive modalities. When employed appropriately, storytelling provides a rich creative experience and offers a wide variety of applications in psychotherapy. By allowing the child to be a storyteller, the child is actively engaged in reparative work of his or her self-esteem. It facilitates the expression of difficult emotions such as worry, anger, and confusion effectively and in a nonconfrontational manner (Gardner, 1974; Kestenbaum, 1985; Lawson, 1987; Silver, 1996; Stirtzinger, 1983; Tanaka, 1992, 2001a, 2001b).

An important consideration in using storytelling is how to bridge the presented story and the child's actual experience of internal conflict. The therapist becomes the mediator of the two. In this chapter, the use of drawing and storytelling in psychotherapy is discussed with examples from the Squiggle Game, Egg Drawing technique, and the Cave Drawing technique.

SQUIGGLE GAME AND STORYTELLING

The Squiggle Game was based on a traditional game for children in England. Winnicott introduced it to the therapeutic domain in his consultation with children. The Squiggle Game later gained worldwide acceptance as an effective art directive (Walrond-Skinner, 1986). Winnicott (1971) pointed out that this technique promotes rapport building between the therapist and child through the exchange of their individual squiggle drawings and the discovery of hidden images in them (Claman, 1980; Nakai, 1982; Tanaka, 1993; Winnicott, 1971; Ziegler, 1976). This guessing game generates playful interaction between the therapist and child. The Squiggle Game promotes the symbolic act of acceptance and acknowledgement of the client's imperfect or unintegrated object by the therapist, thereby facilitating a therapeutic relationship through mirroring the child's drawing.

Based on his concept of the maturation process, Winnicott (1965) explained that infants go through a developmental stage in which they perceive that they create the objects around them and that they are undifferentiated with these objects. Winnicott emphasized the necessity for the "adult" therapist to embrace and provide a holding environment for the "infant" or developmentally arrested child's ideas about the creation. This process, in due course, helps the client to undergo proper separation from the objects and gain objectivity about the outside world (Winnicott, 1968/1989a, 1963/1989).

In the context of play therapy, the Squiggle Game allows for a smooth transition from subjective (projection) to objective experience (the use of an object), and it is precisely this bridging of the two realities that brings therapeutic benefits to the clients. Finally, Winnicott did not intend the Squiggle Game to be used as a guideline for how the interplay of therapist and child client can be facilitated (Winnicott, 1968/1989b). Tanaka saw the potential for narrative interaction in the Squiggle Game. Using the art products from the game, Tanaka facilitated storytelling through making *kamishibai*, a traditional Japanese art of picture card show, or four-frame cartoons (Tanaka, 1992, 1993, 2001a, 2001b). After having two to three sessions with the Squiggle Game, the therapist may elicit narrative expressions by suggesting the child create a story out of those four to six pictures. There are two approaches to this process. The therapist and child may individually create a separate story by selecting their favorite pictures as in parallel play, or collaborate in storytelling by taking turns selecting pictures and adding to the other's story in a random manner. Both approaches are effective in gaining insight to the child's presenting problems within the short time required for a creative exchange.

THE EGG DRAWING AND CAVE DRAWING TECHNIQUES AND STORYTELLING

Tanaka's art therapy techniques, the Egg Drawing and Cave Drawing, are rich in symbolic expression and facilitate storytelling (Tanaka, 1995, 2001a, 2001b). They are two separate art therapy techniques that can be employed individually or together during one session or over the course of treatment repeatedly. Both techniques rely on the active participation of the therapist as the therapist initiates the storytelling through visual and verbal means. To begin, an oval line drawing is presented to the child and the therapist tells the child that this is an egg or a cave opening. These visual and verbal prompts stimulate the active imagination of the child and motivate the child to engage in art expression and storytelling. By encouraging a story, the pictorial space is transformed into symbolic space impregnated with the child's personal meanings. In short, the Egg and Cave Drawings enhance the potential for narratives through specific directives and guided imagery.

The content of the projective art created in the two techniques are the results of two different approaches to the psychological space and thus reflect different aspects of the child. Therefore, having the child create a story from both art products is useful for the therapist to understand the child's psychological state.

ART SUPPLIES

Suggested media for the Egg and Cave Drawings are as follows:

1. Letter-size paper or 8″ × 10″ sketchbook
2. Different grades of pencils ranging from 2B to 6B
3. Eraser
4. Pencil sharpener
5. Fine-tip black markers
6. A set of crayons or color pencils in 24 or 36 colors

APPLICATION OF EGG DRAWING AND CAVE DRAWING TECHNIQUES

For the Egg Drawing, the therapist should follow this directive:

- The therapist first draws an oval shape on a piece of paper.
- The therapist then asks the child client, "What does it look like?" The child may guess that it is an egg; then the therapist would acknowledge it to be cor-

rect. If the child cannot tell, the therapist should suggest that it is an egg. At this point, it is important that both therapist and client recognize the image of the egg together.

- After explaining that something is about to be born, the therapist asks the child to add cracks to the egg.
- When the child draws cracks, the therapist asks, "What is about to be born?" Most of the time, the child will say "a chick." The therapist should respond by saying that "this is a magic egg" and "anything you can think of can come out of it."
- The therapist provides a new piece of paper and directs the child to draw his or her fantasy creation along with the pieces of broken eggshells.
- Finally, the therapist asks the child to color the drawing.

For the Cave Drawing, the therapist should follow this directive:

- Upon completion of an egg drawing, the therapist again draws an oval, slightly larger than the previous one. He or she states that it is not an egg this time.
- The therapist should explain that it is the entrance to a cave. He or she encourages a drawing of the outside world viewed from inside the cave, by saying, "Suppose you live here, what would you see outside?"
- After confirming the client's understanding of the directive, the therapist should ask the client to proceed with the drawing.
- If the child so desires, the therapist should encourage the internal wall of the cave to be colored as well.

When the two drawings are completed, the therapist should ask the child to tell a story using both pictures created from the Egg and Cave Drawings. In general, these two drawing techniques are used together; however, it is possible to employ them individually.

CASE STUDY: L.B.

L.B. is a fair-skinned, small-framed 13-year-old Japanese female who suffered from a long history of sexual and emotional abuse. She was abandoned at birth by her biological parents and was raised by her maternal grandparents. L.B. was allegedly molested by her maternal grandfather from the age of 8 until she sought help this year at a Child Guidance Center at the age of 13. Around the time L.B. reached puberty, she developed a social phobia and school refusal based on her fear that her peers saw her differently. She also presented various symptoms that resulted from the trauma of her sexual abuse such as hypervigilance to the others, sensitivity to touch and loud noises, panic attacks inside the commuter train at rush hours, and chronic somatic complaints.

L.B. described in her early session that her egg drawing (Figure 10.1) depicted a newborn angel who was hiding her face in broken eggshells. In her cave drawing

(Figure 10.2) she drew a thick field of tall grass receding into a mysterious deep forest whose entrance was framed by two rocks in the foreground. She then told the following story titled "The Birth of an Angel."

"Far from where humans live, there was a secret forest. The forest had long lost her guardian angels. The angels guarded the forest and kept humans away. The angels also healed injured people and animals. At the foot of a tree was a golden egg of an unborn angel. 'Crack, crack, crack' crackled the egg. A part of the eggshell peeled off and burst with a blinding silver light. 'Crack, crack,' one piece after another fell off to the ground. Silver light penetrated the golden light of the egg. 'Flap, flap, flap.' When half of the shell fell off, something made a faint sound of flapping feathers. It was of a newborn angel. For a while, the angel was busy moving its wings and airing them dry. 'Phew!' Unable to speak, the angel took a big breath. The egg lost its balance and the angel was thrown out of the egg. Fortunately, she managed to not get hurt as she landed on the soft bed of tall grass. When the angel looked around, there was a cave nearby. The angel decided to hide in the cave for the time being. The pieces of broken egg were taken back to heaven shortly after and was turned into a star."

As indicated in this case illustration, the narrative content that came out of combining storytelling with the Egg and Cave Drawings provided the clinician a deeper

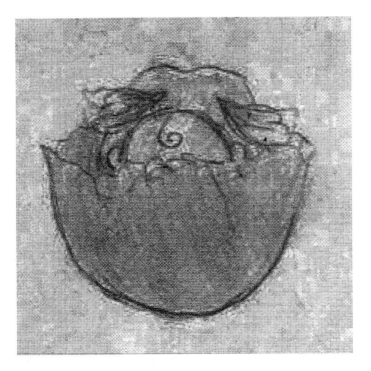

FIGURE 10.1. Egg drawing depicting a newborn angel who was hiding her face in broken eggshells.

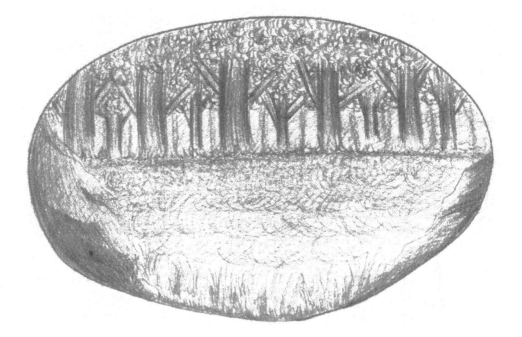

FIGURE 10.2. Cave drawing with tall grass receding into a forest whose entrance was framed by two rocks in the foreground.

understanding of the client's personal meaning. From the story, it may be construed that L.B. is seeking a place of safety. Upon exploration of the angel's function as a healer the author deduced that the angel in the story was L.B.'s wish to heal and felt encouraged about her prognosis.

The symbolism of an angel evolved as L.B.'s therapy progressed. The angel that L.B. drew 6 months later (Figure 10.3) was blindfolded, and her cave drawing (Figure 10.4) depicted a rose and the cemetery. L.B. explained that "the angel was blindfolded so that she would not see the filth of the world." Contrary to what L.B. described, her imagery repeatedly depicted a "single eye," which can have many meanings.

It is apparent that the guardian angel symbolizes L.B. herself who was sexually abused, despite the suggested role of angel as healer. Furthermore, the picture of the rose and cemetery addresses the theme of loss surrounding her mother, whom she had never met, and her own violated sexuality. This process lead to L.B.'s voluntarily writing a short story titled "Funeral" in which she expressed her wish to gain help from her absent mother.

During the ensuing sessions L.B. drew herself as an angel who lay bleeding from its heart and eyes while her one hand gestured toward her skirt drenched in blood and the rest of her body contorted as if she was bound. She titled it "A Wounded Angel." The manifest content of this image is self-blame and helplessness, which are common among victims of incest. It is a self-portrait of someone who is painfully aware of the violated self.

This self-portrait became a pivotal expression as it indicated her courage to face the trauma. It is important to note that around this time, while she developed in-

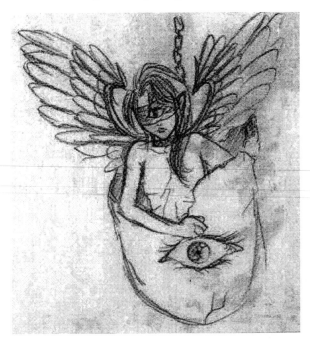

FIGURE 10.3. The blindfolded angel drawn by L.B. 6 months later.

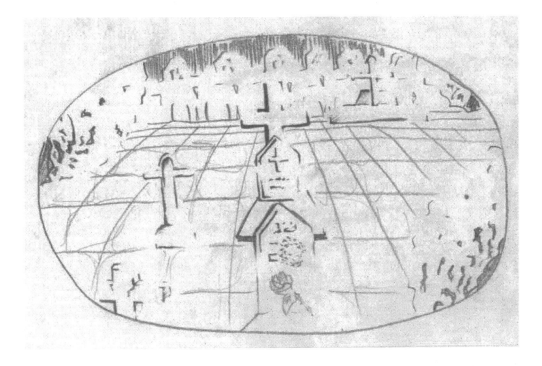

FIGURE 10.4. Cave drawing depicting a rose and cemetery.

creased therapeutic alliance with the clinician, L.B. started to express anger openly toward her grandmother who had failed to protect her from the perpetrator, who was by this time incarcerated.

CASE STUDY: J.Y.

J.Y. is a 12-year-old Japanese male, who was self-referred to the counseling due to presented symptoms of selective mutism and social phobia. J.Y. lived with his biological parents and his younger brother of 8 years in age. J.Y. suffered from dwarfism and therefore had unusually petite stature compared to his peers. Since infancy, J.Y. had received regular hormone injections to promote his physical growth. At the intake J.Y. was shy but cordial toward the therapist. However, his speech was often labored and hardly audible as he became nervous with the interview.

The primary concern that J.Y. presented was a symptom of ophthalmophobia (similar to social phobia in DSM-IV). He reported that he was fearful of his female peers and felt them to be hostile in the way they stared at him. According to school's report, there was no evidence supporting his claim, but J.Y. insisted that at least half the girls in his class gave him "dirty looks." There were some ongoing incidents, however, with a few male peers who persistently teased J.Y. for his physical appearance.

It was evident that J.Y. suffered from poor self-image. In a low-stimuli environment he was capable of expressing himself, but his behavior became inhibited as active interactions with others were required; he lacked assertiveness and was extremely controlling of his emotions in presence of others. J.Y. was motivated to treatment, and art therapy was a preferred modality because he could not participate fully in verbal therapy.

In the second session, art directives of the Egg and Cave Drawings were employed. His first egg drawing was titled "A UFO, Stars, a Watch, a Bus, Shells, and Cherries." The drawing was filled with many of these small objects. In contrast, his first cave drawing depicted molten lava exploding from a volcano. The therapist (Tanaka) was surprised by this expression of anger in contrast to J.Y.'s controlled and relaxed demeanor as he drew the volcano.

J.Y. responded well to art directives and enjoyed coming to therapy. In the course of treatment, he became increasingly self-directed with therapeutic activities and started to express his wish to draw his choice of subject matter. In the middle phase of therapy, the therapist returned to the Egg and Cave Drawing directives for the third time and asked J.Y. to create a story with two art products. J.Y. told a story that took place in outer space.

The egg drawing, titled "Space and Space Ship," depicted a small and faraway galaxy with earth scattered in oblivion of outer space, indicating J.Y.'s tendency to detach and withdraw as his defense (Figure 10.5.) In the cave drawing, titled "An Attack of the Monster Named Ganta," J.Y. depicted a Godzilla-like monster that destroyed the city. His repressed anger and aggression were observed through this picture (Figure 10.6). However, the story from this directive elicited a minimal verbal response from J.Y.: "The monster Ganta laid a huge egg. The egg was colorful. When it hatched, there were many stars inside."

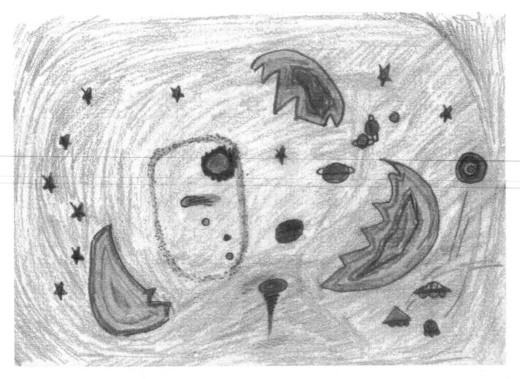

FIGURE 10.5. Egg drawing titled "Space and Space Ship."

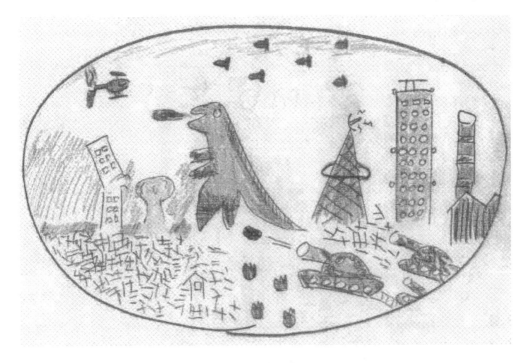

FIGURE 10.6. Cave drawing titled "An Attack of the Monster Named Ganta."

While the constellation of bright stars and vast galaxy in the cave drawing seemed to represent J.Y.'s developing potentials and the story indicated his ability to acknowledge positive aspects of the self (monster), the story itself ignored the monster's aggression and did not touch on the actual fighting scene. This inconsistency of verbal and nonverbal expression was interpreted as an indication of J.Y.'s continued difficulty in verbalization of his feelings despite his increased comfort level in expressing his anger in pictures.

Ensuing sessions consisted of the Egg and the Cave Drawings, Squiggle Game, and Division-Coloring Method (an activity for individuals with handicaps involving coloring in predetermined sections of a paper) with which storytelling was incorporated in nonverbal drawing directives. The increase in written expression was remarkable with the stories he composed for his pictures. His word count went from initial 51 words, 69 for the story mentioned previously, and later increased rapidly to a significant amount of 171, 981, and 1,176 words. Along with this improvement was a parallel progress in his verbal participation in therapy and his involvement with others. J.Y. engaged more actively with verbal interactions and his social phobia subsided gradually.

J.Y. had been diagnosed with dwarfism as an infant and had struggled to thrive. He was rejected and teased by his peers and suffered from terrible inferiority complex. J.Y.'s primary concern of fearing female peers' gazes was interpreted as a projection of his mother's watchful eyes and constant monitoring with his medical condition. It is conceivable that his mother's sadness, frustration, and self-pity with the adolescent's lack of growth were internalized and resulted in J.Y.'s own critical view of himself.

The contents of J.Y.'s drawings were anger and inability to have a proper outlet for self-expression as well as a need for control of feelings and behaviors. Having symptoms of social phobia, J.Y. was intimidated by the format of verbal therapy that required him to deal directly with a therapist. By focusing on the process of art and storytelling J.Y. was able to engage himself to a therapeutic relationship with his therapist.

As J.Y. continued to elaborate on the stories of space, aliens, monsters, and futuristic cities, he developed a relationship with his art and began to own his stories, propelling him to make his internal dialogue explicit. This process assisted J.Y. to come to term with his feelings related to his medical conditions and relationships with peers and family.

J.Y. learned to face his medical predicament as he gained coping skills through mastery of art and storytelling. J.Y. learned to examine and acknowledge his feelings which he could not initially express. His accomplishment came from applying himself in a nonverbal expressive modality that eventually led him to open verbalization and alleviation of his fears and worries.

DISCUSSION

As demonstrated through the case material, children with emotional disorders frequently reveal themes of death, destruction, and rebirth. These themes can indicate a strong desire to change. The clinician's initial task is to recognize this desire and provide a safe, therapeutic space in order to allow for such expression.

The Egg and Cave Drawings techniques provide access to this inner desire, elicit their responses sensitively, and do so in a nonconfrontational manner. The egg drawing is particularly helpful through a paradoxical approach: The child who experienced a trauma or emotional problem takes on an active role in metaphorically breaking the self-image of a fragile egg. This change helps the child experience a sense of control, and at this moment something new is born. The result is a self-determined transformation that is constructive rather than destructive in nature.

The theoretical basis of the egg drawing with its use of a "little" destruction concurs with Winnicott's (1968/1989a) notion that "the destruction plays its part in making the reality, placing the object outside the self" (p. 223). Risk taking is regarded as an essential part of therapy in order for it to be successful. The process of the egg drawing involves the risk-taking process (cracking an egg by the client), which can lead a child to a sense of accomplishment despite the moments of raised anxiety. With repeated employment of the intervention a child may become desensitized to the fear of changing one's personal image (an egg and what comes out of it), thereby engaging in the constant renewal of self-image.

Nonetheless, a word of caution must be made regarding the egg drawing for its paradox. When employing this technique, the clinician must remember that the child who has been traumatized might feel resistant, if not awkward, having been given the directive to purposely destroy a selfobject. Such an experience may exacerbate the child's emotional decompensation. For this reason, sound clinical judgment must be maintained. Although current research indicates that reexperiencing the trauma helps to heal the client, considerations regarding the severity of abuse and appropriate timing in terms of introducing any interventions are critical. The process of this drawing directive can promote trauma reenactment. It may not be appropriate for clients exhibiting behavioral and mental disorganization such as psychosis or the presence of self-injurious behavior. There is a danger of leading the child with metaphorical rehearsal of such actions that need to be contained rather than expressed openly. In general, the egg drawing technique is useful with most populations when the therapeutic relationship is a stable one.

The authors assert that the cave drawing has a wider applicability because of its metaphor of a safe place. The cave, symbolized by an oval frame, functions to set boundaries of real space and therapeutic (pictorial) space. Thus, a comfortable distance is established between a drawer and his or her personal image. This distance allows the clinician to explore the client's wishes and desires safely.

Furthermore, the cave drawing and narrative assist the clinician in evaluating the child during the process of treatment, including his or her limitations represented in symbolical ways. Examples can be seen in the blocks of rock that protect the enchanted forest of the L.B. (Figure 10.2), her bird's-eye view of the cemetery (Figure 10.4), and J.Y.'s comical, movie-like quality of the monster's violence (Figure 10.6).

Whereas the egg drawing examines the child's internal world, the cave drawing most frequently represents his or her fantasy related to conflict and conflict resolution. Storytelling that incorporates these two realities brings greater awareness to the child, who cannot otherwise articulate his or her wishes and insight for solutions. For example, J.Y.'s egg drawing was that of the nebulous, undifferentiated self with lack of boundaries. His cave drawing signified a sense of order and time sequence. Together, the two drawings offered immediate understanding of J.Y.'s predicament with its concrete and cohesive story about the alienated monster.

The techniques mentioned here are not simply projective tests and tools to ascertain information but, rather, methods to bridge the gap from the child's fantasy to reality. The case studies presented here illustrated how the interventions incorporating art and storytelling promoted the child's expression, which led to increased self-awareness and prepared the child for the challenges and changes in life. In summary, therapists should consider the following when applying these two techniques:

1. The Egg Drawing may not be productive or therapeutic with resistant clients unless an appropriate level of therapeutic alliance is established.
2. The Cave Drawing has a greater applicability with wider populations; hence it can be used in the early stages of therapy.

CONCLUSION

Clinical interventions with both verbal and drawing components promote progress in psychotherapy and speech (Gardner, 1974; Kakuyama, 1995). Art therapy, by virtue of the modality, allows for nonverbal communication to make explicit what children cannot verbalize normally. Consequently, art may assist children to verbally express their fantasies and inner thoughts through storytelling.

The quality of the therapeutic relationship between the client and the therapist and the progress of the therapy are reflected in art expression. When a safe holding place for the imagery is successfully established, increased therapeutic alliance is revealed through the change in art expression. With L.B., the core theme in therapy was abuse and abandonment by loved ones. The increased externalization of the wounded self with her angel drawings and stories paralleled L.B.'s growing confidence in the therapist. It is our experience that the richer the therapeutic relationship, the more engrained the story with personal meanings even in the simplest of drawings.

The key point to remember when employing art interventions with a narrative approach is the therapist's attentiveness and ardent effort to communicate through the child's art. There is a therapeutic value in itself if the child enjoyed the session or wants to return for another session. For this reason, the therapist must consider the most abstract and the least threatening art intervention to ease the fear and anxiety of the child. The clinician's goal is not necessarily focused on the completion of the art expression or story but the smooth transition of the phases of therapy and thereby bringing continuity to underlying themes during the course of treatment.

The use of drawing tasks such as Winnicott's Squiggle Game and Tanaka's Egg Drawing and Cave Drawing can be powerful techniques in helping children with emotional problems. The combination of both drawing and storytelling, along with the therapeutic relationship, provide a way for troubled children to express their fears and anxieties through the safety of projection and, in the case of art, nonverbal expression.

REFERENCES

Claman, L. (1980). The squiggle-drawing game in child psychotherapy. *American Journal of Psychotherapy, 34*(3), 414–425.

Gardner, R. (1974). The mutual storytelling technique in the treatment of psychogenic problems secondary to minimal brain dysfunction. *Journal of Learning Disabilities, 7*(3), 135–143.

Kakuyama, T. (1995). Emotional difficulties as a constituent of functional articulation disorders in children. *Proceedings of the 23rd World Congress of the International Association of Logopedics and Phoniatrics* (pp. 129–132). Cairo, Egypt.

Kestenbaum, C. J. (1985). The creative process in child psychotherapy. *American Journal of Psychotherapy, 39*(4), 479–489.

Lawson, D. M. (1987). Using therapeutic stories in the counseling process. *Elementary School Guidance & Counseling, 22*(2), 134–142.

Nakai, H. (1982). Sougo genkai ginmi-hou wo kami shita squiggle [Squiggle technique of Winnicott with mutual limit testing, and facilitation]. *Japanese Bulletin of Art Therapy, 13,* 17–21.

Silver, R. (1996). *Silver drawing test of cognition and emotion.* New York: Ablin Press.

Stirtzinger, R. M. (1983). Story telling: A creative therapeutic technique. *Canadian Journal of Psychiatry, 28*(7), 561–565.

Tanaka, M. (1992). Nagurigaki to monogatari [The mutual storytelling and squiggle game]. *Studies in Clinical Application Drawings, 7,* 147–165.

Tanaka, M. (1993). Squiggle hou no jissai [Practical method of squiggle drawing game] [Special Issue: Squiggle Technique]. *Studies in Clinical Application Drawings, 8,* 19–34.

Tanaka, M. (1995). Tamagoga to Doukutsuga: Rinshobyouga ni okeru daenwaku kuukan no kenkyu [Egg drawing and cave drawing technique: The study of oval boundary technique in clinical drawings]. *Studies in Clinical Application Drawings, 10,* 151–168.

Tanaka, M. (2001a). Approach to art therapy with gender identity disordered adolescents—the significance of narrative elicited through clinical drawings. *Bulletin of Mejiro University Department of Human and Social Sciences, 1,* 85–103.

Tanaka, M. (2001b). On squiggle drawing game with delinquent children: Art therapy and psychopathology of expression (Chapter 2, Expressive Activity and Psychiatric Treatment, Squiggle Drawing Game). *Clinical Psychiatry, Special Volume* (pp. 135–143). Tokyo: Arc Media.

Walrond-Skinner, S. (1986). *A dictionary of psychotherapy: Squiggle Game.* London: Routledge.

Winnicott, D. W. (1963/1989). Fear of breakdown. In C. Winnicott, R. Shepherd, & M. Davis (Eds.), *Psycho-analytic explorations/D. W. Winnicott* (pp. 87–89). Cambridge, MA: Harvard University Press.

Winnicott, D. W. (1965). *Maturation processes and the facilitating environment.* London: Hogarth Press.

Winnicott, D. W. (1968/1989a). The use of an object and relating through identifications. In C. Winnicott, R. Shepherd, & M. Davis (Eds.), *Psycho-analytic explorations/D. W. Winnicott* (pp. 218–227). Cambridge, MA: Harvard University Press.

Winnicott, D. W. (1968/1989b). The squiggle game. In C. Winnicott, R. Shepherd, & M. Davis (Eds.), *Psycho-analytic explorations/D. W. Winnicott* (pp. 299–317). Cambridge, MA: Harvard University Press.

Winnicott, D. W. (1971). *Therapeutic consultations in child psychiatry.* London: Hogarth Press.

Ziegler, R. (1976). Winnicott's squiggle game: Its diagnostic and therapeutic usefulness. *Art Psychotherapy, 3,* 177–185.

CHAPTER 11

Using Drawing in Short-Term Trauma Resolution

William Steele

This chapter presents a structured trauma intervention that relies on reexposure to traumatic memories through drawing, developing a trauma narrative, and cognitive reframing. The intervention discussed is based on a program field tested and researched as part of a 2-year grant project (Steele & Raider, 2001) developed by the National Institute for Trauma and Loss in Children (TLC). Research demonstrated a significant reduction of trauma-specific reactions across all three subcategories of DSM-IV: reexperiencing, avoidance, and arousal (Steele & Raider, 2001). Reduction was seen in the most severe cases (Type II traumas) as well as the least severe (Type I) (Terr, 1991).

These results were not only substantiated by the participating children but also by the independent pre-, post-, and 3-month follow-up evaluations from parents. Field testing took place in both school and agency settings with the intent of developing a program which could be implemented by school counselors and mental health professionals. Structured drawing activities, along with cognitive reframing, were the primary media used for reexposure and initiating the trauma narrative. However, before a discussion of trauma intervention can be initiated it is necessary to understanding what trauma is, how it is induced, and how it manifests itself in children.

TRAUMA REACTIONS IN CHILDREN

In 1994, the American Psychiatric Association acknowledged that children could, in fact, experience posttraumatic stress disorder (PTSD), establishing the following criteria:

1. The person experienced, witnessed, or was confronted with an event or events that involved actual or threatened death or serious injury, or a threat to the physical integrity of self or others. An event need not lead to death for PTSD to be induced. Furthermore, injury need not occur; the threat to one's physical safety can be sufficient to induce trauma.
2. The person's response involved intense fear, helplessness, or horror. Intense fear and helplessness (powerlessness) are the key reactions of trauma. Some children of divorce, given the helplessness of their situation at the time of the divorce, can experience severe PTSD.

Pynoos and Nader (1990); Black, Hendricks, and Kaplan, (1992); Dykman and Buka (1997); and others have substantiated that physical/sexual abuse, murder, domestic violence, random violence, and other forms of assault expose children to all the reactions we once attributed only to adult survivors of war. Children were not involved in the field studies used to develop the American Psychiatric Association's PTSD category and it is therefore limited. In addition to these criteria therapists should consider the reactions observed by Pynoos and Nader (1988), Johnson (1993) and Peterson and Straub (1992), and the World Health Organization's (1992) ICD-9 classification.

PTSD can occur in any child victim. Eth and Pynoos (1985) were two of the first researchers to substantiate that witnesses to violent events were vulnerable to trauma reactions. The closer the physical proximity to the event the greater the intensity of the reactions experienced. There is, however, another level of exposure for those who are neither surviving victims nor witnesses but are related to the victim. Being related to the victim as a family member, a friend, a peer, or someone who goes to the same school as the victim or lives in the same community can create vulnerability to trauma. Schwarz and Kowalski (1991) suggest that one's emotional status at the time of an incident can lead to ongoing memories associated with the incident. Saigh and Bremner (1999) and others strongly suggest that "perceived relatedness" (to victim) coupled with personal vulnerability can leave one exposed to PTSD reactions.

During a training for preschool teachers 6 months after the bombing of the Federal Building in Oklahoma City, one of the teachers told of how the children divided themselves into two groups. One group took the mats they slept on for their naps to one side of the room. They covered themselves with the mats as if they were buried. The other group took two indoor soccer nets to the other side of the room. These children formed pairs and one pair at a time would go to the children hiding under the mats, lift off the mat, and then take their peer over to the soccer net. The different pairs repeated this behavior until all the children were pulled from under the mats and taken to the other side of the room. When all the children were on the other side of the room they switched roles and the rescuers "buried" themselves under the mats and were then "rescued" by the others.

These children, on their own, were rehearsing their ability to rescue one another. They had been exposed to the terror of trauma as witnesses to the Oklahoma bombing via television and perceived themselves to be related to the victims because they were similar in age and in a similar environment.

It is no longer in question that children can, in fact, be affected by the full range of posttraumatic stress. The question becomes, "What type of intervention is going to be most helpful for children exposed to these trauma inducing events?"

TRAUMA INTERVENTION WITH CHILDREN

The major components of intervention with children who have experienced trauma include the following: reexposure to the trauma memories and experiences, developing a trauma narrative or telling of the story, and cognitive reframing. Externalizing the story into a visual representation of the elements of that experience and the cognitive reframing of that experience into one that is manageable are the goals of successful trauma intervention. Drawing is a critical component of both reexposure and telling the story and is discussed later in this chapter. Structure is also an important component that promotes safety and must be maintained throughout the entire process for children to actively participate in trauma intervention.

Reexposure

Reexposing the trauma victims to their experiences is the core component of trauma intervention. Exposure is recognized as the necessary process in helping victims bring their experience into consciousness so it can then be reordered in a way that is manageable. Rachman (1966), Marks (1972), Saigh (1987), and others have used exposure as a core process in helping trauma victims integrate their experience into consciousness. Bessel van der Kolk (van der Kolk, McFarlane, & Weisaeth, 1996, p. 420) states:

> Traumatic memories need to become like memories of everyday experience, that is, they need to be modified and transformed by being placed in their proper context and restructured into a meaningful narrative. The purpose of full exposure is to make the fragments of the traumatic event lose their power to act as conditioned stimuli that reactivate affects and behaviors relevant to the trauma, but irrelevant to current experience.

Likewise, Foa and Kozak (1985) indicate that two conditions are required for the treatment of PTSD and the reduction of fear:

1. The traumatic memories must be reactivated in order to be modified. The ability to decrease fear or anxiety is dependent on the controlled reliving of that fear in a safe environment so as to be able to diminish the response to it.
2. Corrective information must be provided so that the victim can form a new narrative or meaning that places the traumatic memory at the place and time it occurred as opposed to generalizing that experience to everyday life.

Exposure techniques are designed to help the trauma victim realize that the conditioned responses are no longer dangerous and avoidance no longer necessary. The ability to learn to tolerate the intense fear and emotional reactions experienced by a traumatic event is a critical part of recovery (Rothchild, 2001). From here the experience can be modified or reordered into a form that is acceptable and manageable by the victim through a *cognitive restructuring* into a meaningful, integrative narrative. When traumatic memories are not integrated into consciousness, the memories continue to trigger the traumatic state or conditioned responses of avoidance and arousal.

Cognitive Therapy and Reframing

Cognitive therapy (Beck, 1972, 1976; Marks, 1972) facilitates the integration of traumatic memories into conscious memories and present-life experiences. The altering of trauma-driven thoughts is referred to as cognitive reframing.

When a trauma is put into a narrative form inclusive of the details of the experience, these details must then be reordered in a way that is manageable. Once manageable the victim is no longer a victim but a survivor of the experience, in control of rather than reacting to the experience. For example, rather than "this experience has ruined my life and leaves me no choices," cognitive reframing changes that victim position into "I survived this experience and I'll survive others because I have choices." Cognitive reframing, therefore, helps remove those emotions and behaviors that are driven by the dysfunctional thoughts brought about by the trauma.

Cognitive reframing must also address specific-trauma themes as well as any secondary traumatization that may occur if children's reactions are ignored, minimized, or inappropriately responded to by helpers or parents. The intervener must be prepared to reframe the child's reaction to the major themes of trauma—feelings of fear, terror, worry, hurt, anger, revenge, accountability, and victimization.

Drawing

Drawing is used as a form of exposure to assist children in constructing trauma narratives while helping them to relive traumatic memories. Cognitive behavioral psychology has demonstrated "that memories determine the interpretation of the present even when they are not conscious" (Mihaescu & Baettig, 1996, p. 243). Children experience trauma at a sensorimotor level then shift to a "perceptual (iconic) representation at a symbolic level" (Mihaescu & Baettig, 1996, p. 246). "Later, in adult life, these memories are ordered linguistically. When a terrifying incident such as trauma is experienced and does not fit into a contextual memory, a new memory or dissociation is established" (van der Kolk, 1987, p. 289). When memory cannot be linked linguistically in a contextual framework, it remains at a symbolic level for which there are no words to describe it. To retrieve that memory so it can be encoded, given a language, and then integrated into consciousness, it must be retrieved and externalized in its symbolic perceptual (iconic) form.

Drawing is one way to provide a link between dissociated memories and their retrieval into consciousness after which the experience can be translated into narrative form and then reintegrated into the child's past, present, and future life experiences.

Malchiodi (1990, 1998, 2001) states that drawing provides children with an impetus to tell their stories and a way to translate their traumatic experiences into narratives. Riley (1997) observed that the act of drawing is a form of externalization, visible projection of self, thoughts, and feelings.

Pynoos and Eth (1986) relied heavily on drawing as his primary intervention with children traumatized by violence. They indicate that drawing "invariably signifies the child's unconscious preoccupation with the traumatic memory" (p. 316). Drawing provides for an externalization of the experience and through the motor (drawing) and verbal (giving the narrative) actions helps the child move from a passive (internal) powerless involvement with the trauma to an active (external) control of that experience. Once a traumatized child can form a trauma narrative and externalize it in a symbolic fashion the child is able not only to find relief from the terror it created but to regain power over it to the point that energies are no longer spent avoiding and reacting to all the triggers and symptoms created by that trauma.

The use of drawing also has an additional advantage. For children as well as adults, trauma memories are encoded in images because trauma is a sensory experience rather than a solely cognitive experience. For therapists to fully understand the impact of a traumatic incident on a child and to identify the critical trauma references for that child we need to become witnesses to the child's experiences. We must be able to see what children now see related to themselves and to the world around them as a result of their exposure. Drawing provides this opportunity to view the experience and see it as the child sees it. It also provides the stimulus for the child to tell his or her story and in essence make us a witness to the fear, terror, worry, hurt, anger, revenge, accountability, and overall victimization.

In trauma work it is essential to protect traumatized children from losing control. The revisiting of trauma through drawing must be experienced in a controlled fashion so children experience that they, in fact, can gain control out of what has been until now an array of out of control internalized reactions. Not only must the drawing activities be structured, but the media used must also be "containing." An 8″ × 11″ sheet of paper, for example, is far more controllable than is a 3 × 4-foot piece of paper. The larger the format, the greater the potential for losing control. A fine-point colored pencil, for example, is more containing than a jar of finger paints, which novices often discover can quickly move the child from painting the paper to painting the walls as well as the intervener.

KEY COMPONENTS OF INTERVENTION

• Trauma intervention should address the themes of fear, terror, worry, hurt (emotional and physical), anger, revenge, accountability, and victim versus survivor thinking. By focusing on these themes as opposed to the actual symptoms of trauma such as intrusive recollections, intervention defuses the symptoms and level of severity of dysfunctional response triggered by the sensory and cognitive memories of the trauma experience.

• Reexposure, trauma narrative, and cognitive reframing are the theoretical foundations supporting the intervention. With children and adolescents, exposure is accomplished through drawing. The trauma narrative (i.e., the telling of the story) is encouraged and facilitated by asking trauma-specific questions. Cognitive reframing addresses how children relate to the major theses of trauma.

• Trauma-specific questions must be related to the trauma experience, not necessarily to the incident itself. Trauma-specific questions include the following: What do you remember seeing, hearing, or touching? Do you sometimes think about what happened even when you don't want to? Do certain sounds, sights, smells, etc., suddenly remind you of what happened? What would you like to see happen to the person (or thing) that caused this to happen? Do you ever think it should have been you instead? Throughout the intervention process questions are specific to the theme being addressed. Their relevance keeps the child focused on the specific theme, encourages the narrative (story) to be told for each theme, and encourages attention to details. Details of the sensory experience of the trauma are critical in helping to reestablish a sense of control, to provide the therapist with the opportunity to correct any incorrect information (fantasies) the child possesses, and to provide new information. Thus, the processing of details not only helps with control but can also facilitate cognitive reframing.

• The reexperiencing of the traumatic event must be structured so that reexposure to the details and memories does not become an overwhelming flooding into consciousness. The therapist structures slow and progressive detailed reliving, accomplished by presenting structured trauma-specific questions and drawing tasks that address one theme at a time (see "Case Example"). The trauma-specific questions are designed to assist not only in the reexposure but also in the "slow and safe" telling of the story.

Drawing activities should relate to the major themes of trauma. For example, children are asked to draw "what happened," and "what the victim looked like at the time." The purpose of drawing is not to analyze or evaluate but to trigger sensory memories of the trauma. When the child externalizes and "concretizes" experiences in a way that makes us a witness to the experience, it allows the child to regain power over these memories and reorder them in a way that is manageable. Drawings are initiated in a sequential order and in association with specific themes and activities. The instruction is not, "Draw whatever you like." It is specific; for example, "Draw me a picture of what your hurt looks like."

CASE EXAMPLE

Johnny was 10 years old when his older sister, Sally, was brutally murdered by a serial killer. Her body was discovered some 6 months following her murder. A boyfriend was a witness to the murder. He was tied up and unable to help Sally.

One year later Johnny was fighting all the time and preoccupied with such horror characters as Freddie Krueger, and his grades had dropped. His mother reported that prior to the murder Johnny was the "best" youngster of the four children in the family. He was not a witness to the murder yet was understandably exposed to it through his relationship to the victim and through the media's coverage of this high-profile killing.

Johnny was brought in for intervention 1 year following the murder. He had been working with a social worker and had had several visits with a psychiatrist. These clinicians had not discussed the trauma directly, nor had Johnny been asked to draw.

Johnny was first asked to tell what happened. At times he had difficulty actually saying the words he wanted to use to tell his story. He also could not describe what images he was seeing in his mind as he was telling the story. For the first time in 5 months he broke down in tears.

Johnny's physical and emotional reactions were still very intense as if the murder had only just happened. His responses caused many well-meaning adults to tell him it would be better not to think or talk about his feelings. Although this is an understandable reaction, it also protects adults from the terror and powerlessness Johnny's feelings could trigger in themselves. To become a witness to a child's experience, we must be able to see how that child visually defines the experience as well as how he now views himself and the world around him.

Johnny was asked to draw a picture about his experience that he could tell a story about. His drawing (Figure 11.1) is primitive and yet he spent 20 minutes describing the events of the last evening he spent with his sister. He was the last in his family to see her alive. (It does not matter what the trauma victim draws or how he or she draws, just that the victim draws. It is the psychomotor activity of drawing that will begin to trigger the sensory memories of the trauma experience).

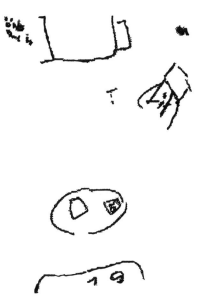

FIGURE 11.1. Drawing of living room where Johnny last saw his sister.

Johnny drew his living room where he, his sister, and her boyfriend were watching television, eating pizza, and having fun the night she left and never returned. It is the starting point of his story, a safe place for him to begin.

In a later drawing (Figure 11.2) Johnny draws a picture that he identified as himself before his sister was murdered. When asked about his mouth he replied, "I'm supposed to be smiling. I need to turn it to a smile." He took a colored pencil and attempted to turn the corners of the mouth upward but was unable to do so.

Many professionals would begin to analyze this behavior and attempt to probe for insight into its meaning. However, analysis and interpretation stop the process and shift back to a cognitive level. Trauma is not a cognitive experience; it is a sensory one. It is important to intervene at a sensory level. Furthermore, only the child can tell us what the drawing means in this process.

Because this drawing (Figure 11.2) was a picture of himself before his sister was killed, Johnny was asked to draw a picture of himself (Figure 11.3) after his sister's murder. In trauma we are always dealing with "then" and "now." "What scared you the most then; what scares you the most now?" are examples of moving between then and now. Again, we avoid interpreting the drawing. It is Johnny who describes how he now feels: powerful yet driven by the terror of horror characters such as Freddie Krueger and Candyman.

Trauma-driven anger or fighting is a response to regaining the sense of power that trauma takes from us. It is a way of not having to experience the overwhelming sense of vulnerability and powerlessness that trauma can create.

When Johnny was asked to draw (Figure 11.4) a picture of his sister dead, he could not quite do it. Instead he drew her in the process of being killed. The two lines going through her body are the arms of the serial killer. At this point he stopped and said he did not want to draw the serial killer. Later, when asked "What scares you the

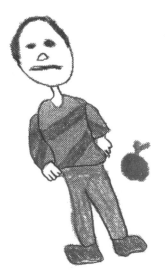

FIGURE 11.2. Self-image before his sister was murdered.

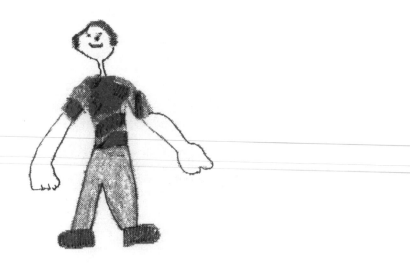

FIGURE 11.3. Self-image after his sister was murdered.

most now?," he told of how he saw the killer in court during the trial and how he now fears the killer will reach out of jail and come kill the rest of his family. Is it any wonder Johnny needs to see and experience himself as powerful?

Because he had not drawn his sister dead, Johnny was again asked to do so. His drawing (Figure 11.5) is the memory he holds of his sister. Hurt is a critical theme to address in trauma intervention. Following this drawing, Johnny was asked, "When you first found out, where did you feel the hurt the most in your body?" His response

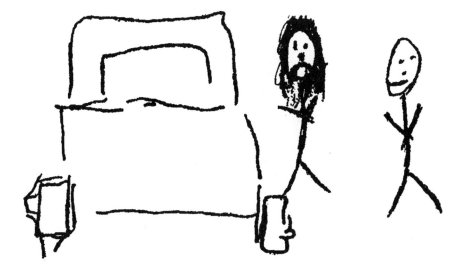

FIGURE 11.4. Drawing of sister being murdered.

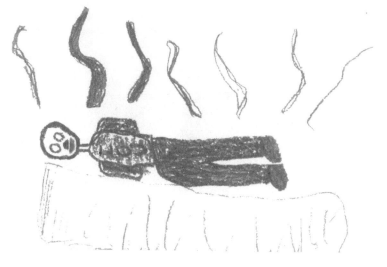

FIGURE 11.5. Drawing of the memory Johnny holds of his sister.

was that he "got a really bad headache." Johnny no longer has headaches, but when he thinks about his sister he "still aches all over."

When participants view Johnny via the videotaped interview of this session, he is no longer choking on his words. He is animated, able to laugh, providing many details without crying or intense reactions. There is a major change from the first 5 minutes of the interview to this part of the process 45 minutes later. The terror, the fear, the sensory struggle are no longer evident.

The intervener then asks Johnny to describe what that hurt was like. He really

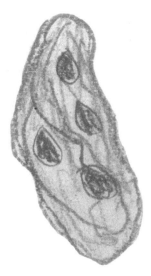

FIGURE 11.6. "This is what that hurt looks like."

cannot describe it. Twenty minutes later when the intervener begins to close the interview, Johnny says, "Wait; you know that hurt we were talking about?" He then picks up a colored pencil and quietly completes another drawing (Figure 11.6). When he is finished he says, "This is what that hurt looks like."

This process actively engages the child in his own healing. As the sensory memories of Johnny's experience are portrayed through drawing and he begins to develop the trauma narrative, he experiences a release of the terror-filled sensations of his experience at the same time that he gains control over them.

Mother reported weeks later that Johnny was "almost like himself again." It should be reported that we never talked about his fighting or other behavioral symptoms, only about his feelings of fear, terror, worry, hurt, anger, revenge, and guilt.

When this process is taught at the Institute, it is difficult for seasoned clinicians to stop analyzing, an attempt at insight. They want to reflect, explore, and interpret feelings that take the child away from his story. Many assume that they cannot ask the child to draw a picture of the person who died, was killed, or was critically injured in the first session. Such an approach may feel safer for the clinician, but children who are living with trauma desperately want an opportunity to have others witness their experience. Exposure through drawing and trauma-specific questions allow this to happen (Steele & Raider, 2001).

CONCLUSION

There are several key reasons why drawing is an important modality in trauma intervention:

- Drawing is a psychomotor activity. Because trauma is a sensory experience, not solely a cognitive experience, intervention must include ways to tap sensory memories of the trauma.
- Drawing provides a safe vehicle to communicate what children, even adults, often have no words to describe.
- Drawing engages children in the active involvement in their own healing. It enables them to move from passive, internal, and uncontrollable reactions to their traumas into an active, directed, controlled externalization of those trauma experiences.
- Drawing provides a symbolic representation of the trauma experience in a language and a format that is external and concrete and therefore manageable.
- The drawing format itself is effective: The paper acts as a container of that trauma. The contained trauma can now be managed at a sensory, tactile level by the child. The child can use it as he or she wants, thereby giving the child a sense of empowerment over the trauma.
- Drawing provides a visual focus on details that encourages children, via trauma-specific questions, to tell their story and to give it a "language" which can then be recorded in a way that is also manageable.
- Drawing provides for the diminishing of reactivity (anxiety) to these memories

through repeated visual reexposure in a medium that is perceived and felt to be safe by the child.

It is not possible to fully describe this trauma intervention model in one chapter. The information here provides a framework and offers guidelines for treating traumatized children. It stresses the importance of having a structured process to create a safe environment. In this safe environment children can reexperience the details of their traumas and tell their stories in order to find relief from the terrors of their experiences and regain a sense of mastery and power over themselves and their environment.

REFERENCES

American Psychiatric Association. (1994). *Diagnostic and statistical manual of mental disorders* (4th ed.). Washington, DC: Author.

Beck, A. T. (1972). *Depression: Causes and treatment.* Philadelphia: University of Philadelphia Press.

Beck, A. T. (1976). *Cognitive therapy and the emotional disorders.* New York: International Universities Press.

Black, D., Hendricks, J., & Kaplan T. (1992). Father kills mother: Posttraumatic stress disorders in the children. *Psychotherapy, Psychosomatic, 57,* 152–157.

Dykman, E. Y., & Buka, S. L. (1997). Prevalence and risk factors for posttraumatic stress disorder among chemically dependent adolescents. *American Journal of Psychiatry, 154,* 752–757.

Eth, S., & Pynoos, R. (Eds.). (1985). *Posttraumatic stress disorder in children.* Washington, DC: American Psychiatric Press.

Foa, E. B., & Kozak, M. J. (1985). Treatment of anxiety disorders: Implications for psychopathology. In A. H. Tuma & J. D. Maser (Eds.), *Anxiety and disorders.* Hillsdale, NJ: Erlbaum.

Johnson, K. (1993). *School crisis management: A hands-on guide to training crisis response teams.* Alameda, CA: Hunter House.

Malchiodi, C. A. (1990). *Breaking the silence: Art therapy with children from violent homes.* New York: Brunner/Mazel.

Malchiodi, C. A. (1998). *Understanding children's drawings.* New York: Guilford Press.

Malchiodi, C. A. (2001). Using drawing as intervention with traumatized children. *Trauma and Loss: Research and Intervention, 1*(1), 21–28.

Marks, I. A. (1972). Flooding (implosion) and allied treatments. In S. Argas (Ed.), *Behavior modification: Principles and clinical applications* (pp. 151–211). Boston: Little Brown.

Mihaescu, G., & Baettig, D. (1996). An integrated model of posttraumatic stress disorder. *European Journal of Psychiatry, 10*(4), 243–245.

Peterson, S., & Straub, R. (1992). *School crisis survival guide.* New York: The Center for Applied Research in Education.

Pynoos, R., & Eth, S. (1986). Witness to violence: The child interview. *Journal of the American Academy of Child Psychiatry, 25,* 306–319.

Pynoos, R., & Nader, K. (1988). Psychological first aid and treatment approach to children exposed to community violence: Research implications. *Journal of Traumatic Stress, 1,* 445–473.

Pynoos, R., & Nader, K. (1990). Children's exposure to violence and traumatic death. Preliminary findings. *Journal of American Academy of Child and Adolescent Psychiatry, 31,* 863–867.

Rachman, S. J. (1966) Studies in desensitization—II: Flooding. *Behavior Research and Therapy, 4,* 1–6.

Raider, M., & Steele, W. (1999). *Trauma response kit: Short-term trauma intervention model evaluation*. Unpublished manuscript, Wayne State University, MI.

Riley, S. (1997). Children's art and narratives: An opportunity to enhance therapy and a supervisory challenge. *The Supervision Bulletin, 9*(3), 2–3.

Rothchild, B. (2001). *The body remembers: The psychophysiology of trauma and trauma treatment*. New York: Norton.

Saigh, P. (1987). In vitro flooding of a childhood post traumatic stress disorder. *School Psychology Review, 16*, 203–221.

Saigh, P., & Bremner, J. (1999). *Posttraumatic stress disorder*. Needham Heights, MA: Allyn & Bacon.

Schwarz, E., & Kowalski, J. (1991). Posttraumatic stress disorder after a school shooting: Effects of symptom threshold selection and diagnosis by DSM-III-R or proposed DSM-IV. *American Journal of Psychiatry, 48*, 592–597.

Steele, W., & Raider, M. (2001). *Structured sensory interventions for traumatized children, adolescents, and parents: Strategies to alleviate trauma*. New York: Edwin Mellen Press.

Terr, L. (1991). Childhood traumas: An outline and overview. *American Journal of Psychiatry, 148*, 10–20.

van der Kolk, B. A. (1987). *Psychological trauma*. Washington, DC: American Psychiatric Press.

van der Kolk, B. A., McFarlane, A. C., & Weisaeth, L. (Eds.). (1996). *Traumatic stress: The effects of overwhelming experience on mind, body, and society*. New York: Guilford Press.

World Health Organization. (1992). *The ICD-10 classification of mental and behavioral disorders: Clinical descriptions and guidelines*. Geneva: Author.

CHAPTER 12

Art and Play Therapy with Sexually Abused Children

Eliana Gil

Sexually abused children are characteristically silent victims. Quelled by manipulative adults or situations beyond their comprehension, they often hesitate to voice their internal distress. Sometimes their "problematic" behaviors reveal underlying concerns and signal a need for protection. Other times, children endure years of suffering, unable or unwilling to compromise their safety or their belief that disclosure will bring feared consequences such as family disintegration, loss of familial love, or harm to self or loved others. Art therapy can offer children substantial opportunities for healing, initially by facilitating communication and later by providing options for working through of painful and complex emotional issues.

SEQUELAE OF SEXUAL ABUSE

In the last three decades the literature on this subject has grown (Conte, 2002). Briere (1992) proposes seven major types of psychological disturbance which are present in most abused adolescents and adults: posttraumatic stress, cognitive distortions, altered emotionality, dissociation, impaired self-reference, disturbed relatedness, and avoidance. In my experience (Gil, 1991), these are symptoms that are also common to young children. Kendall-Tackett, Williams, and Finkelhor (1993), in a review of 40+ empirically sound research studies, identified four major symptoms: posttraumatic stress disorder (fear and anxiety), aggression, depression, and sexually aggressive behaviors. Sexually aggressive behaviors appear to be particularly resistant to therapeutic interventions (Lanktree & Briere, 1995). Friedrich (1995) also encourages a therapeutic focus on development of self, attachment, and affective and behavioral dysregulation issues of great import to growing children. Consumed within these broad categories are other issues commonly associated with child abuse such as sleeping and eating disorders, low self-esteem, inappropriate relational interactions, learning disabilities, and so forth.

Although abused children share common symptoms, their unique and idiosyncratic responses must be carefully assessed putting aside assumptions and expectations that *all* abused children will react in a prescribed fashion. In fact, one thing can be said with certainty: Abused children make unique meaning about their experiences and develop original defensive strategies in order to cope and survive painful life events.

Sexually abused children are exposed to stressful and confusing events that can challenge, debilitate, or render them acutely or chronically vulnerable and helpless (Friedrich, 2002). Abuse can have low to severe impact depending on many variables; generally, impact is greater within longer duration and frequency of the abuse; multiple perpetrators; presence of penetration or intercourse; physically forced sexual contact; abuse at an earlier age; molestation by a perpetrator substantially older than the victim; concurrent physical abuse; abuse with bizarre features; victim's immediate sense of personal responsibility for the molest; and feelings of powerlessness, betrayal, and/or stigma at the time of the abuse (Briere, 1992, pp. 5–6). Chronic sexual abuse by a parent or trusted adult will have the greatest impact on the child and will require mobilization of more sophisticated defensive strategies. The first clinical task, therefore, is to assess the child's distinctive experience.

THE CLINICAL SETTING

Children who enter treatment due to alleged sexual abuse have likely been through a series of verbal interviews by helping professionals. They usually enter the clinical setting hesitant and guarded, unable or unwilling to respond to additional queries about what happened and how they feel. In response to this expectable resistance, I encourage an assessment process that is nondirective, is play based, and does not rely exclusively on verbal communication (Gil, 2002). This approach allows children to develop a sense of comfort and safety as well as to expand their potential to communicate through symbol and language. It also sets the context for subsequent therapeutic work, which obviously will address a range of problematic symptoms (Heineman, 1998; James, 1994).

The play therapy office consists of toys purposefully selected for their symbolic potential (Landreth, 1982). I think of my play therapy office as having "stations," where certain activities can occur: art, sand, puppets, and toys. The art station has an array of pencils, markers, paints, paper, crafts, and an easel. The sand station includes sandtrays, sand, miniatures, and water. Children are encouraged to use as few or as many miniatures as they would like to make a "world" in the sand, or "anything they wish to make" (see, e.g., Mitchell & Friedman, 1994; Homeyer & Sweeney, 1998; Labovitz Boik & Goodwin, 2000). The puppet station offers an array of puppets representing dominance, vulnerability, aggression, docility, and transformation (e.g., a caterpillar that changes to a butterfly). In addition, there are a number of human puppets in different jobs (police, medical) as well as diverse status (e.g., kings and queens, fairy godmother, wizards, or grandparents). I have two toy stations: the nurturing station, which has items such as a dollhouse with animals and ethnically diverse human families, cooking utensils, babies and bathtubs, dishes and silverware, and so forth, and a "reparative" station, which includes symbols of healing such as a medical kit and a hospital. In addition, a number of items such as breast shields, capes, sunglasses, masks, and Nerf swords may provide opportunities for expression of vulnerable and aggressive feelings.

Clinicians introduce children to available materials and activities and invite and allow them to explore and select what they do in the play therapy office. Clinicians express interest and provide unconditional support and genuine concern. They remain emotionally and physically present without imposing an agenda or intruding into the child's experience in the room. The end result is that children's resistance will decrease as they feel valued, safe, and respected by the clinician.

The child's behavior, affect, art, and play are documented by the clinician, who notes what the child does and does not do, toys that are repeatedly selected or avoided, and themes that emerge in the art and the play as well as play experiences that elicit differential affect. Clinicians also help children expand their metaphors by reflecting what is seen and asking clarifying or expanding questions. Often when clinicians ask children to draw self-portraits they may reject images that are not realistic; in doing so, they miss a profound opportunity to learn about the children. Rubin (1984) states: "It is important to keep in mind that self-representations may reflect the way things realistically are, or may be projections of the child's fantasies—they may convey himself as he wishes or fears himself to be, or may represent different facets of his personality" (p. 73). Note in the following example how easily this 6-year-old child communicates difficult emotions:

CLINICIAN: Tell me about the picture you've made.

TONY: This is a squirrel, a tree, and a rock.

CLINICIAN: Mmmhhh.

TONY: The squirrel is behind the rock.

CLINICIAN: Oh, I see. The squirrel is behind the rock. I wonder what that's like, to be behind a rock.

TONY: Good.

CLINICIAN: It's good to be behind the rock. I wonder why.

TONY: The rock keeps him safe. Nobody can see him.

CLINICIAN: What would happen if someone saw the squirrel behind the rock?

TONY: The squirrel would be afraid.

CLINICIAN: Oh, I see. The squirrel would be afraid. I wonder what would make the squirrel feel afraid.

TONY: 'Cuz the kids make fun of him and he doesn't like that.

CLINICIAN: Oh, the kids make fun of the squirrel and the squirrel doesn't like that. How does the squirrel feel I wonder.

TONY: He feels sad.

CLINICIAN: Oh, sad. The squirrel is behind the rock because he thinks that people might make fun of him and then he'll feel sad.

TONY: Yeah, he gets sad and then he gets fightin' mad!

CLINICIAN: So the squirrel has lots of feelings when people make fun of him, sad and fightin' angry.

TONY: Yeah, he gets in trouble when he's mad!

CLINICIAN: So staying behind the rock feels safer to him and he doesn't get in trouble.

TONY: Yeah, it's quiet back there.

CLINICIAN: The squirrel thinks it's quiet behind the rock. Does he like the quiet back there all the time?

TONY: Well, it get's boring sometimes too. He wants to play with his friends.

CLINICIAN: So the squirrel wants to play but sometimes stays behind the rock anyway.

TONY: Yeah 'cuz sometimes I don't have friends. I mean the squirrel doesn't have friends.

CLINICIAN: I wonder what would help the squirrel make friends.

TONY: I don't know. . . .

This is an example of using children's stories, symbols, or metaphors by expressing interest and helping them augment the information initially provided. Several things are worth mentioning: When children draw pictures, unconscious and conscious symbols are selected purposefully. Children create or choose symbols which either possess or are assigned specific traits or attributes. In so doing, children use projection to both distance and address difficult emotional material. By distancing themselves through symbol they buffer themselves from perceptions, cognitions, or affects that feel uncomfortable, overwhelming, or threatening. This "once-removed" approach allows children to address conflictual or perplexing emotional material by exposing themselves incrementally to what is most feared yet compelling. Terr (1990) indicated that traumatized children will either "play it out" or "act it out." In fact, children's willingness and frequent compulsion to literally recreate traumatic events in play has been labeled "posttraumatic play" (Gil, 1999). Rubin (1984) describes the working-through process inherent in posttraumatic play by noting that it is "often accomplished through repetitive confrontations with the feared idea, through drawing or playing out a loaded theme, often with a limited amount of modification" (pp. 85–86).

THERAPEUTIC OPPORTUNITIES AVAILABLE IN ART

Art therapy can assist sexually abused children in many ways: Art allows children to create images that communicate their internal perceptions about self and the world.

According to Naumburg (1987), "Objectified picturization acts then as an immediate symbolic communication which frequently circumvents the difficulties of speech. . . . such symbolic images more easily escape repression by what Freud called the mind's "censor" than do verbal expressions . . . "(p. 2). In addition, when children draw, they do so on paper of specific physical dimensions with set boundaries. Once the images are placed on the space on the paper the child has in essence contained what might otherwise feel staggering. What might be experienced as disorganized or chaotic may then take on qualities of something that is manageable. Random thoughts and feelings might render children overstimulated and confused. Thoughts and feelings "shrunk down" enough to appear within specified dimensions may give children a sense of control. One child who drew a picture of his offender remarked, "He doesn't seem so big and strong now that he's on this paper." He then made himself taller and bigger and captioned the phrase "You can't hurt me anymore big guy."

Making art also permits children to express emotions that might be constricted by feelings of anxiety, fear, confusion, or loyalty conflicts. Angry children afraid to use their voices might be capable of spreading bright red (angry) paint across a piece of paper and may feel some relief from doing so. This may motivate them to try other ways of releasing anger, including using their voices to make sounds, screams, or, eventually, words.

Art also allows clinicians to better understand what children are feeling and what is on their minds. A change in the nature of the image drawn by the child may alert the therapist to a change in perceptions, attitudes, and beliefs. By actively observing children's sequential art we can frequently gauge progress or lack thereof.

Finally, as Malchiodi (1998) asserts, "most children, despite their experiences with painful events, will still find joy in the act of creating art. It may be that through creation of art there is a natural experience of wholeness or working toward wholeness and this, in and of itself, may be what is most important to understand about traumatized children's drawings and their importance in therapy" (p. 137).

CASE ILLUSTRATION

Rosa, an 8-year-old Hispanic girl was referred to me after a medical exam by Sexual Abuse Nurse Examiners at a nearby hospital. The medical findings were congruent with the child's allegation of sexual abuse by her maternal grandfather. Rosa's mother called in crisis, distraught and frightened, eager to come in and discuss her situation. As motivated as she seemed, she canceled her first two appointments, preferring to speak to me by phone.

The mother tearfully described her situation: She and her husband were religious and had been extremely protective of both their children, Rosa and her 5-year-old brother, Jose. The mother noted that her father had come to live with her 2 years earlier, and they had made great sacrifices to accommodate his living with them.

The mother's immediate concerns were twofold: her daughter's virginity and the fact that she could not find a way to tell her husband what had happened to their child. She came to see me after we had spent at least 2 hours on the phone together. I spent quite a bit of our first session in my office discussing her hesitancy to tell her husband whom she described as "a good and sensitive man." Hypothesizing that she could receive needed support from her husband, I explored her concerns. She described being terrified that her husband would have a violent response and attempt to kill her father. Interestingly, Rosa's father had no history of any violence whatsoever, making me speculate that it was the mother's own constrained rage that she feared. In addition, she was worried that her husband would view their female child as "damaged," being traditional in his view that women should be virgins when they marry.

The mother and I discussed her fears and she was receptive to my suggestions, particularly my offer to meet with her husband immediately so he could be informed about Rosa's sexual abuse. I noted that Rosa was young and there was no reason to believe that Rosa would automatically have long-term physical or emotional problems, particularly if responses were swift, sensitive, and appropriate. The mother called her husband from my office and he agreed to join her, sensing something was terribly wrong. My next appointment had been canceled, and I was able to accommodate a joint parental session straightaway.

I assisted the mother in the process of telling her husband what had happened and predictably Father was shocked and concerned. He held his wife as she cried, and reproached her for not telling him earlier and then turned to me for information. "Is she injured?" "Is she going to be okay?" "How will this affect her future? She's so little, so young, so tender, how does she understand this?" I told him that the worst was over now and that at this point we would concentrate on helping Rosa recover. I also told him that children's resiliency is remarkable and it was reasonable to expect Rosa to survive these experiences. Finally, the question arose: "Is she still a virgin?" I told him that I was not a medical doctor but that I had been assured by the nurses that her injuries would heal quickly. "She's so young," I told him, "by the time she marries it is likely that this will be a very remote memory and her body will be completely healed." After this initial session I scheduled an appointment to meet with Rosa. The mother and father left hand in hand and brought Rosa to each of her subsequent appointments. I encouraged them to take their daughter in their arms and tell her that they were very sorry that grandfather had hurt her and they were very proud of her for telling them so they could put an end to the abuse.

Treatment with Rosa

Rosa was initially shy and quiet but after the first two appointments she was filled with anticipation and excitement about coming to the play therapy office. I did a combination of nondirective and directive work with her, starting with a tour of the play therapy room and an invitation to do whatever she wanted. In the first session she explored freely moving from one thing to another. She was interested in the sandtray and miniatures and placed two large spiders and a dinosaur in the sand as well as an insect hiding behind a "wall" (see Figure 12.1).* In addition, she buried a well, rendering it "dry," and a casket was buried next to a tombstone. She commented that the dead person was her "good grandfather" who had died and was buried in her country. She commented that she cried whenever she thought of him dying. I was impressed with her ability to express her emotions and commented, "It sounds like you miss your grandfather who died and that he was a good grandfather to you." She nodded her head affirmatively. I did not ask more but was struck by her choice of multiarmed insects and how the tray seemed somewhat barren and threatening as well as sad.

The next session Rosa asked if she could paint and stated, "I'll make a picture of me!" I set up the easel, paints, and brushes and offered Rosa a choice of paper (she picked 11″ × 14″ rather than standard 8½″ × 11″ or the larger 18″ × 24″). She made a small figure on the bottom right-hand side of the page (Figure 12.2). The rather large oblong arms seemed disconnected from the body and she encapsulated her self-portrait with a bright red square shape which she then colored in with purple and rectangular green and black shapes. The black rectangle sits directly on top of her figure, giving the picture an interesting look. When she finished her picture she said, "This is me and I'm inside my house. There's a black cloud inside my house." "Oh," I responded, "there's a black cloud inside your house." She sat back in her chair and said in a quiet voice, "I don't like my room because my *abuelito* [grandfather] would do bad things to me in my bed." "I'm sorry to hear that," I said. "It sounds like you had one grandfather who was very good to you and one grandfather who did bad things." "Yeah," she said, "and I'm scared he's going to come and get me." Rosa and I then discussed her fear that her grandfather was going to kill her because she told. The more she talked the more I realized that her grandfather had made many serious threats that had rendered this child helpless and terrified. Rosa seemed to have opened the floodgates and talked about her grandfather with great disdain. "He made me touch his *palomita* and he told me I should lick it and kiss it and I did." "That's okay Rosa," I told her, "when grandfathers tell their granddaughters to do something, they obey them because they're little and the grandfathers are the adults. He was wrong to ask you to touch his *palomita* and you didn't do anything wrong." She looked at me through tears and said, "*Abuelito* told me that God knew I was a bad girl and that he was mad at me." She then added, "He told me that my mommy and daddy will be mad at me when they find out what I did and that I was bad."

I was internally enraged to hear the type and level of manipulation that this man had used to ensure this child's silence. Rosa looked sad and confused and I held her hand and told her that her grandfather had done bad things to her (her language) and that she was a good little girl and God and her parents loved her very much. I continued to reassure her that her parents held her grandfather responsible because he knew that it was wrong for him to touch her. "What's more," I added, "your parents want to take good care of you and make sure this doesn't happen to you again."

*As an art therapist I find sand therapy an easy transition. In fact, I view the creation of sand scenarios as parallel to creating an art product. Interestingly, some children who cannot or will not draw are able and willing to use miniatures to create pictures in the sand. These pictures have the added dimension of being three-dimensional and vibrant. The scenario has a "life" similar to that found in artwork.

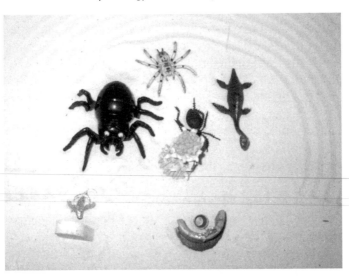

FIGURE 12.1. Sandtray with two large spiders, an insect hiding behind a "wall," and a dinosaur.

Later we agreed that her mother should join us and I encouraged Rosa to tell her some of what we had discussed. She prefaced her comments with "Mami, please don't cry, okay?" Rosa was well on her way to healing, letting months and months of preoccupation and fear come forward, eliciting clarity of response, reassurance, support, and nurturing from those around her. As they left, I commented that perhaps the cloud in her room would not feel so heavy and dark anymore. She smiled.

During the next two sessions I invited Rosa to work on a project developed by

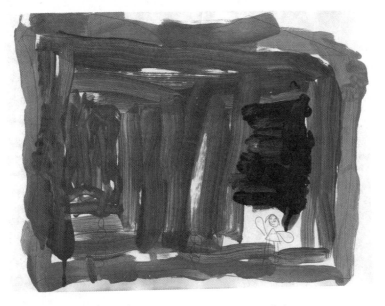

FIGURE 12.2. Painting with a small figure.

Sobol and Schneider (1996) which consists of children building a "safe environment" for an animal miniature. I chose to recommend this project based on the picture she had made in which she appeared confined in her room. The encapsulation in Rosa's self-portrait can be interpreted in two ways: She might feel the need to feel safe with reinforced boundaries or she might feel imprisoned and constricted. I wanted to give her an opportunity to transform the image by asking her to make a safe environment which I assumed might have a quality of freedom rather than containment. Rosa chose a dog, commenting that she always wanted to have a dog but the landlord would not let her family keep one. She picked the dog, placed it on a small cardboard plate (see Figure 12.3), and proceeded to build it a safe world in which the dog's needs were met (she included food, water, a soft bed, and toys to play with). She also made a toy phone (included later) so that the dog could talk to friends and parents as well as call for help when needed. She was pleased with her product and rushed out of the office to show her parents what she had created—our difficult previous session had been followed with a session full of mastery and satisfaction.

In the following two sessions Rosa returned to the sand and miniatures making wedding scenarios. The first week she poured some water to make the sand wet and malleable. She liked the sensation of wet sand and talked about the beaches in her country and how much she enjoyed going to the beach with her "good grandfather." She was obviously enjoying these memories and suddenly constructed a wedding (Figure 12.4) with a bride and groom, bridesmaid, best man, and a small pet dragon who was there to take care of everyone. A fairy godmother took center stage to take care of the bride and groom. Finally, Rosa selected a two-headed dragon and reflected, "That dragon is kind of scary and he can scare people but nobody knows he's there so they're okay." I guessed that Rosa was struggling with how reliable her sense of safety was. Rosa's grandfather had fled the country after the abuse surfaced and although she was happy that he was not a present threat, she had recently told her

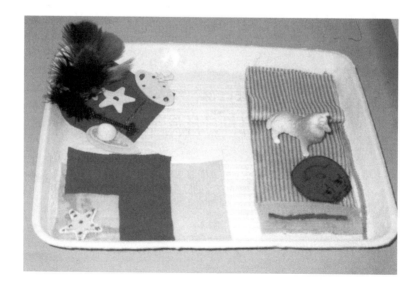

FIGURE 12.3. Safe world in which the dog's needs were met.

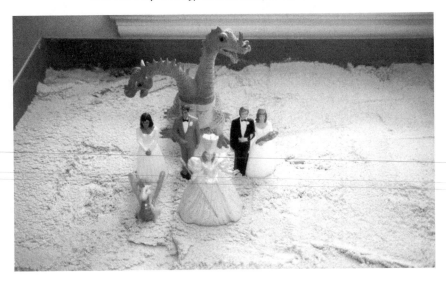

FIGURE 12.4. Sandtray depicting a wedding with a bride and groom, bridesmaid, best man, a small pet dragon who was there to take care of everyone, a two-headed dragon, and a fairy god-mother.

mother that maybe he would "sneak back" when no one was looking. Rosa and I talked a little about the wedding and what it was like to know that the bride and groom might be in danger. She said she did not know what would happen but came to the next session ready to create another sand world. Figure 12.5 shows an expanded version of the wedding scene with a great many more animals lined up parallel to the two-headed dragon. "Now," she said, "he can't do bad things because the elephants will stop him . . . they are very, very strong." This appeared to be Rosa's way of stating the obvious: Her parents would be there no matter what dangers the future would bring. She was also careful to place some baby birds and mothers in birds' nests and said that the parents were taking care of their babies, helping them grow, and finding good food to eat. She laughed and we took a picture of her sand scenario for her to take home.

Rosa was making progress and seemed comfortable with me. She had told her mother that she wondered why God had let this happen to her and her mother and I discussed how to respond. I realized that it would be important to let Rosa know that sexual abuse happens to lots of children and that they often feel they have done something wrong. I selected a book titled *No, No, and the Secret Touch* (Patterson & Feldman, 1993) and read the book to Rosa. I also played an audiotape that accompanies the book and I played it to Rosa's delight. She absolutely loved the book and often stated, "I felt that way," identifying with the little seal (who is sexually abused by her uncle), or "I know she's scared but she should tell her mom and dad . . . they'll help her." Rosa had made such a positive identification with the little seal in the story that the next week I surprised her with a project which she thoroughly loved: I had purchased a set of seal parents and a baby seal and invited her to make another safe environment. Her parents tell me that to this day she says "good night" to the seal family.

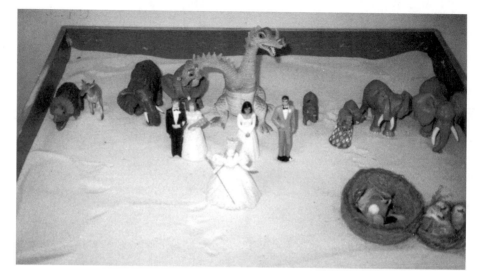

FIGURE 12.5. Sandtray with an expanded version of the wedding scene with more animals lined up parallel to the two-headed dragon.

Following this work which directly addressed the sexual abuse, I invited Rosa to make another self-portrait and she did so willingly. This second self-portrait (Figure 12.6) was made on larger paper and the color scheme changed. Rosa placed herself on a grassy field with patches of flowers growing underfoot. She made a "very warm sky" with orange saying that the sun was so hot it made a "cloud" of heat. I noticed that the cloud overhead in her original picture which she described as "heavy and dark" was now replaced by a warm cloud which was "helping the flowers to grow." I also noted that Rosa's arms were now connected to her body and she had her feet firmly planted on the ground. She said her arms were outstretched because she was welcoming the warm sun. I felt this picture showed progress in Rosa's emotional state and reflected her new view of the environment as nurturing and safe.

At this point, Rosa's parents felt that she was now "more herself" and they wanted to resume their lives and put the abuse behind them. We had a family meeting in which we openly discussed what had occurred, everyone's reactions to the abuse, current feelings about grandfather, and what each person thought would happen in the future. I'll never forget Rosa's last statement in this meeting: "Even though *abuelito* is not here and the police can't punish him, God will punish him when he gets to heaven." Parents asserted that God would indeed punish grandfather for hurting her and the session ended.

At our termination session Rosa brought a cake she had baked for me and we each had a piece on small plates with small eating utensils. After our meal she rushed to make a final tray. The wedding scene appeared again, this time a double wedding complete with flower girls, fairies, wizards, and an array of guests, mostly four-legged (Figure 12.7). Rosa stood back and said, "This is my wedding and this is my mom and dad. There are lots of nice people at the wedding and lots of love to go

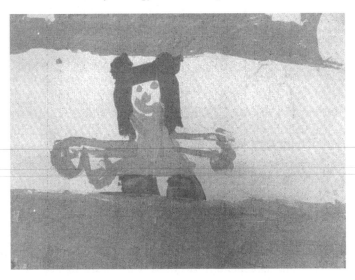

FIGURE 12.6. Painting of self on large paper.

around." She smiled and said, "This is my good *abuelito*'s place because he will be with me when I get married."

I reviewed with Rosa the work she had done in treatment, chronicling her initial disclosure, medical exam, and visits with me. I showed her pictures of all her work and she smiled as she recognized them, copies of which she had taken home. She offered many insights about her work and about the lessons she had learned.

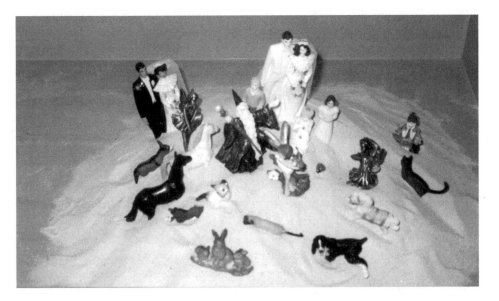

FIGURE 12.7. Sandtray of a double wedding with flower girls, fairies, wizards, and an array of guests, mostly four-legged.

Summary

Rosa experienced child sexual abuse by a loved and trusted family member who threatened and confused her. As a result, she had become more and more frightened to tell her mother what was happening convinced that she had been a bad and sinful girl who her mother and indeed God himself, would reject and punish.

Rosa had a series of acute responses to the abuse including nightmares, hypervigilance, and depression. After the disclosure she still felt tormented by a number of cognitive distortions which needed to be directly addressed.

My therapy with Rosa included individual and conjoint family sessions. An early sandtray scenario in combination with a spontaneous self-portrait allowed me to understand some of Rosa's concerns: fear, feelings of entrapment, and a desire to protect and shield herself from danger.

Rosa used art to show what perhaps she could not yet conceptualize or verbalize: She had a dark cloud overhead and important questions persisted and preoccupied her in spite of her physical safety. Rosa's ability to externalize concerns that were initially difficult to put into words allowed me to respond more directly to her unique apprehension.

The sand scenarios which I viewed as another type of externalization again suggested impending danger and threat. Rosa was able to face the fear that the bride and groom could not see, but she mobilized resources to stand by her side and provide rescue (the elephant family). By changing her initial scenario, and through the creation of "safe" environments, Rosa would now "take in" the possibility of safety and protection and eventually images of resiliency, protection, and nurturing appeared in abundance (fairies, wizards, pets). In addition, she clearly expressed her renewed reliance on her parents as she placed them at her own wedding (representing future orientation) and included her dead grandfather whom she obviously cherished.

Rosa's parents cooperated with the therapy process fully. They observed the relief Rosa experienced after verbalizing, crying, and expressing herself through art, crafts, and sand therapy. They valued her art products highly and helped Rosa care for them.

Several cross-cultural issues emerged in my work with Rosa, including the fact that the concept of therapy is unfamiliar to many Hispanics and there may be a tendency to feel uncomfortable trusting in, or relying on, people outside the family. Our phone conversations were necessary steps in building sufficient trust for Rosa's mother to come to my therapy office.

In addition, because therapy is an unfamiliar idea, it is important to explain what it is and is not and the potential benefits that can occur. Many Hispanic clients believe that children should "forget" abuse and never discuss the issue openly as talking about it or thinking about it only causes suffering. It may take a while to help parents recognize that although forgetting and placing abuse experiences in the past are long-term goals once they have been processed, the immediate goals are to make sure the child has a chance to ask questions, clarify thoughts, and express what may be a broad range of thoughts and feelings. Parents also need to comprehend how to be helpful to their children and how to respond to specific questions about sexuality.

Finally, Hispanic families often turn to the church and prayer as a logical and powerful resource. In this case, the parents were encouraged to make use of this trusted emotional asset. The fact that Rosa eventually relegated the role of justice to God clearly indicated her reliance on a higher power.

CONCLUSION

Sexually abused children deserve age-appropriate opportunities to recover from highly stressful and confusing experiences (Klein, 2001). Art and play therapy are universal activities that most children view as outlets for expression and which are perceived as inviting and low stress. These activities allow children to make intolerable feelings tolerable, make chaotic and disorganized thoughts more contained and therefore manageable, and process emotions in a once-removed stance that facilitates identification, projection, and working through of difficult or conflictual thoughts and feelings. Art and play are windows into the child's perceptions of self and the world in which he or she lives. When children reflect and respond to the images, symbols, and metaphors they create, their first glimpse of positive change (transformation) may become available—imagining change is the first step to creating positive change.

REFERENCES

Briere, J. N. (1992). *Child abuse trauma: Theory and treatment of the lasting effects.* Thousand Oaks, CA: Sage.

Conte, J. R. (Ed.). (2002). *Critical issues in child sexual abuse.* Thousand Oaks, CA: Sage.

Friedrich, W. F. (2002). *Psychological assessment of sexually abused children and their families* Thousand Oaks, CA: Sage.

Friedrich, W. N. (1995). *Psychotherapy with sexually abused boys: An integrated approach.* Thousand Oaks, CA: Sage.

Gil, E. (1991). *The healing power of play: Working with abused children.* New York: Guilford Press.

Gil, E. (1999). Understanding and responding to post-trauma play. *Association for Play Therapy Newsletter, 17*(1), 7–10.

Gil, E. (2002). Play therapy with abused children. In F. W. Kaslow (Ed.) & R. F. Massey & S. D. Massey (Vol. Eds.). *Comprehensive handbook of psychotherapy* (Vol. 3, pp. 59–82). New York: Wiley.

Heineman, T. V. (1998). *The abused child: Psychodynamic understanding and treatment.* New York: Guilford Press.

Homeyer, L. E., & Sweeney, D. S. (1998). *Sandtray: A practical manual.* Canyon Lake, TX: Linda Press.

James, B. (1994). *Handbook for treatment of attachment-trauma problems in children.* New York: Lexington Books.

Kendall-Tackett, K. A., Williams, L. M., & Finkelhor, D. (1993). The impact of sexual abuse on children: A review and synthesis of recent empirical studies. *Psychological Bulletin, 113*(1), 164–180.

Klein, N. (2001). *Healing images for children: Teaching relaxation and guided imagery to children facing cancer and other serious illnesses.* Watertown, WI: Inner Coaching.

Labovitz Boik, B., & Goodwin, E. A. (2000). *Sandplay therapy: A step-by-step manual for psychotherapists of diverse orientations.* New York: Norton.

Landreth, G. L. (1982). Recommended play therapy materials. In G. L. Landreth (Ed.), *Play therapy: Dynamics of the process of counseling with children* (pp. 153–154). Springfield, IL: Charles C Thomas.

Lanktree, C. B., & Briere, J. (1995). Outcome of therapy for sexually abused children: A repeated measures study. *Child Abuse and Neglect, 19*(9), 1145–1155.

Malchiodi, C. A. (1998). *Understanding children's drawings.* New York: Guilford Press.

Mitchell, R. R., & Friedman, H. S. (1994). *Sandplay past, present and future.* New York and London: Routledge.

Naumburg, M. (1987). *Dynamically oriented art therapy: Its principles and practice.* Chicago: Magnolia Street.

Patterson, S., & Feldman, J. (1993). *No, no and the secret touch.* Greenbrae, CA: National Self-esteem Resources and Development Center.

Rubin, J. A. (1984). *Child art therapy: Understanding and helping children grow through art.* New York: Van Nostrand Reinhold.

Sobol, B., & Schneider, K. (1996). Art as an adjunctive therapy in the treatment of children who dissociate. In J. L. Silberg (Ed.), *The dissociative child: Diagnosis, treatment and management* (pp. 191–218). Lutherville, MD: Sidran Press.

Terr, L. (1990). *Too scared to cry.* New York: Harper & Row.

CHAPTER 13

Drawings in Forensic Investigations of Child Sexual Abuse

Marcia Sue Cohen-Liebman

Forensic investigations encompass a distinct and defined methodology with regard to process and procedure. The practice and theory of art therapy have been incorporated in forensic investigations in recent years (Cohen-Liebman, 1994, 1997, 2002; Gussak & Cohen-Liebman, 2001). This integration has emerged due to art therapists' demonstrating the value of art therapy to those in a position to assess demand (Smart, 1986) and is proving to be pragmatically sound within a forensic context. Art therapists are participating as experts in forensic arenas and presenting evidentiary material in the form of drawings to courts both civil and criminal (Cohen-Liebman, 1994; Levick, Safran, & Levine, 1990; Lyons, 1993; Rickert, 1996) and drawings are being admitted as evidence in child sexual abuse litigation (Malchiodi, 1990). The intrinsic and ameliorating benefits of drawings within investigative interviews of children are the subject of recent exploration (Cohen-Liebman, 1999, 2002), as is the utility of drawings as judiciary aids (Cohen-Liebman, 1995, 2002).

FORENSIC INVESTIGATIONS

Forensic investigations are fact-finding endeavors that merit meticulous and thorough inquiry. Forensic assessments differ from standard mental health evaluations. Procedures support a psycholegal orientation and are dictated by circumscribed practice. Forensic interviewers adhere to specific standards when facilitating a fact-finding process. Findings from empirical studies guide and inform forensic interview practices (Reed, 1996).

National organizations have published guidelines for the evaluation of children who may have been abused (American Academy of Child and Adolescent Psychiatry, 1990; American Professional Society on the Abuse of Children, 1990). The central component of a child sexual abuse investigation is an interview of the alleged victim by a highly skilled child interview specialist or law enforcement agent. Frequently, child abuse interviews are conducted at multidisciplinary interviewing centers that promote interagency collaboration and team cooperation in an effort to minimize repetitive interviews while maximizing the information provided by the child (Cohen-Liebman, 1999; Davies et al., 1996; Sheppard & Zangrillo, 1996; Sorenson, Bottoms, & Perona, 1997). Investigative interviews often are conducted according to guidelines, although different communities subscribe to distinct interview guidelines or protocols (Bourg et al., 1999; Carnes, Wilson, & Nelson-Gardell, 1999; Davies et al., 1996; Myers, 1998; Poole & Lamb, 1998; Reed, 1996; Sorenson et al., 1997; Yuille, Hunter, Joffe, & Zaparniuk, 1993). Component parts may vary, yet the content is comparable not only in this country but abroad as well (Cheung, 1997; Cohen-Liebman, 1999; Davies et al., 1996; Monteleone, 1996; Poole & Lamb, 1998). Effective interviewing techniques and best practice for investigative interviews have been the focus of study in recent years.

Civil proceedings such as custodial matters may require the skills of forensic evaluators commissioned by the court to conduct a neutral and objective evaluation. The process may involve the parents/guardians and the child(ren) who are the subject of the dispute. The objective of a court-ordered process is to assist the court in decision making by providing objective information and informed opinions (American Academy of Child and Adolescent Psychiatry, 1990). The expert is essentially charged with the task of explaining behavioral and psychological findings in language that is applicable to the court and useful in the decision-making process. Specialized competence is required, as is familiarity with state laws (American Psychological Association, 1994).

FORENSIC ART THERAPY

Forensic art therapy is developing into a specialization within art therapy extending the practical application of the field beyond the traditional realms of evaluation and treatment (Cohen-Liebman, 1997). Forensic art therapy integrates art therapy practice and theory within a legal context and with standard forensic procedure and protocol. It is used for fact-finding purposes and is investigative in nature rather than interventive (Cohen-Liebman, 1997, 2002; Gussak & Cohen-Liebman, 2001). Forensic art therapy uses creative expression in the elicitation of information pertinent for fact finding or investigative purposes. Forensic art therapy assists in the resolution of legal matters that are in dispute (Gussak & Cohen-Liebman, 2001).

Forensic art therapy is practiced in a nontraditional setting that is outside the parameters of clinical practice. Clients are referred by a system involved in a legal dispute or engaged in an investigative function such as law enforcement, prosecution, child protection, or judiciary (e.g., judge or mediator). Such clients often come involuntarily and may be remanded by the court or an investigative body to participate in an interview or evaluation. Forensic art therapy is distinct from art therapy practiced within a forensic setting (e.g., prisons or detention centers) (Cohen-Liebman & Gussak, 1998; Gussak & Cohen-Liebman, 2001), but because of the scope of this brief chapter, these differences are not addressed here.

The forensic art therapist does not assume the role of advocate or adversary but, rather, retains a neutral, objective stance. The process and resultant information are communicated to an investigative team and findings may be presented at court requiring testimony by the therapist, necessitating knowledge of legal tenets, case law, and ethical issues.

FORENSIC VERSUS CLINICAL PROCEDURES

There are inherent differences between investigative and clinical approaches to interviewing children regarding sexual abuse. The purpose of the clinical evaluation of child sexual abuse according to the American Academy of Child and Adolescent Psychiatry (1990) guidelines is to determine whether abuse has occurred, if the child needs protection, and if the child needs treatment for medical or emotional problems. In the assessment of allegations of child sexual abuse, the goal of the interviewer is to gather information in a nonthreatening manner while minimizing secondary trauma that can be induced by systemic intervention.

In contrast, a forensic process addresses legal issues and obtains information to assist with legal determinations (Haralambie, 1999; Mannarino & Cohen, 1992). A central objective of a forensic interview is to obtain information in an effort to ascertain whether abuse occurred (Reed, 1996) and to procure information in a manner that is objective, developmentally sensitive, comprehensive, and forensically defensible (Cohen-Liebman, 1999; Davies et al., 1996). Additional goals of the interview include corroboration of the data collected, the exploration of alternate hypotheses, and the assessment of suggestibility, credibility, and competency. Competency is defined as a child's ability to testify in court in a reliable, meaningful manner, whereas credibility refers to the child's truthfulness and accuracy (American Academy of Child and Adolescent Psychiatry, 1997).

In a forensic process, the interviewer adopts a neutral stance and refrains from interviewer bias. The interviewer is an advocate for the facts and is considered a truth seeker. Adherence to prescribed forensic procedure is mandatory in order for the process to be legally defensible in court.

In contrast, a therapeutic relationship is not neutral and is predicated upon an empathetic response by the therapist. Thus, subjective interpretations and nonspecific accounts are acceptable. The manner in which data are collected is not integral to the process. In a clinical process a general idea of abuse is sufficient whereas in a forensic process details are imperative (Raskin & Esplin, 1991). In a forensic context, the task is to gather information and discern the truth through the acquisition of factual material while the clinician provides support and intervention usually after the investigative process is complete. Validation of thoughts and feelings is an integral part of a clinical process. In contrast, a forensic process is centered around objectivity, fact finding, and truth seeking. Forensic practice is governed by ethical and legal practices that extend to collection and preservation of data.

DRAWINGS AND FORENSIC INVESTIGATION

Drawings can assist the interviewer in achieving many of the goals associated with the investigative process. Drawings have been identified as enhancing and increasing the productivity of the interview process (Farley, 1987). A child's experience can be expressed pictorially through a drawing which can later serve as evidentiary material (Burgess, Hartman, Wolbert, & Grant, 1987; Cohen-Liebman, 1995; Gussak & Cohen-Liebman, 2001). Information derived from drawings can assist the investigative team in the determination of additional measures and interventions.

Drawings are considered novel, scientific evidence and are subject to a special admissibility hearing in some jurisdictions (Cohen-Liebman, 1994). Drawings have been identified as an ancillary support for interviewers (Poole & Lamb, 1998) and a means of eliciting information regarding allegations of sexual abuse (Schetky & Green, 1988). Human-figure drawings have been identified as helpful to interviewers in eliciting information from children (Haralambie, 1999). Children may lack the cognitive capability or the verbal capacity to articulate their abusive experiences. They also may be too embarrassed or ashamed to discuss the abuse. Research studies (Kelley, 1984) indicate that often children who have been reticent to discuss their experiences may become more open and verbal after drawing the abuse. On occasion, a child may ask to show rather than tell what happened. Such a depiction may enhance disclosure and signal additional elements to explore.

Faller (1996) identified a number of authors who offered suggestions regarding specific drawing tasks that might elicit information relevant to sexual abuse. The American Academy of Child and Adolescent Psychiatry (1997) guidelines state that the usefulness of drawings lies in the affect and information they elicit and certain characteristics that may be suggestive of sexual abuse. They indicate that drawings are helpful in forensic assessments. The American Professional Society on the Abuse of Children (1990) addresses the use of drawings within the psychosocial evaluation of sexual abuse and provides suggestions for drawing tasks within a forensic evaluation. Conte, Sorenson, Fogarty, and Dalla Rosa's (1991) survey to assess the use of free or nondirected drawings in the evaluation of sexual abuse yielded an 87% positive response. Drawings are frequently cited as valuable for the development of rapport (Bourg et al., 1999; Davies et al., 1996; Friedrich, 1990). Haugaard and Reppucci (1989) contend that a child's depiction of an abuse scene decreases concern regarding possible influence. The clinical application of spontaneous drawings has also been addressed (Cohen-Liebman, 1995; Faller, 1996; Friedrich, 1990; Schetky & Green, 1988).

Drawings are frequently categorized in the same manner as anatomically detailed dolls. Some research identifies these aids as least suggestive and most useful when used for recall and demonstration purposes after a child has made a verbal disclosure (American Professional Society on the Abuse of Children, 1995; Bourg et al., 1999). Drawings are considered similar to dolls for discussion and demonstration of anatomy (Bourg et al., 1999; Davies et al., 1996). Bourg et al. (1999) discuss the use of dolls and various media to offer assistance with regard to a child's understanding of forensic concepts because it is often easier for a child to demonstrate understanding rather than provide a verbal explanation.

Many authors concur that care should be taken in the interpretation of drawings (American Academy of Child and Adolescent Psychiatry, 1990; Burgess & Hartman, 1993; Cohen-Liebman, 1995, 1999; Farley, 1987; Friedrich, 1990; Hibbard, Roghmann, & Hoekelman, 1987; Malchiodi, 1998; Schetky & Benedek, 1992; Sorenson et al., 1997). Interviewers are cautioned not to interpret or overinterpret drawings in an effort to determine the likelihood of sexual abuse.

ADVANTAGES OF DRAWINGS IN FORENSIC INVESTIGATIONS

Drawings offer significant advantages in a forensic context:

1. As interviewing tools, drawings are used in a supportive capacity in the investigation of a legal matter.
2. In the capacity of charge enhancement, drawings provide contextual information that can contribute to the determination of charges as well as the identification of additional arenas to investigate.
3. Drawings as judiciary aids provide evidentiary material that is admissible in a judicial proceeding (Cohen-Liebman, 2002; Gussak & Cohen-Liebman, 2001).

DRAWINGS AS INTERVIEWING TOOLS

Interviewing tools are referred to as aids, media, tools, or props. These tools include, but are not limited to, free play, drawings (both free or nondirected and anatomical), and anatomically detailed dolls. Pros and cons associated with the incorporation of interviewing tools have been delineated from differing perspectives and generally they have been regarded with secondary significance as supportive elements within forensic interviews. Myers (1998) states that during investigative interviews and courtroom testimony, props are often used to help children describe events.

Drawings and drawing materials as interview tools or investigative implements can help facilitate the development of rapport and establish trust between the child and the interviewer. Often a variety of media are selected in advance of the process, providing the child with a choice of materials. The art materials connote a child-friendly process, and the ability to self-select materials encourages a sense of empowerment. These tools may serve as a stimulus for both the interviewer and the child to explore material that is both manifest and latent. Material that is initially presented through drawings may serve as a catalyst for eventual disclosure of information and provide details that may be salient to the investigation. Drawings can stimulate and focus conversation, provide structure to the process, and be used to explore related topics and issues.

Cohen-Liebman (1999, 2002) has expanded on the notion of drawings as interview tools through exploration of the role drawings contribute within an investigative process. The inclusion of drawings within an investigative interview format was examined in combination with the Common Interview Guideline (CIG) developed by Cohen-Liebman for child sexual abuse investigators in the city of Philadelphia (Cohen-Liebman, 1999, 2002). The author identified intrinsic benefits associated with the integration of drawings within the investigative format as well as the inherent advantages for the child, the team, and the process. Drawings integrated within the phases of the CIG assist in the attainment of the specified goals and objectives. Drawings were demonstrated to supplement and complement the five phases of the CIG identified as Rapport Building, Developmental Assessment, Anatomy Identification, Fact-finding, and Closure.

Regardless of the manner in which drawings are included as interviewing tools, verbalization by the child is integral. Several authors advocate that verbal descriptions be sought by the child for clarification and explanation purposes, thus alleviating an assumptive stance by the interviewer (Farley, 1987; Sorenson et al., 1997). Bourg et al. (1999) state that communication with tools cannot effectively substitute for statements, but they can provide value for clarity when verbalization is limited. Children may be asked to explain the subject matter contained in the drawing or they may be asked to show what happened next.

Drawings as interview tools help in culling information to assist in the comprehension of developmental levels and associated spheres including social, emotional, and cognitive. This information is integral for the interviewer in addressing the needs of the child while adhering to forensic practice. Suggestibility and accuracy, fundamental components within the interview process, can be addressed and clarified through the child's own depictions.

Drawings are valuable as an interview tool in anatomy identification and allow for identification of sexual and nonsexual body parts. Some children have difficulty identifying sexual parts through direct body demonstration and such a request may provoke stress or encourage a traumatic reaction. The use of a client-generated picture or diagram allows for distillation of anxiety and stress as well as a concrete and permanent record that is objective.

Case Example

A 6-year-old boy was interviewed following allegations that he was molested by a 19-year-old male. The child presented with speech difficulties and displayed a possible tic disorder or a neurological problem for which he was scheduled for further evaluation. He proceeded to make a spontaneous drawing which he referred to as an alien. He was asked to use his drawing to assess anatomy identification. He identified nonsexual body parts and sexual body parts on the figure. When asked if he had similar body parts he reported that he had two private parts, and he proceeded to make a second figure which he referred to as himself with a monkey ear. He identified buttocks through the use of a marker. Finally, he drew a picture of a figure which he stated was his mother. Although he did not have terminology for private parts, he indicated that girls (his mother) have a different private part than boys (see Figure 13.1).

In this case, spontaneous drawings served several purposes. They provided an opportunity to assess developmental and skill levels as well as establish rapport. They also provided a way to assess anatomy identification that was client directed and spontaneous. The drawings also encouraged further exploration of related issues including the allegations. Through the drawings the child was able to convey what the alleged perpetrator did to him. He also discussed the use of force and confirmed his verbal statement by pointing to the buttocks he drew. He also verbally stated what the alleged perpetrator did.

DRAWINGS AS CHARGE ENHANCEMENTS

Charge or forensic enhancements are details or elements of an event that may contribute to the determination of charges. Charge enhancements are identified as

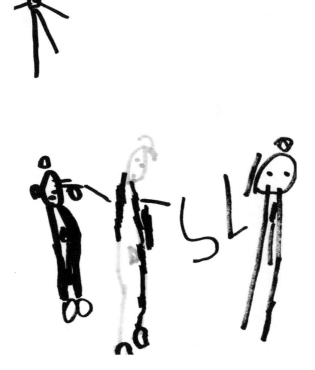

FIGURE 13.1. Drawing by 6-year-old boy molested by 19-year-old male.

threats, bribes, rewards, coercion, pressure, physical harm, restraint, force, weapons, abduction, pornography, photography, sexual aids, media including television, cable or videos, mapping (a diagram of the scene/event), witnesses (observers), additional participants, and additional victims. These elements may be integral in obtaining and providing the basis for the acquisition of a search warrant in conjunction with verbal descriptions.

Charge enhancements can surface in the content of drawings. Children may depict elements of their abusive experience, including situational and contextual information, that may contribute to the direction of additional investigation and eventual prosecution. The information imparted through a graphic depiction may influence the filing of charges in tandem with a verbal confirmation or statement that lends credence to the depiction or in which the picture corroborates a verbal statement.

Figure 13.2 is an example of a drawing that depicts situational and contextual material. Drawn by a 6-year-old girl, the child attempted to depict her abusive experience, which occurred on a school bus. The drawing is indicative of the location of the abuse (on the school bus). It also provided information regarding how the perpetrator, an upper classman, took her to a seat in the back of the bus where he molested her before returning her to her seat in front behind the bus driver. The child's verbal associations provided additional information in tandem with the drawing which supported charges. Finally, it provided a map or diagram of the scene.

Disclosure drawings are characterized by Cohen-Liebman (1999) as including

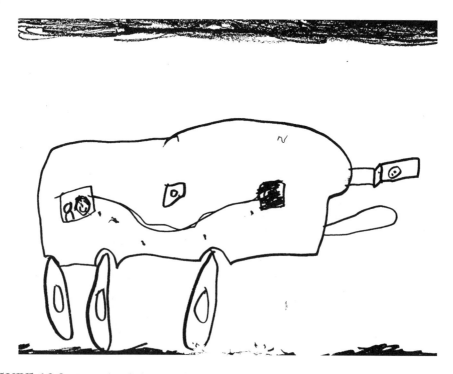

FIGURE 13.2. Example of charge enhancement: Drawing by a 6-year-old girl of the place (a school bus) where the abuse happened.

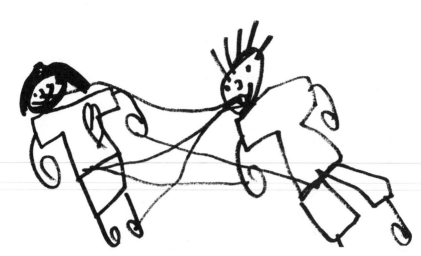

FIGURE 13.3. Example of charge enhancement: Drawing depicting the sexual abuse of a 7-year-old girl.

salient and significant information pertaining to the child's experience of abuse and may support charges. These drawings can support and expand on a verbal account thus promoting corroboration.

Figure 13.3 is a disclosure drawing. The drawing was made by a 7-year-old girl. The line extensions provided the child with an ego-syntonic way to communicate the types of abuse perpetrated against her.

DRAWINGS AS JUDICIARY AIDS

Drawings have been identified as evidentiary material. A representative sampling from the various disciplines addresses the viability of drawings as judiciary aids and as a support to facilitate testimony (Burgess et al., 1987; Cohen-Liebman, 1995; Farley, 1987; Malchiodi, 1990; Veltkamp & Miller, 1994). In some states, statutes have been written that specifically provide for the use of drawings to assist the child witness at the discretion of the court (Haralambie, 1998). The child's identification of pictorial elements demarcates a drawing as a piece of evidence that is legally and clinically convincing and also renders it admissible in court (Faller, 1993).

In the capacity of judiciary aids, drawings can evoke a profound and intense response by both judge and jury. Because they are client generated, drawings afford an objective and developmentally congruent statement that is reflective of the child's experience. Often the emotional response and level of traumatization are also characterized in the drawings made by children. Whether in isolation or combination, factual material and emotional response can have a significant impact on a legal proceeding.

If an investigative process proceeds to a judicial hearing, the interviewer may be called into court to present evidentiary material as a witness. In this capacity, the presentation of drawings may be offered to support the conclusions and findings of the interviewer. The propensity of drawings to function as judiciary aids is considerable (Burgess, McCausland, & Wolbert, 1981; Kelley 1984; Landgarten, 1987; Miller, Veltkamp, & Janson, 1987). They may contain the effects of the abuse; details of situational factors contributing to the abuse; the content of the abuse, depicting who, what, when, where, and how; provide details pertaining to the setting, participants, observers, and other victims; help rule out alternate explanations; and offer corroboration and clarification of verbal statements.

Case Example

A report was received by Child Protective Services (CPS) alleging that a 7-year-old girl had disclosed to her mother that her father had lifted up her nightie and put his finger in her cookie (vagina). The child was referred for an investigative interview. The Interview Center has a strict policy prohibiting the entry of anyone suspected to be an alleged perpetrator. The father brought the child to the center and gained access to the building. In an effort not to provoke additional stress for the child, a quick decision was made to allow the father to remain in the lobby while his daughter was interviewed. The child presented as highly agitated and anxious. She denied the allegations. It was not until the child was brought back to the center for a second interview the following week that the impact of the father's presence was comprehended. During the time interval between the appointments, the child had been removed temporarily from the care of her parents and placed in a shelter. The parents were making reciprocal accusations and both were contending that they had custody. Thus, in an effort to resolve some of the child protective issues, the child was placed in a residential facility.

The child was brought to the center by the child protective worker for the next appointment. Upon entering the interview room the child disclosed that she was afraid to tell previously because her daddy told her not to say anything. She expressed that she was afraid he would not take her to nice places if she told. She spontaneously disclosed that her daddy promised to buy her a pet and clothing and take her to the zoo if she did not tell what happened. The child was emotionally fragile, agitated, and upset. She indicated that she did not want to discuss the allegations, but she was willing to depict the abuse graphically. She proceeded to make a series of drawings illustrating the alleged activity. This means of communication appeared to provide her with a cathartic release for associated thoughts and feelings. The child discussed the allegations in detail for the first time.

Through a succession of drawings she was able to depict her account of what transpired during a single abusive incident. The drawings, poignant and compelling, convey the gravity of the child's emotional and physical discomfort. Based on the information obtained in conjunction with collateral investigation, the report of sexual abuse was substantiated by the child protective worker. The father was also charged criminally. At the criminal proceeding, however, the drawings and the corresponding report were not allowed into evidence. In fact, only one question was asked of the interviewer on the witness stand, "Did Mr. Z come to the center?" Other than being informed that there were concerns regarding the possible backlash if the interviewer's extensive report was admitted into evidence, no plausible explanation was offered regarding the sequestration of the material. As a result, the jury never saw the drawings made by the child. The alleged perpetrator vehemently denied on the witness stand that he had been to the center. The criminal and child protection systems conduct parallel investigations and may reach different conclusions based on their respective burden of proof. Despite the CPS finding, the alleged perpetrator was found to be not guilty by the criminal justice system.

In response to the finding by CPS, the alleged perpetrator appealed and was granted a hearing. During this proceeding which was conducted with a hearing officer, the drawings were presented and discussed individually. In addition to the attorneys, the hearing officer asked specific questions regarding the use of drawings as well as the depictions contained in the drawings. Several months passed before a decision was made. The interviewer received a phone call from the city solicitor in which she relayed the hearing officer's decision to uphold the finding of sexual abuse. The city solicitor acknowledged the role the drawings contributed as well as the information imparted by the interviewer as significant in the decision to uphold the original indicated finding. The drawings in effect communicated the child's experiences while demonstrating the intrinsic role they served within the investigative process and as judiciary aids.

CONCLUSION

The literature indicates that sole reliance on a child's drawing as confirmation of sexual abuse is not plausible at this time (Cohen-Liebman, 1995; Levick, 1986; Malchiodi, 1990, 1998). Although empirical data are not available to conclusively support graphic indicators as the sole indication of sexual abuse, consensus is evident with regard to the use of drawings within the assessment or investigation of sexual abuse in an ancillary or adjunctive capacity (Cohen-Liebman, 1995; Poole & Lamb, 1998). Drawings have been used in the evaluation and assessment of sexual abuse most often in the form of interview aids, props, and communication tools. They can provide assistance in the assessment and evaluation of sexual abuse for forensic purposes. Drawings created within the context of an investigative interview provide data for both investigative and prosecutorial purposes while minimizing interviewer interpretation due to the integration within the fact-finding process.

Drawings employed in combination with other investigative processes may yield additional information which may provoke further exploration. An investigative interview which includes drawing tasks can provide insight into a child's coping skills, level of trauma, emotional reaction to the abuse, and, in many cases, abuse-specific information (Cohen-Liebman, 1999).

Proponents of multidisciplinary investigations support the use of drawings within the investigative interview format. The increased acceptance of drawings in investigative interviews is due, as Smart (1986) states, to the recognition of the field of art therapy and its expansion and collaboration with other disciplines. Forensic use of drawings extends the potentialities inherent in the modality beyond traditional application and signifies the interface of art therapy within the judicial arena.

REFERENCES

American Academy of Child and Adolescent Psychiatry. (1990). *Guidelines for the evaluation of child and adolescent sexual abuse.* Washington, DC: Author.

American Academy of Child and Adolescent Psychiatry. (1997). Practice Parameters for the forensic evaluation of children and adolescents who may have been physically or sexually abused. *Journal of the American Academy of Child and Adolescent Psychiatry, 36*(10), 37S–56S.

American Professional Society on the Abuse of Children. (1990). *Guidelines for psychosocial evaluation of suspected sexual abuse in young children.* Chicago: Author.

American Professional Society on the Abuse of Children. (1995). *Guidelines for use of anatomical dolls during investigative interviews of children who may have been sexually abused.* Chicago: Author.

American Psychological Association. (1994). Guidelines for child custody evaluations in divorce proceedings. *American Psychologist, 49,* 677–680.

Bourg, W., Broderick, R., Flagor, R. Kelly, D. M., Ervin, D. L., & Butler, J. (1999). *A child interviewer's guidebook.* Thousand Oaks, CA: Sage.

Burgess, A. W., & Hartman, C. R. (1993). Children's drawings. *Child Abuse and Neglect, 17,* 161–168.

Burgess, A. W., Hartman, C. R., Wolbert, W. A., & Grant, C. A. (1987). Child molestation: Assessing impact in multiple victims. *Archives of Psychiatric Nursing, 1*(1), 33–39.

Burgess, A. W., McCausland, M. P., & Wolbert, W. A. (1981). *Children's drawings as indicators of sexual trauma. Perspectives in Psychiatric Care, 19*(2), 50–57.

Carnes, C. N., Wilson, C., & Nelson-Gardell, D. (1999). Extended forensic evaluation when sexual abuse is suspected: A model and preliminary data. *Child Maltreatment, 4*(3), 242–254.

Cheung, K. F. M. (1997). Developing the interview protocol for video-recorded child sexual abuse investigations: A training experience with police officers, social workers, and clinical psychologists in Hong Kong. *Child Abuse and Neglect, 21*(3), 273–284.

Cohen-Liebman, M. S. (1994). The art therapist as expert witness in child sexual abuse litigation. *Art Therapy: Journal of the American Art Therapy Association, 11*(4), 260–265.

Cohen-Liebman, M. S. (1995). Drawings as judiciary aids in child sexual abuse litigation: a composite list of indicators. *The Arts In Psychotherapy, 22*(5), 475–483.

Cohen-Liebman, M. S. (1997, November). *Forensic art therapy.* Preconference course presented at the annual conference of the American Art Therapy Association, Milwaukee, WI.

Cohen-Liebman, M. S. (1999). Draw and tell: Drawings within the context of child sexual abuse investigations. *The Arts in Psychotherapy, 26*(3), 185–194.

Cohen-Liebman, M. S. (2002). Art therapy. In A. P. Giardino & E. A. Giardino (Eds.), *Recognition of child abuse for the mandated reporter* (pp. 227–258). St. Louis: G. W. Medical.

Cohen-Liebman, M. S., & Gussak D. (1998). *Investigation versus intervention: Forensic art therapy versus art therapy in forensic settings.* Paper presented at the annual conference of the American Art Therapy Association, Portland, OR.

Conte, J., Sorenson, E., Fogarty, L., & Dalla Rosa J. (1991). Evaluating children's reports of sexual abuse: Results from a survey of professionals. *American Journal of Orthopsychiatry, 61,* 428–437.

Davies, D., Cole, J., Albertella, G., McCulloch, L., Allen, K., & Kekevian, H. (1996). A model for conducting forensic interviews with child victims of abuse. *Child Maltreatment, 1*(3), 189–199.

Faller, K. (1993). *Child sexual abuse: Assessment and intervention issues.* Washington, DC: U.S. Department of Health and Human Services, National Center on Child Abuse and Neglect.

Faller, K. (1996). *Evaluating Children Suspected of having been sexually abused: The APSAC Study Guides 2.* Thousand Oaks, CA: Sage.

Farley, R. H. (1987). Drawing interviews: An alternative technique. *The Police Chief, 54*(4), 37–38.

Friedrich, W. N. (1990). *Psychotherapy of sexually abused children and their families.* New York: Norton.

Gussak, D., & Cohen-Liebman, M. S. (2001). Investigation vs. intervention: Forensic art therapy and art therapy in forensic settings. *American Journal of Art Therapy, 40*(2), 123–135.

Haralambie, A. M. (1999). *Child sexual abuse in civil cases: A guide to custody and tort actions.* Chicago: American Bar Association.

Haugaard, J. J., & Reppucci, N. D. (1989). *The sexual abuse of children: A comprehensive guide to current knowledge and intervention strategies.* San Francisco: Jossey-Bass.

Hibbard, R. A., Roghmann, K., & Hoekelman, R. A. (1987). Genitalia in children's drawings: An association with sexual abuse. *Pediatrics, 79*(1), 129–137.

Kelley, S. J. (1984). The use of art therapy with sexually abused children. *Journal of Psychosocial Nursing, 22*(12), 12–18.

Landgarten, H. (1987). *Family art psychotherapy.* New York: Brunner/Mazel.

Levick, M. F. (1986). *Mommy, daddy, look what I'm saying.* New York: M. Evans.

Levick, M. F., Safran, D., & Levine, A. (1990). Art therapists as expert witnesses: A judge delivers a precedent-setting decision. *The Arts in Psychotherapy, 17,* 49–53.

Lyons, S. (1993). Art psychotherapy evaluations of children in custody disputes. *The Arts in Psychotherapy, 22*(2), 153–159.

Malchiodi, C. A. (1990). *Breaking the silence: Art therapy with children from violent homes.* New York: Brunner/Mazel.

Malchiodi, C. A. (1998). *Understanding children's drawings.* New York: Guilford Press.

Mannarino, A. P., & Cohen, J. A. (1992). Forensic versus treatment roles in cases of child sexual abuse. *The Pennsylvania Child Advocate Protective Services Quarterly, 7*(4), 3–7.

Miller, T. W., Veltkamp, L. J., & Janson, D. (1987). Projective measures in the clinical evaluation of sexually abused children. *Child Psychiatry and Human Development, 18*(1), 47–57.

Monteleone, J. (1996). *Recognition of child abuse for the mandated reporter.* St. Louis: G.W. Medical.

Myers, E. B. (1998). *Legal issues in child abuse and neglect practice.* Thousand Oaks, CA: Sage.

Poole, D. A., & Lamb, M. E. (1998). *Investigative interviews of children: A guide for helping professionals.* Washington, DC: American Psychological Association.

Raskin, D. C., & Esplin, P. W. (1991). Statement validity assessment: Interview procedures and context analysis of children's statements of sexual abuse. *Behavioral Assessment, 13,* 265–291.

Reed, L. D. (1996). Findings from research on children's suggestibility and implications for conducting child interviews. *Child Maltreatment, 1*(2), 105–120.

Rickert, C. M. (1996). Art Therapy. In J. A. Monteleone (Ed.), *Recognition of child abuse for the mandated reporter* (pp. 59–80). St. Louis: G.W. Medical.

Schetky, D. H., & Benedek, E. (1992). *Clinical handbook of child psychiatry and the law.* Baltimore: Williams & Wilkins.

Schetky, D. H., & Green, A. H. (1988). *Child sexual abuse: A handbook for health care and legal professionals.* New York: Brunner/Mazel.

Sheppard, D. I., & Zangrillo, P. A. (1996, March–April). Coordinating investigations of child abuse. *Voices,* 21–25.

Smart, M. (1986). Expanded work settings for art therapy. *Art Therapy, 3,* 21–26.

Sorenson, E., Bottoms, B., & Perona, A. (1997). Handbook on intake and forensic interviewing in the children's advocacy center setting. Washington, DC: Office of Juvenile Justice and Delinquency Prevention.

Veltkamp, L. J., & Miller, T. W. (1994). *Clinical handbook of child abuse and neglect.* Madison, CT: International Universities Press.

Yuille, J. C., Hunter, R., Joffe, R., & Zaparniuk, J. (1993). Interviewing children in sexual abuse cases. In G. Goodman & B. Bottoms (Eds.), *Child victims, child witnesses: Understanding and improving testimony* (pp. 95–116). New York: Guilford Press.

CHAPTER 14

An Art Therapy Approach to Attention-Deficit/ Hyperactivity Disorder

Diane S. Safran

In the past 20 years, the number of children diagnosed with attention-deficit/ hyperactivity disorder (AD/HD) has increased as have their needs (Barkley, 2000; Robin, 1998). The primary treatment, medication with or without behavior therapy, has proven to be extremely helpful. However, medication is not always a treatment option because of either medical reasons or resistance to the idea of medication by parent or child. It also does not address the social skills deficits, such as impulsivity and hyperactivity, found in so many children with AD/HD (Jensen et al., 2001). The goal of this chapter is to help mental health providers understand the significance of art therapy in helping children with AD/HD develop social skills and to more fully understand this disorder.

KEY FEATURES OF AD/HD

The diagnosis attention-deficit disorder, with or without hyperactivity, is a recent one. It was first included in DSM-II (American Psychiatric Association, 1967). It is now seen as a neurologically based disorder, which affects both learning and behavior (Zametkin, 1995), frequently affecting school performance. It is frequently mislabeled as laziness, or stubbornness, and also frequently misdiagnosed and misunderstood. The current definition in the fourth edition of *Diagnostic and Statistical Manual of Mental Disorders* (DSM-IV; American Psychiatric Association, 1994) of

AD/HD now takes into account the cognitive processing problems that are behind these behavior problems. Girls are less frequently diagnosed or misdiagnosed (Nadeau, Littman, & Quinn, 1999; Nadeau & Quinn, 2002).

Like so many of the disorders defined by DSM-IV, AD/HD, the designation used throughout this chapter, is frequently comorbid with other disorders such as learning disabilities, anxiety, depression, and conduct disorder. It has many individual manifestations but has several clear components: inattention, impulsivity, and hyperactivity.

Inattention

Inattention or distractibility is common with most children with AD/HD who also experience a bombardment of distractions (Hallowell & Ratey, 1994). Art therapy is focused on finding ways to redirect the energy required to maintain attention so that it can be applied to listening, learning, and productively using the learned information. Inattention can take other forms, such as daydreaming. One boy's picture in art therapy depicts his brain "flying out the window" (see Figure 14.1). This drawing was in response to the question about why school was so difficult for him. He was a quiet, highly defensive, and underachieving student who was resistant to verbal therapy and, like many students with AD/HD, had been labeled lazy. Through art therapy he found a nonverbal vehicle to explain how he felt about the impact of AD/HD on his life.

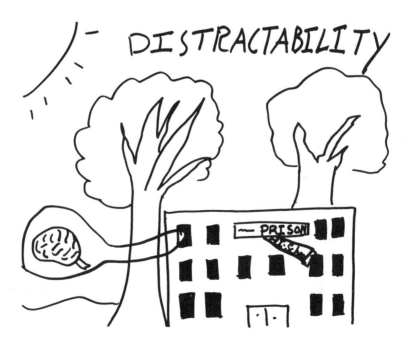

FIGURE 14.1. Drawing of "distractability."

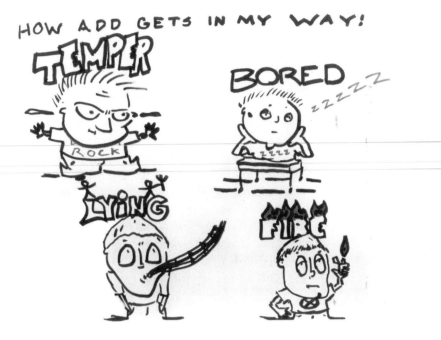

FIGURE 14.2. "Impact of AD/HD on you."

Impulsivity

Impulsivity, essentially acting or talking without thinking of the consequences, is a basic feature of AD/HD. Children with AD/HD often have high expectations and are surprised when they are not able to accomplish them. This sets in motion a "failure chain" and rather than learning from a mistake, they repeat it over and over again.

Impulsivity can lead to other problems, such as lying or stealing. A boy's drawing of the "Impact of AD/HD" on him clearly illustrates his impulsivity (see Figure 14.2). He was frequently in trouble for acting without thinking (such as setting his shower curtain on fire to see what would happen).

Hyperactivity

Hyperactivity includes externally visible symptoms, such as motor activity, restlessness, nail biting, and hair twirling, and is also evident through sleeplessness, talkativeness, overactive imagination, or a flood of ideas that the child is unable to prioritize. In art therapy, hyperactivity can manifest as filling up a drawing with random scribbles, the inability to stop activity, or even intrusion on others' artworks.

ADVANTAGES OF ART THERAPY
WITH CHILDREN WITH AD/HD

Art therapy has many benefits as a treatment modality, and in work with children with AD/HD there are several specific advantages: (1) it is a child-appropriate activity, (2) it uses visual learning skills, (3) it lends structure to therapy, and (4) it gives children a way to express themselves. The product of art therapy, the art itself, provides the child with an immediate and visual record of those feelings or ideas. Because the person with AD/HD often has difficulty remembering what has been learned, artwork becomes a way to reencounter feelings or thoughts, thus making learning easier.

Art expression is preverbal; in other words, it does not rely solely on words. Individuals whose vocabulary may be inadequate to express intense feelings such as rage may be able to use nonverbal communications in therapy to explain these feelings. For individuals with AD/HD, art can be used to help others to understand their experiences that cannot be explained with words alone. Students' drawings are extremely effective in helping teachers and administrators more clearly understand the significance of the impact of AD/HD. One middle school boy's experience clearly illustrates this point. When asked what school was like for him, he drew himself as a small boy behind bars. He titled this drawing "Being in school is like being in jail!" When I attended a meeting with administrators and teachers at his school, they described him as being deliberately disruptive. It had never occurred to any of them that he had AD/HD. The impact of viewing his drawing and learning that he had been newly diagnosed with AD/HD set an entirely different tone to the meeting. Rather than being angry with him, they set about establishing a program that would help him be successful in school. The teachers later told me that his drawing had more impact on their understanding of this child than anything I could have told them.

Art therapy is most useful when combined with psychiatric observation, psychological testing, individual and/or group therapy, and educational support. This is crucial to understanding and working with the myriad problems experienced by the AD/HD population (Ellison, 2000).

ART-BASED ASSESSMENT OF AD/HD

Art expression may also be used as a means of assessment (DiLeo, 1973), in addition to the standard assessment instruments for AD/HD. In evaluating children with AD/HD, I prefer the following art-based assessments: Kinetic Family Drawing (KFD; Burns & Kaufman, 1972), House–Tree–Person-Drawing (HTP) (Buck, 1978; Hammer, 1967), the Silver Drawing Test (Silver, 2000), and the Levick Emotional and Cognitive Art Therapy Assessment (LECATA; Levick, 1998). These tests can provide information about the child's ability to organize and use space, as well as the child's ability to plan and sequence the steps required in drawing. Other techniques, such as Draw-A-Person-In-the-Rain (Oster & Gould, 1987) and the scribble technique (Cane, 1951; Naumburg, 1966) can also be helpful in making clinical observations.

Engaging the child in art expression also provides an opportunity to evaluate comorbid problems as well as other cognitive factors that may interfere with performance. Sometimes the way a child handles art materials suggests that an occupational therapy evaluation is needed. I constantly assess children throughout the art therapy experience, from how they come into the room and where they sit—alone or in the group. The drawings during the assessment phase and treatment become part of the patient's evaluation documentation and are available for review by other professionals as background material for diagnosis.

THE THERAPY PROCESS

Art therapy, whether in a group or individual sessions, offers particular benefits to children with AD/HD (Henley, 1998). Art is an activity and children are familiar with activities in school. Activities require listening skills, the ability to focus on a single task, planning and organization, and sharing space and materials. Because art therapy encourages spontaneous behavior, it also provides a way of observing and assessing children on medication for AD/HD. The therapist will have a chance to see the threshold and possible rebound of the medication, and its efficacy, helping the child's physician fine-tune his or her medication dosage (Epperson & Valum, 1992).

The art therapy space should have at least a couple of walls of white homosote or a similar substance so it is easy for children to tack up their work. Chairs with arms provide a defined boundary preventing predictable invasion of others space. Using paper 18″ × 24″ provides a defined space on which to work. Scented markers are recommended because the smells intrigue the children and the manner in which they react to the markers adds another element and can therefore be helpful in assessing distractibility and the time required for refocus. Felt pens and colored pencils provide more structure than paint clay or oil pastels. These children are stimulation seekers. They require predictability, consistency, and structure to be successful.

It is important that the therapist keep in mind that children may act impulsively and become impatient and restless. The child's age must also be taken into account along with any developmental issues. Children under 6 years old will naturally have a shorter attention span, and with AD/HD lack of attention is exaggerated (Rubin, 1978). One needs to develop activities geared to their abilities, keeping drawings simple and time frames for completing them short. If the session is coming at the end of a long day of school, this also needs to be considered.

Each session is structured in three parts. I begin with a review of the rules and most important points and discoveries made during the prior session, discussing insights or situations that have occurred since the last session. I then introduce a new concept regarding AD/HD that may be affecting the child and have the children draw it. The final part of the art therapy session is for sharing drawings through observation and discussion, leading to closure, which includes a review of the process and progress of the session.

GROUP ART THERAPY

Art therapy groups for children with AD/HD are an effective method for the treatment of AD/HD patients and may be more successful than individual treatment alone. The goals of art therapy groups are (1) to improve self-awareness; (2) to improve social skills; (3) to continue to educate children about AD/HD; (4) to build self-esteem; (5) to teach children skills and strategies to become more successful in school, at home, and with their peers; and (6) to practice these skills within the safety of their group. Individual goals are established for each group member, in addition to common goals (Safran, 2002).

Art therapy groups run for 8 weeks. In the first session I begin by establishing rules to aid the children in having a successful group experience. During this session they learn that they all have AD/HD and the definition of the diagnosis, and they introduce themselves with a drawing. As mentioned, all sessions focus on one facet of AD/HD, such as core symptoms. The child is then asked to draw, for example, "How has AD/HD affected you at school?" Time is specifically allotted to discuss these drawings, and themes emerge during group discussion. For example, most children with AD/HD have difficulty in school and their drawings depict concerns such as inability to concentrate, impulsive behavior, anger toward unsympathetic teachers and teasing classmates, poor grades, and feelings about the inappropriate expectations of both teachers and parents.

In the second session the children see a video on AD/HD and I ask them to draw "How do you feel about having attention-deficit/hyperactivity disorder?" The youngsters take a few minutes to talk about how they feel before they begin to draw. They are then asked to make a drawing that shows how they really feel about having AD/HD so that even I, as an adult who hardly know them at all, can understand clearly. This experience encourage trust of the therapist and their peers. Many of them answer that question with drawings and comments such as "I'm not happy, "It's not fair" or "It makes me angry." Others say, "I feel frustrated," "I feel different," or "I don't feel normal." They are beginning to learn how to express their feelings in a group setting without being guarded, silly, or defensive. Most AD/HD youngsters feel that their differences cause others to victimize them. In this session, my emphasis is on the idea of not being a "victim." This is a moment when the children truly begin to communicate their feelings through their drawings.

In the following sessions I talk about the impact of AD/HD on school and homework, friendships, and family members. The children also learn about medication and what it can and cannot do. In each session they do a drawing involving the topic. One boy, in response to the question of how AD/HD affects him, drew "Reversed Sleeping Habits" (see Figure 14.3). His drawing illustrates a frequent problem in children with AD/HD—difficulty settling down and falling asleep—a problem that contributes to fatigue, inattention, irritability, sleep disorders, and, possibly, failure in school.

Group members come to understand each other as they explore the impact of AD/HD on each person's social and academic performance. They also move from individual drawings to group projects in which they execute their ideas together. It is often through their work on murals (Harris & Joseph, 1973) that they make important discoveries about their right to communicate their feelings, especially when the actions of others directly affect them or the cooperative group activity. Group activity provides an opportunity to listen, to learn how to negotiate, to share ideas, and to work together in a cohesive manner. Problems, such as impulsivity, become a point of group discussion and children are able to finally recognize the impact of their actions on the very people—peers—with whom they are trying to develop a relationship. Learning is facilitated because the children are struggling with similar issues; in a classroom setting the child with AD/HD is often made to feel like the "wrong" or "bad" one.

Children often do not know how to go about building a friendship with someone their own age. Their tireless but often inappropriate efforts usually end in failure, self-disparagement, and further isolation. Art therapy groups give them a chance to work on these skills. The idea that they can actually tell another group member that his or her behavior or comments hurt or upset them is usually met with disbelief. But as they work together on art projects, the youngsters are provided ample opportunities to express their feelings to others through art and words. For example, one girl had scribbled many different colors together, in a chaotic conglomeration. Her picture displayed graphically what it feels like to be bombarded by multiple senses and feelings simultaneously, but she had a difficult time describing what she was feeling with words. I said, "There are lots of feelings here, layer upon layer of feelings. Do other people in the group feel that way at times?" Discussing what is apparent in one child's drawing, with that child and the entire group, helps everyone relate to what the person drew and the feelings exposed in the drawing. It also makes it acceptable for others in group to share their individual feelings, both visibly in their artwork and verbally in group discussion.

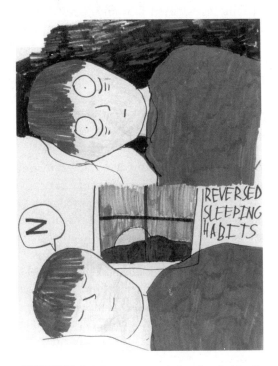

FIGURE 14.3. "Reversed sleeping habits."

Art also provides an area in which children can shine. Many children with AD/HD are creative, and group art therapy gives them a chance to discover that others can admire them, providing a positive experience.

CASE EXAMPLE: BILL

From the very beginning of his life Bill had been motorically active, which got him into trouble every day with people in authority and his own peers. Like many children with AD/HD, Bill had learning disabilities as well as an auditory processing problem. His hyperactivity, impulsivity, and intense sensitivity caused him to no longer trust himself to do the right thing, to say the right thing, to feel the right sensation, or to be the right person. As a result, he became mute.

Bill was 9 years old when he was referred to me. When Bill and I first met, he was experiencing a great deal of difficulty at home and in school. His home life was terrible. He made no connections to people inside or outside his family. His behavior was explosive and disruptive. At school, he had a history of consistent school failure. This began at age 3, when a nursery school asked his parents to remove him. As a young child Bill exhibited no deductive reasoning ability or any fear of being hurt. He did whatever entered his mind. He also had a high threshold for pain.

When we met, Bill had been involved in a series of extremely impulsive school playground episodes including choking another classmate during an outburst. His teachers were angry with him and punished him. His parents were frustrated with him and punished him. His sister hated him and blamed him for ruining the entire family's life. His grandparents were confused and did not understand him. His pediatrician told his parents to spank him harder. Bill's parents took him to a variety of mental health professionals, but nothing seemed to work. By the time Bill came to me he was mute. I was just another person in a long line that included his pediatrician, an allergist, neurologist, pediatric cardiologist, homeopath, nutritionist, neuropsychologist, and child psychiatrist. The psychiatrist referred him to me—an art therapist—based on the fact that Bill did not respond to any "talking therapy." Not even play therapy worked with Bill.

Bill and I began the treatment by getting acquainted through art. Bill's impulsivity was readily apparent in his drawings. He was a very capable young artist, comfortable with materials and art making, and with our agreement that he did not have to talk about his artwork. When Bill "talked," we heard only a series of monosyllabic mumbling. During these early sessions it was completely unrealistic to encourage him to elaborate verbally about his drawings, or anything else for that matter. In Bill's initial art therapy sessions he drew how he felt and how his AD/HD was affecting his life. He drew about school, about kids teasing him and refusing to play with him, and about how his teachers yelled at him. He drew how his AD/HD affected his brother, sister, and parents and how he felt incompetent and stupid. Those drawings were a gift to his family. His parents began to see that he was hurting. For the first time they saw visible evidence of a child struggling with the world in which he found himself (see Figure 14.4).

Bill was 11 years old when I asked him to join an art therapy group consisting of

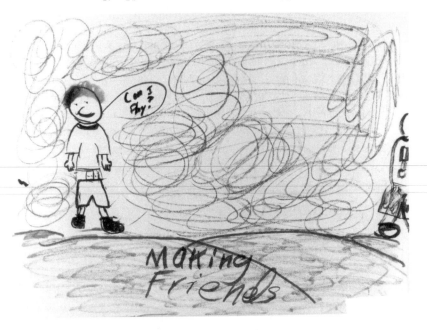

FIGURE 14.4. "Making friends."

children his age. All of them had school and home-related problems in addition to problems with impulsivity. I suggested to Bill that his group goal might be to learn to regulate or control his impulsivity. In retrospect, the achievement of that goal was his greatest success during the several years we worked together.

A major lesson for Bill in dealing with impulsivity took place when the group began to work on its first mural. The group members had already recognized Bill as impulsive but also a skilled artist. The group members were to draw an island and add to it what they needed to feel safe and comfortable. But before the group had a chance to process the suggestion, Bill jumped up and drew the island in the center of the large sheet of mural paper. At once, and without discussion or warning, the whole group had to deal with an island about which no group member had given their input, and that was immediately seen as inadequate in size to contain the drawings of all members of the group.

In a following individual session Bill and I used that experience to process what had happened and the impact of that single impulsive act on each member of the group, including Bill. Even though he could not talk about his feelings at that point, each member had only to look at him to understand how he felt. His body betrayed his feelings of shame, anger, and embarrassment. Bill's ears turned beet red. He hated that about himself, because his body spoke spontaneously for him. This provided the group members with an opportunity to discuss with Bill their feelings in a nonhostile manner and also demonstrated to each member the impact of impulsivity on others.

In art therapy I always recorded Bill's recent successes through his drawings. This made a lasting impression on this fragile young man and impressed his parents

and siblings as well. Bill and I worked together over a period of years both individually and in an art therapy group. He slowly regained his will to talk and was later
able to use medication, which his body learned to tolerate. In one of Bill's later drawings he showed a picture of medication being a treasure—his treasure. He monitors
his medication, understands the value of it, and knows how it has helped him to focus, control his impulsivity, and change his life. Bill understands that he will continue
to struggle with AD/HD, that it is part of him, and part of who he is. Through his
drawings, Bill was able to express his pain and through his art therapy group experience learn new strategies to cope with his AD/HD.

ART THERAPY WITH FAMILIES OF CHILDREN WITH AD/HD

Art therapy can also be helpful for the parents and siblings of children with AD/HD.
The child's artwork is a crucial piece of information for parents and family. As the
case of Bill demonstrates, having parents review their child's drawing helps them understand that there may be much more going on within the child than a parent may
realize.

Because the family is so adversely affected by AD/HD, it is often important to
give everyone in the family a chance to participate in therapy. Family members try to
cope with their reactions to AD/HD behavior which they consider to be lazy, defiant,
stubborn, incompetent, irresponsible, selfish, passive–aggressive, or narcissistic as
well as heartbreaking. Each person needs attention to become part of a healthy, functioning family. All members need help to learn to communicate in a way that does
not promote defensiveness, and family art projects provide an effective means of doing so (Riley & Malchiodi, 1994).

In working with families, cooperative art activities are effective. For example,
the therapist may ask the family to draw a mural depicting a family boat trip.
Though it sounds simple, everyone must decide on such things as where they are going, what kind of a boat they will take, what provisions to pack, what the weather
will be like, and who will draw what. The central idea of a family art task is to look
at the strengths and weaknesses of each family member in order to understand AD/
HD's impact on everyone. The therapist will observe who says what, who helps
whom, who participates and who does not, whose ideas are acceptable, who is the
antagonist and who acts as peacemaker, who is the first to give up, who takes leadership, and what happens when frustration takes place.

It is important for the therapist to highlight key themes for family members. For
example, if the most impulsive family member drew a boat that was too small to
reach the destination or packed lots of fun stuff but none of the necessities for the
trip, family members can discuss how that makes them feel and how impulsivity or
impatience affects the entire family. Group projects such as family murals clarify family dynamics along with the family's responses to their art experience. The therapist
may discuss the project as a family unit or, if the children are quite young, might talk
with the parents alone. Occasionally, it can be helpful to meet with siblings alone
(Landgarten, 1987).

It is not unusual for parents of children with AD/HD to feel ineffective. For example, in one family of three children, in which the youngest, a 5-year-old boy, had AD/HD, the family relinquished their power to him in order to prevent conflict. When asked to draw an island and how they would all live together on it, the parents had planned to show a tropical resort, but the 5-year-old child with AD/HD wanted soldiers and tanks. The mother decided she would not draw at all, while the father tried unsuccessfully to dissuade the son. The oldest girl became so frustrated she stopped participating entirely. The middle child tried to get his mother to draw. In the end, the family divided the island so everyone could have his or her way. But the entire island ended up being surrounded by army troops and barricades and no one was in control. All along the parents missed the signs that their 5-year-old was acting like a family dictator while looking for one parent to set limits and establish boundaries.

This brief example demonstrates that art therapy can be extremely useful in providing a view into a family dynamic that is often difficult to understand through words alone. Sometimes parents will just sit back and let youngsters make every important decision about a drawing. Perhaps the parents are tired of endless conflicts; perhaps they deem it necessary for their children to feel part of the democratic process. It is far more helpful for parents to work together to slow down the child with AD/HD. It is a good sign when families devise methods for getting off the island. In less healthy families, the water is filled with sharks and the island dotted with wild animals and active volcanoes. They cannot imagine a safe place where everyone enjoys each other's company.

Family art therapy sessions also give parents a chance to practice being more assertive and setting clear limits for their children. They give children a chance to learn how to correctly respond to their parents new "executive" status. The therapist is in the position to capitalize on the family's art therapy experience as a way to identify, address, and integrate new habits and skills into the family structure.

CONCLUSION

Art therapy is an active form of therapy that provides a kinesthetic and visual approach to learning for children with AD/HD. It is a viable tool for enhancing the skills that children with AD/HD require in order to be successful. Children learn more about their disorder through drawings, and this enhances their self-esteem.

Art therapy groups provide AD/HD children with an opportunity to learn from each other. Sharing their drawings and thoughts becomes a vehicle for change and at the same time enhances self-worth. Families of children with AD/HD can benefit from family art therapy. Joint drawings or murals provide parents, siblings, and the child with AD/HD with a voice to express the experience of AD/HD and its impact on family dynamics. The art products become powerful tools for the therapist to understand, intervene, and assist children and parents in effectively coping with this disorder.

One of Bill's final drawings depicted "What I like about having AD/HD." Bill drew a picture of his creativity, high energy, sports involvement, and friendliness. Bill, like so many children in art therapy, came to see AD/HD not as a curse but possibly as an advantage, and certainly not something to be ashamed of.

REFERENCES

American Psychiatric Association. (1967). *Diagnostic and statistical manual of mental disorders* (2nd ed.). Washington, DC: Author.

American Psychiatric Association. (1994). *Diagnostic and statistical manual of mental disorders* (4th ed.). Washington, DC: Author.

Barkley, R. (2000). *Taking charge of ADHD*. New York: Guilford Press.

Buck, J. N. (1978). *The House–Tree–Person technique*. Los Angeles: Western Psychological Services.

Burns, R. C., & Kaufman, H. S. (1972). *Actions, styles, and symbols in Kinetic Family Drawings*. New York: Brunner/Mazel.

Cane, F. (1951). *The artist in each of us*. New York: Pantheon.

DiLeo, J. H. (1973). *Childrens' drawings as diagnostic aids*. New York: Brunner/Mazel.

Ellison, P. (2000). Building social skills in children with AD/HD: A multimodal approach. *CHADD AD/HD Resource Manual*, pp. 68–70.

Epperson, J., & Valum, L. (1992). The effects of stimulant drugs on the art products of ADHD children. *Art Therapy: Journal of the American Art Therapy Association*, 9(1), 36–38.

Hallowell, E. M., & Ratey, J. J. (1994). *Driven to distraction*. New York: Pantheon Books.

Hammer, E. (1967). *Clinical applications of projective drawings*. Springfield, IL: Charles C Thomas.

Harris, J., & Joseph, C. (1973). *Murals of the mind*. New York: International Universities Press.

Henley, D. (1998). Art therapy as an aid to socialization in children with ADD. *American Journal of Art Therapy*, 37, 2–12.

Jensen, P., Hinshaw, S., Swanson, J., Greenhill, L., Conners, C., & Arnold, L. (2001). Findings from the NIMH multimodal treatment study of AD/HD (MTA): Implications and applications for primary care providers. *Journal of Developmental and Behavioral Pediatrics*, 22(1), 60–73.

Landgarten, H. B. (1987). *Family art psychotherapy: A clinical guide and casebook*. New York: Brunner/Mazel.

Levick, M. (1998). *The Levick Emotional and Cognitive Art Therapy Assessment*. Dade County Public Schools Clinical Art Therapy Department, Dade County, FL.

Nadeau, K. G., Littman, E., & Quinn, P. O. (1999). *Understanding girls with AD/HD*. Silver Springs, MD: Advantage Books.

Nadeau, K. G., & Quinn, P. (2002). *Understanding women with AD/HD*. Silver Springs, MD: Advantage Books.

Naumburg, M. (1966). *Dynamically oriented art therapy*. New York: Grune & Stratton.

Oster, G. D., & Gould, P. (1987). *Using drawings in assessment and therapy*. New York: Brunner/Mazel.

Riley, S., & Malchiodi, C. A., (1994). *Integrative approaches to family art therapy*. Chicago: Magnolia Street.

Robin, A. L. (1998). *ADHD in adolescents*. New York: Guilford Press.

Rubin, J. A. (1978). *Child art therapy*. New York: Van Nostrand Reinhold.

Safran, D. (2002). *Art therapy and AD/HD: Diagnostic and therapeutic approaches*. London: Jessica Kingsley.

Silver, R. (2000). *Art as language*. New York: Brunner-Routledge.

Zametkin, A. J. (1995). *AD/HD today: Clinical wisdom for the practitioners: The biologic basis of AD/HD*. Deerfield, IL: Discovery International.

CHAPTER 15

Art Therapy with Children Who Have Autism and Their Families

Robin L. Gabriels

Understanding young children who have autism can be initially perplexing and mysterious. Because these children do not seem to understand or know how to interact with others, they present a challenge to the parents and the professionals who attempt to engage and teach them. Therefore, gaining a clearer understanding of this disability is imperative for the development and implementation of effective intervention practices.

Autism was first described and named by Leo Kanner in 1943. He defined autism as being an early form of childhood schizophrenia (Wing, 1997). Although autism is no longer recognized as such, the behavioral symptoms Kanner first described in autism are similar to the symptoms that define autism today in the fourth edition of the *Diagnostic and Statistical Manual of Mental Disorders* (DSM-IV, American Psychiatric Association, 1994) and ICD-10 (World Health Organization, 1992). Autistic disorder is a severe developmental disability with onset of behavioral symptoms before 3 years of age. The symptoms involve impairments and delayed development within the domains of social interaction and communication along with repetitive, stereotypical, and restrictive (e.g., need for routines) behavioral patterns.

One of the most baffling aspects of autistic disorder is the fact that children differ in the degree of symptom presentation across all areas implicated in the diagnosis. For example, these children can range in social presentation from being aloof to being actively interactive but inappropriate in their interaction attempts. They can also range in their communication abilities from being nonverbal to being verbal, but idiosyncratic in their use of language (Dalrymple, Porco, & Chung, 1993). There are several other symptoms associated with autism, which also vary in severity across children. These can include unusual sensory responses, problems with motor skills, significant cognitive delays (with higher cognitive functioning in restricted areas), self-injurious behaviors, along with abnormalities in attention, eating, sleep, and mood. In addition, research has demonstrated that children with autism have impairments in the areas of motor imitation (Stone, Ousley, & Littleford, 1997), functional/symbolic play (Libby, Powell, Messer, & Jordan, 1998), generalizing skills/concepts (Koegel, Koegel, & Parks, 1995), and generating imaginative creativity (Craig & Baron-Cohen, 1999; Happe & Frith, 1996). An estimated 35–45% of individuals who have autism also have a seizure disorder, and approximately half of these individuals begin to have seizures in puberty (Happe & Frith, 1996). Mental retardation is also present in individuals who have autism approximately 70–75% of the time, and an estimated 50% of individuals with autism do not develop communicative speech (Wakschlag & Leventhal, 1996).

Areas of strength identified in many individuals who have autism include good rote memory and visual–spatial/problem-solving skills (Happe & Frith, 1996). There have been reports of some individuals with autism who have savant skills in artistic ability (Cox & Eames, 1999; Gardner, 1982). Hou et al. (2000) compared the artwork of six artistic savant children who also had features of pervasive developmental disorder with nonartistic savant children with autism. The artwork of these savants indicated several common features, such as showing a preference for using a single art medium and limited variation of artwork themes. Of note, several features common in autistic disorder, such as attentiveness to visual detail, intact rote memory and visual–spatial skills, and tendency toward obsessive interest and compulsive repetition, assisted in their production of successful artwork (Hou et al., 2000).

ETIOLOGY AND DIAGNOSIS

Although the exact etiology of autism is unknown at present, the field has come a long way from the previous theories of this disorder, which attributed autism to a disturbance in the child's ability to bond with his or her parents (Wing, 1997). Autism is now recognized as a neurodevelopmental disability, having an organic basis involving differences in brain structures and the way the brain processes and integrates information. Current research is providing information about the implications of these structural differences on the brain function, behavior, and learning styles of this population. Recent genetic research indicates that there may be a genetic link associated with the etiology of autism, and it appears that several genes may be implicated in the disorder rather than just one particular gene (Whaley & Shaw, 1999).

The variability of autism symptom presentation and the possibility of its co-occurrence with medical, environmental, and cognitive factors complicate the diagnosis of autism. Therefore, it is crucial that this diagnosis be made after considering the assessment findings of a multidisciplinary team of professionals (e.g., psychologist, physician, speech–language pathologist, and occupational or physical therapist) who are familiar with the diagnosis of autism (Filipek et al., 1999).

TREATMENT ISSUES

There are many approaches and programs available for working with children who have autism, not all of which have been substantiated by research. In the 1950s, psychodynamic approaches were prevalent and were based on the premise that autism was caused by inadequate parenting. However, research has not demonstrated the effectiveness of this approach and autism is now recognized as a neurodevelopmental disorder (Schreibman & Anderson, 2001). Biological interventions (e.g., drug, vitamin, and nutrition) are also currently under investigation (Whaley & Shaw, 1999). Both behavioral and developmental research have implications in the treatment of children with autism. Behavioral research has demonstrated the positive effects of applying behavior-learning theory techniques to the treatment of various cognitive, imitation, language, behavior, and social deficits associated with autism. Likewise, developmental research offers insight about typical patterns of skill accusation and prerequisites needed before attaining higher-level skills (Schreibman & Anderson, 2001). These approaches assist children with autism in their home and school environments. For example, behavior-learning principles help to provide them with predictable and understandable cause-and-effect/trial-and-error learning environments. Given the specific needs of children with autism, behavioral cause-and-effect learning must be made explicit by breaking down tasks into smaller components and teaching new skills in a structured setting with minimal distractions using a reward/incentive system specific to the child's interests. A number of programs are available that emphasize different aspects of behavioral learning theory and vary in the intensity and focus of the application of these principles. For example, Lovaas (1981) developed an intensive, one-to-one, discrete trial teaching (DTT) program format that directly applies principles derived from operant behavior learning theory (e.g., positive reinforcement, shaping, chaining, task analysis, errorless learning, prompting, and modeling) to teach specific skills. In addition, functional analysis techniques provide a means to better understand problematic behaviors, thus assisting in the process of developing effective behavior intervention plans (O'Neill, Horner, Albin, Storey, & Sprague, 1990). The TEACCH (Treatment and Education of Autistic and Related Communication Handicapped Children) program emphasizes cognitive-behavioral and developmental approaches involving both structured and incidental teaching techniques along with organizing the physical environment to assist in a person's ability to understand the environment and work independently (Schopler, Mesibov, & Hearsey, 1995). Other programs, such as Greenspan's Floor-Time model, stress incidental/cause-and-effect teaching within a developmental framework. This involves both following the child's lead and creating interactive opportunities with the child (Greenspan & Weider, 1998).

Regardless of the program emphasis, research has demonstrated that intensive and comprehensive early intervention programs are effective for improving the outcomes of children who have developmental disabilities in general (Ramey & Ramey, 1998). Specifically, the variable outcomes reported across programs with children who have autism, combined with the variations in brain and biological correlates of autism, suggest that an approach tailored to fit the individual needs of the child and family may be most effective (Corchesne, Yeung-Courchesne, & Pierce, 1999). Finally, given the heterogeneous nature of this population and variable treatment outcomes, individuals with autism may be best served if therapists can individually prescribe treatments by integrating an understanding of developmental and behavior learning theory, research, and techniques (Schreibman & Anderson, 2001). From this developmental and behavioral knowledge base, the therapist can then branch out into a child-directed approach to effectively engage the child and set up creative opportunities for skill generalization and learning. Of note, Temple Grandon (1998), a successful and independent professional adult diagnosed with autism as a child, advocates for therapists and educators to pay attention to children's specific interests and cultivate them as a foundation for interaction and learning.

THE ROLE OF ART THERAPY IN EARLY INTERVENTION

The role of art therapy (i.e., helping clients with self-expression and self-understanding through the use of symbolic imagery) is somewhat different with children who have autism (Oster & Gould, 1987). Young children with autism tend to lack the basic skills required in the areas of attention, play, communication, cognition, imitation, generalization, and motor coordination to understand and engage in the world. Therefore, art therapy needs to be adapted to the strengths and needs of these children. Art media, tools, and activities can be used to interest and engage this population in order to build on their visual–spatial strengths and at the same time develop foundation academic, art, play, and social skills. After the child has developed these foundation skills, the therapist can introduce a variety of social-art experiences to assist in skill generalization and social skill development.

Anderson (1994) discusses the importance of "art-centered learning" for children with disabilities. This type of learning involves incorporating an educational curriculum within the context of art activities. Anderson's approach is similar to the educational "whole language approach," which "is based on the premise that children learn best when instruction is not broken down into subject areas" (Anderson, 1994, p. 105). The art therapist can be a valuable addition to a multidisciplinary team of therapists and educators in a variety of settings (e.g., school groups or individual sessions). Overlapping treatment approaches enable professionals to address the multiple overlapping needs of children with autism.

SENSORY PROCESSING AND ART THERAPY

Some children and adults with autism have difficulties with sensory modulation including tendencies to over- or underreact to sensory stimuli (McIntosh, Miller, Shyu, & Hagerman, 1999). The connection between how the brain processes sensory information and its impact on an individual's learning and behavior has been described by sensory integration theory (Ayres, 1972). Specifically, this theory attempts to explain how neurobiologically unexplained motor coordination and sensory processing problems may affect some children's mild to moderate learning and behavior problems. The implications of this theory for intervention suggest that enhanced sensory integration/processing and learning can result from providing meaningful sensory experiences (Fisher & Murray, 1991).

The tendency for some children with autism to become preoccupied with sensory-based activities can be a useful advantage for the therapist. Sensory materials can entice a child with autism to engage with new materials and interact with others, including the child's peers. However, it is important for the therapist to be aware of the impact sensory materials (e.g., visual, auditory, tactile, and smell) can have on the child's sensory systems. Given this, the therapist should consult on a regular basis with the child's occupational or physical therapist regarding the specific sensory issues and needs of the child. This information will be necessary for averting potential behavioral upsets that may result when a material is intolerable to a child with a specific sensory sensitivity. In addition, ongoing consultation with an occupational or physical therapist who has a specialty in sensory integration can assist the therapist in developing a systematic plan for desensitizing a child to overstimulating or aversive materials.

Some sensory activities can be soothing or have particular interest to the child with autism. However, the therapist needs to consider whether the activity of choice is either inappropriate and/or repetitive. For example, a child might enjoy watching his or her saliva slowly drip down a vertical surface. In this instance, the therapist might first consider the visually appealing sensory nature of this activity for the child and then decide to introduce the child to a more appropriate medium and activity, such as making dripping paint pictures. Awareness of the sensory needs and issues particular to the child can guide the therapist in choosing materials and activities that can redirect socially inappropriate sensory activities to those that promote positive social interaction.

BUILDING FOUNDATION SKILLS

Motor Skills

Treatment research has indicated that motor planning problems are decreased when an individual with autism is provided with many opportunities to practice motor movements and when complex motor tasks are broken down into small steps and then paired with a sequence of visual cues (Rogers, 1999). Along with motor planning difficulties, this population also has difficulties with motor imitation (Stone et al., 1997).

Art therapy can provide an arena for the child with autism to practice motor coordination and imitation skills through a variety of activities such as cutting, gluing, drawing, and painting. It is important to first have the child master these skills during one-on-one instruction before expecting the child to participate in a multistep art project and/or a group activity setting. Teaching basic tool use and drawing imitation skills has implications for later writing skills (Wolery & Brookfield-Norman, 1988). (For specific suggestions about teaching foundation fine motor skills to children with disabilities, see Bruni, 1998). When teaching foundation motor skills to a child with autism, it is necessary to prepare materials in such a way that the task objectives are clearly defined with visual cues (e.g., drawing a line across a strip of paper to indicate where the child should cut or preparing a dried glue boundary around simple shapes to provide the child with a physical cue to color within the form). This kind of preparation can help avoid negative behaviors that can result when a child is faced with incomprehensible tasks and expectations. Additionally, a child is more likely to engage in a new motor skill task (e.g., cutting), if there is an inherently reinforcing aspect to the task, such as snipping straws and watching pieces fly across the room.

Even after the child has mastered basic fine motor skills, some children with autism may initially resist the novel experience of task generalization or become distressed by having to perform physically challenging motor tasks. To address these problems, the therapist should focus on activities that are inherently motivating or topics of particular interest to the child. Children with autism have specific preferences just as typical children do. However, these preferences may involve exclusive interests (e.g., cartoon characters) and may be unusual or nonsocial in nature (e.g., vacuum cleaners). If an activity can initially capture a child's interest, the child can begin to understand that these difficult motor activities provide a means to an end and thus have a purpose. For example, one 4½-year-old boy was motivated to engage in a variety of motor coordination activities in order to create a house for his favorite Christmas cartoon character (Figure 15.1). During this activity, he cut out and glued on the house and Christmas tree. He was further enticed to squeeze the glue bottle so

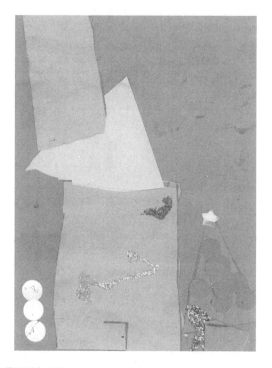

FIGURE 15.1. Collage of Christmas cartoon character.

that he could sprinkle on some much-desired glitter to decorate the house and to peel off dot stickers to create a snowman.

Cognitive Skills

As previously mentioned, although a majority of the autistic population meets IQ and adaptive behavior score criteria for mental retardation, many have strengths in the area of visual–spatial skills. The therapist can use these strengths to increase understanding and generalization of a variety of cognitive concepts. Several cognitive preacademic skills can be targeted by the therapist (e.g., categorical concepts of matching identical objects, pictures, pictures to objects, colors, shapes, and size) (Anderson, 1994). Other preacademic reading and math skills to target include matching letters, words, pictures to words, numbers, and numbers to quantities (Wolery & Brookfield-Norman, 1988). As a general rule, art activities and art teaching tasks need to be presented with clear visual cues that define task objectives. The TEACCH program offers many ideas for organizing materials to assist with task comprehension (Schopler, Reichler, & Lansing, 1980). For example, one art activity is to have the child match and then glue precut shapes onto another paper that has a matching predrawn shape outline. This kind of task can be varied to involve matching and sorting other items such as letters, colors, numbers, and later more complex concepts of picture categories. It is important when introducing this kind of sorting/matching task to first provide the child with only one item to match in order to decrease the possibility of error and/or confusion on the part of the child.

After the child has mastered simple cognitive conceptual tasks (e.g., matching identical objects, pictures/shapes, pictures to objects, letters, and numbers), the therapist can increase complexity by introducing more items to match and sort and can vary the task with different materials for generalization of concepts. For example, shape-matching tasks can be expanded to have a child match a variety of predrawn shapes to create a favorite animal, character, or object (Figure 15.2). After the picture is complete, the child can trace the name of the character or his or her own name as a way of incorporating letter/word-writing skill practice. An example of a color discrimination concept generalization task might be to introduce color mixing art activities, such as painting with the three primary colors (red, blue, and yellow), so that the child can discover new colors as they overlap on the paper (Anderson, 1994). Number and letter sequencing concepts can be generalized to having the child complete simple dot-to-dot drawings to make a favored character or object.

The structure of the art therapy room, including limiting the amount of visually distracting materials on the wall, can lend itself to promoting child focus along with development of preacademic skills such as prereading and categorization/sorting skills. For example, the therapist can introduce sight word reading by taping picture/word labels onto objects and art materials (e.g., chair, table, door, paint, and brushes) around the room (Anderson, 1994). Also, the therapist can incorporate sorting tasks, such as sorting crayons versus scissors into separately marked bins, into a clean-up routine. The TEACCH system offers a helpful model for structuring and organizing successful classroom settings for children who have autism (Schopler et al., 1995).

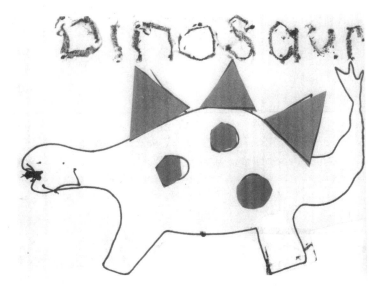

FIGURE 15.2. "Dinosaur."

Social/Communication Skills

One of the most problematic aspects of communication for individuals with autism, regardless of their verbal abilities, is an impaired understanding of the social pragmatics of language. This involves an understanding of how language, eye contact, and gesture relate to and affect the social environment (Rogers, 1999). Autism intervention principles derived from developmental literature indicate that preverbal communication skills (e.g., gesture and eye contact) are necessary for the later development of intentional verbal communication and that words should be associated with preverbal communication skills (Wetherby & Prizant, 1999). The cognitive and language impairments along with the sensory preoccupation interests of a child with autism can also have a negative impact on their ability to interact with and be understood by others (Lord, 1995). Social skills deficits have been considered a core characteristic of autism. These deficits can be evidenced in a child as early as 12 months of age and they persist throughout adulthood (Olley & Gutentag, 1999). In young children with autism, social deficits are apparent in their lack of "joint attention skills—the ability to share attention with another person" (Sigman & Kim, 1999, p. 283). This includes a lack of responsive social smiling and use of eye contact and/ or gesture to engage others. In addition, children with autism tend to engage in limited amounts of symbolic play and attend less to other people than do their peers (Sigman & Kim, 1999).

The visual nature of art therapy materials and techniques can bolster the process of mapping words onto actions to enhance word understanding for children who have autism, thus affecting their level of social interaction. For example, as a child is creating art, the therapist can pair each of the child's actions with a simple single word about the action. Also, art activities can be a motivating and interesting way for children with autism to demonstrate and practice their word knowledge. One 7-year-old boy with minimal verbal skills engaged in an art task of pasting precut body parts onto a predrawn figure (Figure 15.3). The task involved the therapist labeling the body part as she handed it to the child to put on (e.g., "Put ears on"). This task was interesting to this child and he correctly placed (without assistance or visual cues) all body parts in their appropriate location on the figure, including the hair. Prior to this task, this child had refused to demonstrate his knowledge of the meaning of body part words when given directions, such as "Point to your nose."

There is a paucity of literature regarding inclusive art-centered activity groups for children who have autism, despite the fact that these types of groups have potential value for enhancing social and academic skills along with providing artistic vocational skill competency. Schlein, Mustonen, and Rynders (1995) demonstrated a need for structured social inclusion activities by showing how 15 elementary school children with autism were integrated into unstructured school activities (e.g., recess and lunch). These children rarely had interactions with their nondisabled peers in these settings. However, positive interactions between two groups increased when they were included together in structured community art activities. When developing art-centered activity groups, these authors stress the importance of preparing nondisabled peers to engage peers who have autism as well as preparing children with autism by first teaching them basic art skills. In addition, it is important to choose art activities that encourage cooperation and interaction; for example, creating a large puzzle together (Schlein et al., 1995).

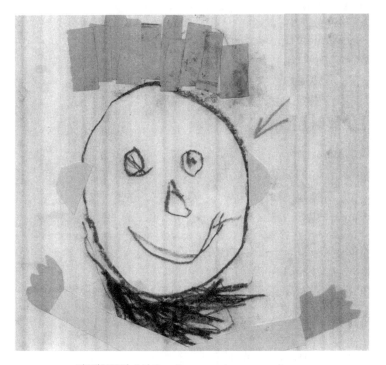

FIGURE 15.3. Construction paper figure.

USING ART THERAPY TO ENHANCE SOCIAL SKILLS IN OLDER CHILDREN AND TEENS WITH AUTISM

Art-centered activity groups designed specifically for people with autism can also provide supportive social environments for older children, teens, and adults with autism. Exposure to and mastery of various media can be the first target goal for the group and then group members can engage individually or in small groups in the art-making process. Following this, group members can display and talk about their creations. The visual nature of the art produced can provide an effective cue to promoting successful conversation. One teen group engaged in an individual photography activity in which the teens were first taught basic principles of photography and then given opportunities to take pictures of their environment. Group members later displayed their photos and talked about how their pictures captured things that are important to them and how they see the world (L. Marcus & B. Bianco, personal communication, May 24, 2000). An example of an interactive group task is a pass-around-picture activity in which each group member chooses a different colored marker and begins to draw a picture. After a few minutes, group members pass their pictures to the person to their right and then spend a few more minutes adding something to the other group member's picture. Group members are cautioned to be considerate of other's drawings and try to add things to their pictures that continue the theme begun by the original drawer. This passing and drawing process continues until all pictures have been returned to their original owners. Following this process, group members take turns sharing what they added to each person's drawing. Within this discussion, group members can be encouraged to identify their rationale for adding certain drawings to particular pictures and to receive feedback about this in an effort to illuminate the importance of thinking about or considering another person's desires and preferences.

ART THERAPY WITH FAMILIES OF CHILDREN WITH AUTISM

A child's diagnosis of autism can be devastating and overwhelming to parents. Initially, parents may react to their child's diagnosis with feelings of depression and helplessness, wondering what this diagnosis means for their child's future as an adult. The complex nature of the diagnosis of autism can also challenge natural parenting instincts, leaving parents feeling anxious and uncertain about how to differentiate which of their child's behaviors are specific to autism and which are common to typical development. The myriad professionals needed to treat their child can also stress the family system, due to the resulting lack of privacy from therapy scheduling demands.

Riley and Malchiodi (1994) discuss the advantages of multifamily art therapy groups to assist families with a disabled family member to share coping strategies and gain support from others. These kinds of art therapy groups promote family cohesiveness by providing a means to include all family members at their various levels of developmental ability. An example of a beginning multifamily art group activity might be the creation of a family coat of arms on which family members draw, write, or use collage materials to identify unique aspects about their family, such as coping strategies, individual members' roles and contributions, and support systems. Families can later exhibit their creations to the entire group. Other activities include the child with autism by engaging the family in an art-making activity with an art medium already familiar to the child. These particular activities can take place either in multifamily group or in individual family therapy settings. For example, one family engaged in drawing a family portrait. The nonverbal 7-year-old child with autism began the activity by drawing a person, which his family labeled as himself. Following this, this child watched with an uncommon amount of interest and attention as his brothers and mother took turns drawing themselves and verbally labeling the features they added. Figure drawings and other additions, such as trees, were labeled with words to promote communication and prereading skills. Toward the conclusion of this activity, the child with autism wanted to color in his family members' figures. He also willingly participated with his family in drawing a large rainbow at the top of the picture. At the end of this activity, family members identified a sense of pride and accomplishment at having successfully worked together.

Treatment providers also need to be sensitive and alert to individual needs and strengths of siblings. Providing supportive art therapy groups for siblings to draw and talk about their positive and negative feelings and experiences about living with their sibling who has autism can help decrease stress levels and increase their use of positive coping strategies. For example, in an art therapy sibling group, an 8-year-old girl drew several pictures about what it was like to have a brother with autism. In one picture she described the importance of taking responsibility of her sibling by writing, "If you want some advice I can tell you some. If you have an autistic brother or sister and your mom and dad tell you to watch them then you should always have your eye on them no matter where they are or they might get into trouble." In another picture (Figure 15.4), this same sibling depicted a frustrating situation when she had to clean up after her brother who inadvertently created a mess. About this picture she wrote, "My brother made me mad when he made the games fall all out of the cabinet and I had to clean up the mess." These pictures elicited a discussion from other siblings in the group about their similar experiences and feelings and ways to cope.

CONCLUSION

Art therapy can serve a valuable role as part of multidisciplinary interventions to assist young children who have autism in the development and generalization of foundation skills needed in the areas of preacademics, art, play, and socialization. In addition, the sensory nature of art media can entice children with autism to engage with others. After these basic foundation skills are developed, art activities can be used to promote meaningful social interactions for children with autism and their peers and family members. Art therapy group activities can also provide a forum for siblings and parents to garner support from each other to identify better ways to cope with the child who has autism.

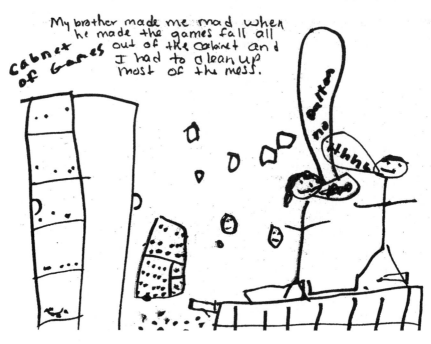

FIGURE 15.4. Drawing representing sibling frustration.

ACKNOWLEDGMENTS

I am indebted to my friends and colleagues in the autism field for sharing their expertise and editorial suggestions: Dina Hill, PhD, Kjesti Johnson-Easton, MA, and Lenita Hartman.

REFERENCES

American Psychiatric Association. (1994). *Diagnostic and statistical manual of mental disorders* (4th ed.). Washington, DC: Author.

Anderson, F. E. (1994). Art-centered education and therapy for children with disabilities. Springfield, IL: Charles C Thomas.

Ayres, A. J. (1972). *Sensory integration and learning disorders*. Los Angeles: Western Psychological Services.

Bruni, M. (1998). *Fine motor skills in children with down syndrome: A guide for parents and professionals*. Bethesda, MD: Woodbine House.

Courchesne, E., Yeung-Courchesne, R., & Pierce, K. (1999). Biological and behavioral heterogeneity in autism: Roles of pleiotropy and epigenesis. In S. H. Broman & J. M. Fletcher (Eds.), *The changing nervous system* (pp. 292–340). New York: Oxford University Press.

Cox, M., & Eames, K. (1999). Contrasting styles of drawing in gifted individuals with autism. *Autism: The International Journal of Research and Practice, 3*(4), 397–409.

Craig, J., & Baron-Cohen, S. (1999). Creativity and imagination in autism and asperger syndrome. *Journal of Autism and Developmental Disorders, 29*(4), 319–326.

Dalrymple, N., Porco, B., & Chung, J. (1993). *Instructional modules on autism*. Bloomington, IN: Indiana University, Institute for the Study of Developmental Disabilities.

Filipek, P. A., Accardo, P. J., Ashwal, S., Baranek, G. T., Cook, Jr., E. H., Dawson, G., Gordon, B.,

Gravel, J. S., Johnson, C. O., Kallen, R. J., Levey, S. E., Minshew, N. J., Ozonoff, S., Prizant, B. M., Rapin, I., Rogers, S. J., Stone, W. L., Teplin, S. W., Tuchman, R. F., & Volkmar, F. R. (1999). The screening and diagnosis of autistic spectrum disorders. *Journal of Autism and Developmental Disorders, 29,* 439–484.

Fisher, A. G., & Murray, E. A. (1991) Introduction to sensory integration theory. In A. G. Fisher, E. A. Murray, & A. C. Bundy (Eds.), *Sensory integration theory and practice* (pp. 3–25). Philadelphia, PA: F. A. Davis.

Gardner, H. (1982). *Art mind, and brain: A cognitive approach to creativity.* New York: Basic Books.

Grandon, T. (1998). Teaching tips from a recovered autistic. *Focus on Autistic Behavior, 3*(1), 1–8.

Greenspan, S. I., & Wieder, S. (1998). *The child with special needs: Encouraging intellectual and emotional growth.* Reading, MA: Addison-Wesley.

Happe, F., & Frith, U. (1996). The neuropsychology of autism. *Brain, 119*(4), 1377–1400.

Hou, C., Miller, B. L., Cummings, J. L., Goldberg, M., Mychack, P., Bottino, V., & Benson, D. F. (2000). Artistic savants. *Neuropsychiatry, Neuropsychology, and Behavioral Neurology, 13*(1), 29–38.

Koegel, R. L., Koegel, L. K., & Parks, D. R. (1995). "Teach the individual" model of generalization: Autonomy through self-management. In R. L. Koegel & L. K. Koegel (Eds.), *Teaching children with autism: Strategies for initiating positive interactions and improving learning opportunities* (pp. 67–78). Baltimore: Paul H. Brookes.

Libby, S., Powell, S., Messer, D., & Jordan, R. (1998). Spontaneous play in children with autism: A reappraisal. *Journal of Autism and Developmental Disorders, 28*(5), 487–496.

Lord, C. (1995). Facilitating social inclusion: Examples from peer intervention programs. In E. Schopler & G. B. Mesibov (Eds.), *Learning and cognition in autism* (pp. 221–240). New York: Plenum Press.

Lovaas, I. (1981). *Teaching developmentally disabled children: The me book.* Baltimore: University Park Press.

McIntosh, D. N., Miller, L. J., Shyu, V., & Hagerman, R. J. (1999). Sensory modulation disruption, electrodermal responses and functional behaviors. *Developmental Medicine and Child Neurology, 41,* 608–615.

Olley, J. G., & Gutentag, S. S. (1999). Autism: Historical overview, definition, and characteristics. In D. B. Zager (Ed.), *Autism identification, education, and treatment* (pp. 3–22). Mahwah, NJ: Erlbaum.

O'Neill, R. E., Horner, R. H., Albin, R. W., Storey, K., & Sprague, J. R. (1990). *Functional analysis of problem behavior: A practical assessment guide.* Sycamore, IL: Sycamore.

Oster, G. D., & Gould, P. (1987). *Using drawings in assessment and therapy: A guide for mental health professionals.* New York: Brunner/Mazel.

Ramey, C. T., & Ramey, S. L. (1998). Early intervention and early experience. *American Psychologist, 53*(2), 109–120.

Riley, S., & Malchiodi, C. A. (1994). *Integrative approaches to family art therapy.* Chicago: Magnolia Street.

Rogers, S. J. (1999) Intervention for young children with autism: From research to practice. *Infants and Young Children, 12*(2), 1–16.

Schlein, J. S., Mustonen, T., & Rynders, J. E. (1995).Participation of children with autism and nondisabled peers in a cooperatively structured community art program. *Journal of Autism and Developmental Disorders, 25*(4), 397–411.

Schopler, E., Mesibov, G. B., & Hearsey, K. (1995). Structured teaching in the TEACCH system. In E. Schopler & G. B. Mesibov (Eds.), *Learning and cognition in autism* (pp. 243–268). New York: Plenum Press.

Schopler, E., Reichler, R. J., & Lansing, M. (1980). *Individualized assessment and treatment for autistic and developmentally disabled children (Vol. 2): Teaching strategies for parents and professionals.* Baltimore, MD: University Park Press.

Schreibman, L., & Anderson, A. (2001). Focus on integration: The future of the behavioral treatment of autism. *Behavior Therapy, 32,* 619–632.

Sigman, M., & Kim, N. (1999). Continuity and change in the development of children with autism. In S. H. Broman & J. M. Fletcher (Eds.), *The changing nervous system: Neurobehavioral consequences of early brain disorders* (pp. 274–291). New York: Oxford University Press.

Stone, W. L., Ousley, O. Y., & Littleford, C. D. (1997). Motor imitation in young children with autism: What's the object? *Journal of Abnormal Child Psychology, 25*(6), 475–485.

Wakschlag, A. S., & Leventhal, B. L. (1996). Consultation with young autistic children and their families. *Journal of American Academy of Child and Adolescent Psychiatry, 35*(7), 963–965.

Wetherby, A. M., & Prizant, B. M. (1999). Enhancing language and communication development in autism: Assessment and intervention guidelines. In D. B. Zager (Ed.), *Autism: Identification, education, and treatment* (pp. 141–174). Mahwah, NJ: Erlbaum.

Whaley, K. T., & Shaw, E. (Eds.). (1999, July). *National early childhood technical assistance system (NECTAS) resource collection on autism spectrum disorders.* Chapel Hill, NC: NECTAS.

Wing, L. (1997). The history of ideas on autism; Legends, myths and reality. *Autism: The International Journal of Research and Practice, 1*(1), 13–23.

Wolery, M., & Brookfield-Norman, J. (1988). (Pre)academic instruction for handicapped preschool children. In S. L. Oldom & M. B. Karnes (Eds.), *Early intervention for infants and children with handicaps: An empirical base.* Baltimore: Paul H. Brookes.

World Health Organization. (1992). *The ICD-10 classification of mental and behavioral disorders: Diagnostic criteria for research.* Geneva: Author.

CHAPTER 16

Medical Art Therapy with Children

Tracy Councill

Medical applications of art therapy are a natural extension of the use of art therapy with psychiatric populations. The fundamental qualities that make the creative process empowering to children in general can be profoundly normalizing agents for those undergoing medical treatment. When the ill child engages in art making, he or she is in charge of the work—the materials to be used; the scope, intent, and imagery; when the piece is finished; and whether it will be retained or discarded. All these factors are under the child artist's control. Participating in creative work within the medical setting can help rebuild the young patient's sense of hope, self-esteem, autonomy, and competence while offering opportunities for safe and contained expression of feelings.

Art therapy has been used with a variety of pediatric medical populations, including cancer, kidney disease, juvenile rheumatoid arthritis, chronic pain, and severe burns (Malchiodi, 1999). When medical art therapy is included as part of team treatment, art expression is used by young patients to communicate perceptions, needs, and wishes to art therapists, mental health professionals, child life specialists, and medical personnel. It is extremely useful in assessing each young patient's strengths, coping styles, and cognitive development. Information gathered through artworks can be invaluable to the medical team as it seeks to treat the whole person, not just the disease or diagnosis.

WHAT A MEDICAL DIAGNOSIS MEANS

The diagnosis of a serious illness or injury is a catastrophic blow to the young patient and the family's fundamental sense of trust and well-being. The onset of a serious illness is often experienced as a bolt out of the blue, robbing the child and family of the normal routines and functional illusion that bad things happen to other people. Though adults may become ill as a result of destructive lifestyle choices or the aging process, children are expected to grow and flourish. Although some serious disorders result from a hereditary cause, and the family may be somewhat prepared when they manifest in a child, many other diseases occur without explanation. For example, most childhood cancers are diagnosed unexpectedly and without a known cause: A cell in the body is manufactured incorrectly and the replication of that error becomes the process of disease.

In his famous book, *When Bad Things Happen to Good People*, Kushner (1989) explores the universal human wish for an explanation for misfortune. Painful as they are, guilt and self-blame offer the comfort of an explanation. During my early years as an art therapist with pediatric cancer patients, I worked with an 8-year-old boy whose play and artwork evolved around the theme of punishment. The characters in his art and play were always being punished, though what they had done wrong was never clear. After working with him for some time without movement from this constant theme, I decided to interpret his play and art expressions to him in words. "You know," I said, "doctors and nurses don't know exactly why kids get cancer, but they do know it isn't their fault. Cancer isn't a punishment, it's when a person's cells don't work right." He stopped what he was working on, looked me straight in the eye and said, "So you mean I got sick for nothing?" "Well, kind of," I said, "but we do know it isn't your fault." In my effort to replace what I felt was a mistaken assumption with a compassionate truth, I had challenged his explanation. Though he had heard these words before from his doctors and nurses, our work together in art and play allowed him to consider for the first time an alternative explanation for his guilt.

The hospital setting itself can be a source of both hope and distress to the ill child and his or her family. Though naming a condition and beginning treatment offer hope for cure and relief from suffering, the medical environment itself can feel like a foreign land. Medical terminology is a new language that must suddenly be mastered. The hospitalized patient, surrounded by the sights, smells, sounds, and rhythms of the medical environment, may feel transplanted into an alien culture (Spinetta & Spinetta, 1981). A visit from the art therapist, a grown-up who brings art materials and an invitation to draw or paint, instead of needles or pills to swallow, can be instantly comforting to a frightened child. Whether that first encounter leads to an expressive piece of artwork or just a few simple marks, it can establish a meaningful link to life outside the hospital and provide a concrete way to respond to the hospital experience.

ART-BASED ASSESSMENT WITHIN THE MEDICAL SETTING

There are some general considerations in assessing medically ill children. Theories of personality and cognitive development are fundamental and a therapist with a good command of these concepts can be invaluable to the parents and the medical team in helping them anticipate and meet the ill child's needs along the way. For example, knowing that a toddler, who is beginning to assert some independence and identity, may react to treatment with fits of anger and regression can help parents decide how best to respond to their little one's behavior. The school-age youngster, who may become demanding, irritable, and emotionally labile in the face of his or her loss of relative independence, can make use of creative strategies to use words and symbols to express feelings and assert mastery. Generally, the older the child, the greater the emotional impact of the losses associated with serious illness. Older children have more independence to lose, and yet they have likely developed a broader range of interests and strategies for meeting life's challenges than have their younger counterparts. The capable therapist adapts art materials and processes to many levels of sophistication so that any young participant can find a creative voice through art.

In the medical environment, it is also important to understand how children of various ages think about their bodies and about the concept of death. For example, young children may regard the body as a bag of blood and fear that venipuncture for a blood test will cause all their blood to flow out. They can be reassured by a simple explanation of how blood flows through the body and by drawing a picture of what the body looks like inside. I sometimes use a body tracing as a starting point for a life-size collage, asking children to place red ribbons inside the outline where the blood goes, plastic bubble wrap for lungs, popsicle sticks for bones, and so on. This exercise helps the therapist to understand the child's perceptions and provides the opportunity to offer information that may correct misunderstandings and allay fears.

Most young children believe that death is reversible. They tend to be more concerned about being abandoned by their caregivers than about dying. Young children are often preoccupied with fears of bodily harm and physical integrity. They may understand that death is permanent, but they often interpret illness or death as a punishment. Older children generally have a more sophisticated understanding of death, but it is normal for adolescents to believe themselves to be invincible. Coping with the demands of illness and treatment may push young people to emotional maturity beyond their years, resulting in a sense of being "different" from their peers.

Susan Bach (1990), a Jungian analyst who for many years collected pictures drawn by hospitalized children, has developed a system of analyzing children's artwork to aid in understanding disease processes and predicting eventual outcomes and children's experiences of death and dying. She feels that certain graphic messages point to processes of physical healing or degeneration, stemming from the child's "inner knowingness" of the state of his body and his fate (p. 185). Her work presents a fascinating interpretation of symbols, colors, and pictorial composition, challenging the therapist to remain open to the expression of children's unconscious wisdom through art expression.

One of the great values of art therapy is its capacity to call attention to the patient's strengths. Elinor Ulman, in her work with the chronically mentally ill, stressed an appreciation of the patient's strengths as part of the personality assessment (Ulman & Levy, 1975). Understood as a way of discovering strengths, art therapy can be a bridge from the sad and lonely places of illness to the joy of human connection and understanding.

For example, a 7-year-old leukemia patient experienced an idiosyncratic reaction to medication that caused her to exhibit strange seizure-like episodes with repetitive motions and verbalizations, arising spontaneously and resolving without intervention. Her symptoms did not easily fit the expected pattern of organic etiology, so I was asked to contribute to the assessment, specifically to determine whether she was pretending to have these "fits" to get attention. In one of the art evaluation sessions, she created a dramatic marker drawing of an opera singer in Verdian costume, mouth open wide, occupying center stage. The story she told about the picture was that the singer had been kidnapped and held captive deep in the woods. She was singing as loudly as she could so her lover would come and rescue her (Figure 16.1). The picture was reassuring in its sustained attention, integrated composition and sure execution, suggesting that her cognitive functions remained intact.

The main character's placement on center stage might well suggest attention-seeking behavior, but the most compelling aspect of the picture was its unmistakable cry for help: A frightened and lonely figure stood alone in the woods, waiting to be rescued. Whether or not her seizures bought her secondary gains, she was able to use graphic media to send a message to the health care team that she needed and wanted their help. Through consultation with other institutions, her condition was soon di-

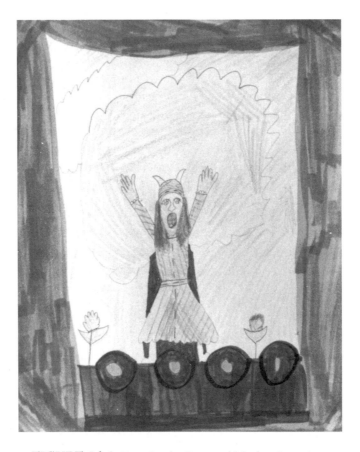

FIGURE 16.1. Drawing by 7-year-old leukemia patient.

agnosed as a rare side effect of a particular medication. Her medications were changed, and the strange episodes no longer occurred.

Art therapists have developed many methods of evaluating personality through art, but the limitations of the medical environment, especially the difficulty of securing a private space for a long period, can make some art-based assessments difficult to administer. Based on my experience with pediatric cancer patients, I suggest the following art-based assessments as a prelude to treatment:

- Clinical assessments such as those developed by Rubin (1984), Kramer (Kramer & Schehr, 1983), and Ulman (Ulman & Levy, 1975) can yield a wealth of information, especially if there is concern that the child may have underlying psychopathology beyond adjustment to illness. Rubin (1984) emphasizes spontaneous artwork and careful observation in her Diagnostic Art Interview. Kramer recommends encouraging the child to try a variety of art media in an open-ended art interview, evaluating the child's approach to the media as well as his or her reflections on the artworks produced. Ulman's personality assessment tool may be used with older teenagers and young adults. It combines "free pictures" and directed tasks to elicit information about the client's ability to organize his or her thoughts into visual expression, as well as eliciting pictures with meaningful content.
- The Child Diagnostic Drawing Series (CDDS), developed by Sobol and Cox (1992), is another procedure that combines free drawings and directed tasks. The authors are collecting data in an effort to statistically validate the interpretation of their instrument. This measure may have the added benefit of scientific measurement in addition to interpretation in the context of the art therapy literature—an important consideration when art therapy is part of medical research. These assessments are perhaps the best known and most used in the field of art therapy, but they all require an extended period of uninterrupted time.

There are two one-drawing measures that may yield important information about medical patients:

- A drawing of Person Picking an Apple from a Tree (PPAT) (Gantt, 1990; Lowenfeld & Lambert-Brittain, 1975) is useful in evaluating coping ability and resourcefulness. This drawing asks the child to depict someone solving a problem—picking an apple from a tree—and expresses strategies children may employ when encountering obstacles in real life.
- A drawing of a bridge going from one place to another and including oneself on the bridge (Hays & Lyons, 1981) can yield information about the patient's perception of the present and expectations of the future. This can be an important question for patients facing life-threatening illnesses or making the transition to home following a long hospital stay.

Both of these drawing tasks are ways to encourage metaphoric expressions about life experiences, as opposed to full personality assessments. They must be reserved for patients who can accomplish recognizable representations and generally are no younger than 5 years of age.

Assessment of patients' adjustment to illness and/or injury is an important aspect of medical art therapy. Valerie Appleton (2001) has developed an Art Therapy Trauma and Assessment Paradigm for use with young people who have experienced traumatic burn injuries. She proposes four stages, each characterized by specific psychosocial issues, art themes, and graphic features. Her model is based on stages of emotional reactions to trauma identified by Lee (1970), but Appleton has expanded them to include the following art therapy goals: Stage I. Impact: Creating Continuity, Stage II. Retreat: Building a Therapeutic Alliance, Stage III. Acknowledgment: Overcoming Social Stigma and Isolation through Mastery, and Stage IV. Reconstruction: Fostering Meaning. With such a model as a framework, art therapists can better understand the significance of clients' graphic messages and assess their progress in adapting to life circumstances that have been changed by traumatic injury.

Evaluating artistic development is essential to any therapist working with children. It is important for the therapist to recognize the developmental stages in children's artwork and possible indications of pathology, from emotional distress to organic brain damage. Although there is no formal assessment to evaluate children's artistic development, therapists should be familiar with *The Child's Creation of a Pictorial World* (Golomb, 1992). This volume is an excellent reference on development and art, as are Lowenfeld & Lambert-Brittain's (1975) *Creative and Mental Growth* and Gardner's (1980) *Artful Scribbles: The Significance of Children's Drawings*. Spontaneous pictures, too, can help the art therapist understand the patient's strengths, skills, and understanding, especially when children discuss the meaning of their artwork with the therapist.

There is no one correct way to assess medical patients through art. It is important that therapists receive training in how to administer and interpret specific assessments and that they remain open to the multidimensional meanings and interpretations supplied by the client.

ART THERAPY WITH PEDIATRIC PATIENTS

Art therapy is beneficial to children for many reasons, but there are several reasons that are particularly compelling with pediatric patients.

Rebuilding a Sense of Well-Being

Making art, the uniquely human act of creating meaning out of formless materials, can be a powerful vehicle for rebuilding the medical patient's sense of well-being. Offering familiar materials with the skilled therapist's support can reassure the ill child that he or she is still a person with a great deal to offer. Edith Kramer (1979) recognized the intrinsic power of the artistic process to bring order to the chaos within. When a child is ill, words often fail, either because the child's vocabulary does not match the experience or because the ill child feels he must protect the adults around him from his feelings (Bluebond-Langner, 1978).

Engendering Hope

Snyder et al. (1997) theorize that "children who think hopefully can imagine and embrace goals related to the successful treatment of their physical problems . . . children with health problems need to focus upon new goals, find alternative ways to do things, and muster the mental energy to begin and continue treatment regimens" (pp. 400–401). Creating art is a safe vehicle for self-expression: It can start from just a squiggle or a line, and it is the artist who decides what to include, when the work is finished, and what it means. In particular, art therapy with physically ill children helps them practice the hope-engendering process of creating art. The child and the therapist work together to choose materials, set goals, and plan the means to achieve them. The finished product is tangible evidence that the ill child can accomplish a great deal. This kind of achievement helps transform the ill child from the passive victim of a disease into an active partner in the work of getting well.

Gaining a Sense of Mastery

Art therapy can be used to help young patients gain a sense of mastery over troubling events. As treatments become more effective, the medical community is learning more about the impact of illness and treatment on those who are cured of their disease. In the study of childhood cancers, there is a growing body of literature about "late effects," the long-term effects of cancer treatment on young survivors. Posttraumatic stress disorder is increasingly being appreciated in cancer survivors and their parents, especially at times of developmental transition (Rourke, Stuber, Hobbie, & Kazak, 1999). The disorder is characterized by a cluster of reexperiencing, avoidance, and arousal symptoms associated with experiencing or witnessing an event that is perceived as a threat to the bodily integrity of the self or a loved one (American Psychiatric Association, 1994). According to Rourke, "a model of posttraumatic stress, in which cancer and treatment are seen as life-threatening events with the potential for precipitating trauma reactions, appears to explain the ways in which child and adolescent survivors of cancer and their parents react to diagnosis and treatment" (Rourke et al., 1999, p. 130). Stuber, Cristakis, Houskaamp, and Kazak (1996) suggest that supportive intervention, both during and after treatment, can diminish the traumatic effects of treatment and help patients better integrate their experiences.

In a long-term research project aimed at promoting integration of traumatic experiences, Chapman, Morabito, Ladakakos, Schrier, and Knudson (2001) describe a study of an art therapy intervention targeted specifically to reduce symptoms of PTSD in children treated at a large, urban hospital trauma center. Chapman's procedure, the Chapman Art Therapy Treatment Intervention or CAATI, is designed for "incident-specific, medical trauma to provide an opportunity for the child to sequentially relate and cognitively comprehend the traumatic event, transport to the hospital, emergency care, hospitalization and treatment regimen, and posthospital care and adjustment" (p. 101).

When art therapy can be offered during treatment, difficult experiences can be described in art, encouraging steps toward mastery of troubling feelings. One 7-year-old being treated for cancer developed a highly contagious infection that required her to be isolated from other patients for a period of several months. The infection was not dangerous to those with normal immune function, but it posed a significant threat to other clinic and hospital patients. She was not well enough to attend school, go to movies, play sports, and take part in many other activities during her medical treatment, so the added isolation from others at the outpatient center was a powerful loss for her.

Though her therapists were able to develop ways to work with her safely without spreading the infection, she attempted less and less in art as the period of isolation wore on. When she was finally free of the infection and could rejoin the waiting-room art sessions, her first creation was an elaborate clay sculpture of an igloo, complete with an Eskimo to inhabit it, a dog, a supply of food, and a fire to keep him warm. (Figure 16.2) As she explained it, "he has everything he needs, but no people." Her work seemed a detailed and matter-of-fact reflection of her experience of prolonged isolation. Other patients in my experience have depicted procedures they found anxiety-provoking, especially diagnostic scans and radiation therapy. These procedures may be especially troubling to children because they must be alone during treatment and the forces acting on their bodies are both invisible and intangible. Drawing the treatment setting, the machinery used, and sometimes themselves receiving the treatment gives them the opportunity to revisit the experience and assert mastery over it by bringing it into the shared reality of therapist and client (Figure 16.3).

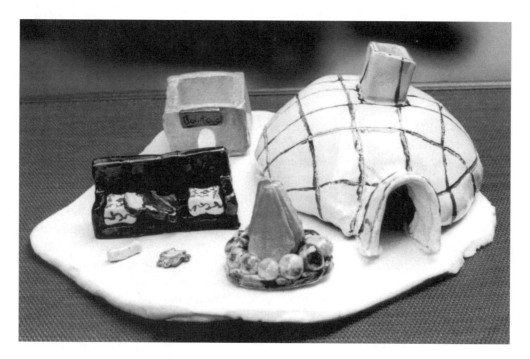

FIGURE 16.2. Clay sculpture of an igloo by young patient.

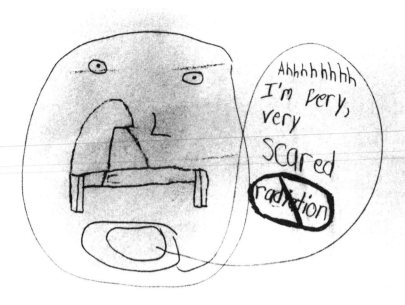

FIGURE 16.3. Drawing of the radiation therapy machine.

MIND–BODY CONSIDERATIONS

For the past decade or so there has been a great deal of emphasis on the relationship between physical well-being and emotional states. *Healing and the Mind* (Moyers, 1993) helped these concepts reach a larger audience. Practitioners in many disciplines, from doctors of conventional medicine to specialists in acupuncture and biofeedback, have explored the complex interrelationships between illness, healing, and the unconscious messages that inform our perceptions of the self and the world. For example, minimizing the perception of pain through self-hypnosis and dissociation has been at the core of natural childbirth education for many years and is routinely employed to help patients who experience chronic pain. Mobilizing the immune system by expressing emotions and avoiding illness by positive thinking are the subjects of both serious scientific inquiry and supermarket tabloids. The new emphasis on preventive medicine and education to encourage healthy lifestyle choices has helped normalize ideas that once seemed far-fetched.

The power of art therapy to support affective expression, assist clients in experiencing feelings of mastery and relaxation, and help individuals develop and practice their own healing meditations has integrated the principles of mind–body and the discipline of art therapy. For example, art therapist Carol DeLue (1999) studied the physiological response of school-age children to the task of creating mandala drawings. Using biofeedback techniques, she concluded that simply drawing within a circular outline produces a physiologically measurable relaxation response. Relaxation has long been linked to reducing the subjective experience of pain and increasing cooperation with medical procedures.

Dr. Bernie Siegel (1990) and many others write of the significance of self-discovery in the resolution or improvement of cancers in adults. Adults with cancer often reflect on their life histories, priorities, and relationships, usually in anticipation of death. Sometimes it is reported that these individuals discover and reintegrate long-denied aspects of themselves, and in some instances spontaneous remission of their cancer follows. Carmen Zammit (2001) reports on such a case study using art therapy as a medium to facilitate the patient's journey of self-reclamation and the corresponding spontaneous and durable remission of the patient's cancer. She describes a process whereby adults may use the creative process to gain insight into life choices that contribute to illness and make changes that facilitate health.

Children's illnesses are likely not related to lifestyle choices and problems in intrapsychic development, yet the artwork of ill children most often speaks from an intuitive place of wisdom. Susan Bach (1990) advances a system of interpretation of graphic messages in the artwork of ill children that she feels can predict treatment outcomes based on visual cues in their drawings. In a stunning example from my own work, a young boy drew a one-legged "Anger Monster" during a period of remission from his leukemia. I was so impressed by the drawing that I asked our medical team to evaluate his leg. No problem could be detected at that time, but two years later the boy's cancer returned in the form of a lesion in his right leg—matching the spot where the drawn Anger Monster's leg had been cut off. Spontaneous artwork may add useful information to medical evaluations, both as an indicator of emotional adjustment and a graphic representation of physical symptoms.

A boy of 9 who would eventually die from a brain tumor created a painting of a bright blue and orange butterfly and inscribed it "I'm Healthy!" The butterfly was his contribution to the annual Pediatric Oncology Art Exhibit that year, but it reflected a medical status contradictory to objective measures. His tumor was not responding well to treatment, but it would grow slowly, allowing him several years of life marked by a gradual loss of functioning. When he painted his butterfly, he was aware that his tumor was still growing despite aggressive treatment, but his artwork spoke with authority about his experience of himself. There was a marked contrast between his perception of himself as a whole person and the scientific measure of his condition. His resilient personality, his family's support, and his work in art therapy enabled him to experience and affirm his healthy self in the midst of years of struggle with cancer. This perception helped him maintain a core sense of self-esteem and well-being even as he lost many cognitive and physical functions.

Medical illness can place profound stress on patients and their family systems. Treatment for a chronic illness may go on for many years, requiring adaptation by every member of the family. The health within the family system prior to diagnosis is a well-documented predictor of the child's adaptation to illness and treatment. A 1998 study of families of patients with sickle cell disease links behavioral problems in child patients with caregivers' self-ratings of hostility, anxiety, and depression (Ievers, Brown, Lambert, Hsu, & Eckman, 1998).

Access to medical care itself can be a significant family stressor. It is not uncommon for patients to temporarily relocate to a medical center far from home where some specialized treatment is available. A 7-year-old boy in just such a situation exhibited very fragile defenses, withdrawing in tearful regression and noncompliance with medical treatment whenever he felt frustrated or out of control. The concerted efforts of the art therapists and the entire health care team, including supporting his mother in devising new strategies for setting limits on her son, enabled this angry and frightened boy to find more effective strategies for managing and expressing his emotions. He and his mother together made many expressive sculptures in clay during the course of his treatment, including a 10-inch-high sculpture of a volcano. He caused the volcano to erupt at many clinic visits using baking soda, vinegar, and red tempera paint to create a satisfyingly dramatic discharge of metaphorical lava.

Investigators have documented increased compliance with medical regimens by those who receive education about their medications and encouragement to take responsibility for administering them (Richardson, Shelton, Krailo, & Levine, 1990). Creating art can also be a powerful component of caring for oneself. Art media can be used to develop representations of an individual's relaxation cues: A drawing of a safe place can be a comforting addition to the hospital room, and a cue to practice taking an imaginary journey to that safe place when being in the hospital feels overwhelming.

Chronic pain patients can diminish the isolation they often feel when their pain seems unappreciated by the medical team by creating their own pain scales, locating their pain within body outlines, or creating images to symbolize their pain. Creating a visual representation of their experience, and perhaps even discussing it with health care providers, can bridge the gap of frustration that patients often feel when their symptoms do not abate despite pharmacological intervention.

When materials can be made available, patients can enhance the treatment environment by creating their own mobiles, tabletop fountains, or other artwork for use as distraction during painful procedures or as aids to relaxation. Displaying children's art in the treatment space can promote feelings of pride, acceptance, and safety, encouraging children to forge alliances with the medical team because they feel they are known and appreciated as whole human beings.

CONCLUSION

Children coping with medical conditions face many physical and emotional challenges. They must at times relax developmentally appropriate defenses to allow medical intervention and endure long periods of isolation from peers, school, and home. Simultaneously, they must somehow accept the idea that treatments that are at least unpleasant and often painful are working for their benefit.

Art therapy brings familiar materials and the universal language of visual expression to the foreign land of medicine. Through artwork and a sensitive therapist, ill children can respond to their situation with meaning and purpose. Judy Rubin (1984) conveys a profound trust in the ability of children to find ways to use the creative process to heal themselves. When art therapy is available to ill children, many pathways can be found to offer emotional support and connection in very stressful circumstances.

Art therapy in the medical setting offers the potential for humanizing the health care experience and empowering patients to engage their intuitive, creative wisdom in the work of getting well. Listening to patients and helping them find ways to tap their inner resources through art expression is the cornerstone of art therapy. Medical art therapy offers a modality that is at once comforting, challenging, and enjoyable, giving children hope and a voice in expressing their experience of serious and life-threatening illness.

REFERENCES

American Psychiatric Association. (1994). *Diagnostic and statistical manual of mental disorders* (4th ed.). Washington, DC: Author.

Appleton, V. (2001). Avenues of hope: Art therapy and the resolution of trauma. *Art Therapy, 18*(1), 6–13.

Bach, S. (1990). *Life paints its own span*. Einsiedeln, Switzerland: Daimon Verlag.

Bluebond-Langner, M. (1978). *The private worlds of dying children*. Princeton, NJ: Princeton University Press.

Chapman, L., Morabito, D., Ladakakos, C., Schrier, H., & Knudson, M. M. (2001). The effectiveness of art therapy intervention in reducing posttraumatic stress disorder (PTSD) symptoms in pediatric trauma patients. *Art Therapy, 18*(2), 100–104.

DeLue, C. (1999). Physiological effects of creating mandalas. In C. Malchiodi (Ed.), *Medical art therapy with children* (pp. 33–49). Philadelphia: Jessica Kingsley.

Gantt, L. (1990). *A validity study of the formal elements of an art therapy scale for diagnostic information in patients' drawings*. Unpublished doctoral dissertation, University of Pittsburgh.

Gardner, H. (1980). *Artful scribbles: The significance of children's drawings*. New York: Basic Books.

Golomb, C. (1992). *The child's creation of a pictorial world*. Los Angeles: University of California Press.

Hays, R. E., & Lyons, S. (1981). The bridge drawing: A projective technique for assessment in art therapy. *The Arts in Psychotherapy, 8*, 207–217.

Ievers, C. E., Brown, R. T., Lambert, R. G., Hsu, L., & Eckman, J. R. (1998). Family functioning and social support in the adaptation of caregivers of children with sickle cell syndromes. *Journal of Pediatric Psychology, 23*(6), 377–388.

Kramer, E. (1979). *Childhood and art therapy*. New York: Schocken.

Kramer, E., & Schehr, J. (1983). An art therapy evaluation session for children. *American Journal of Art Therapy, 23*, 3–12.

Kushner, H. (1989). *When bad things happen to good people*. New York: Avon.

Lee, J. M. (1970). Emotional reactions to trauma. *Nursing Clinics of North America, 5*(4), 577–587.

Lowenfeld, V., & Lambert-Brittain, W. (1975). *Creative and mental growth* (6th ed.). New York: Macmillan.

Malchiodi, C. A. (Ed.). (1999). *Medical art therapy with children*. London: Jessica Kingsley.

Moyers, B. (1993). *Healing and the mind*. New York: Doubleday.

Richardson, J. L., Shelton, D. R., Krailo, M., & Levine, A. M. (1990). The effect of compliance with treatment on survival among patients with hematologic malignancies. *Journal of Clinical Oncology, 8*(2), 356–364.

Rourke, M. T., Stuber, M. L., Hobbie, W. L., & Kazak, A. E. (1999). Posttraumatic stress disorder: Understanding the psychosocial impact of surviving childhood cancer into young adulthood. *Journal of Pediatric Oncology Nursing, 16*(3), 126–135.

Rubin, J. (1984). *Child art therapy*. New York: Van Nostrand Reinhold.

Siegel, B. S. (1990). *Love, medicine and miracles.* New York: Harper & Row.

Snyder, C. R., Hoza, B., Pelham, W. E., Rapoff, M., Ware, L., Danovsky, M., Highberger, L., Rubenstein, H., & Stahl, K. (1997). The development and validation of the children's hope scale. *Journal of Pediatric Psychology, 22*(3), 399–421.

Sobol, B., & Cox, C. T. (Speakers). (1992). *Art and childhood dissociation: Research with sexually abused children* (Cassette Recording No. 59-144). Denver, CO: National Audio-Video.

Spinetta, J. J., & Spinetta, D. (1981). *Living with childhood cancer.* St. Louis, MO: Mosby.

Stuber, M. L., Cristakis, D. A., Houskaamp, B., & Kazak, A. E. (1996). Post-trauma symptoms in childhood leukemia survivors and their parents. *Psychosomatics, 37*(3), 254–261.

Ulman, E., & Levy, B. (1975). An experimental approach to the judgment of psychopathology from paintings. In E. Ulman & P. Dachinger (Eds.), *Art therapy in theory and practice* (pp. 393–402). New York: Schocken.

Zammitt, C. (2001). The art of healing: A journey through cancer, implications for art therapy. *Art Therapy, 18*(1), 27–36.

CHAPTER 17

Using Art Therapy to Address Adolescent Depression

Shirley Riley

The years between the onset of puberty and the final stages of adolescence magnify traits that can be channeled into art therapy activities (Allen, 1988). Narcissistic focus, issues of power between teens and adults, and exploration and questioning of values can be expressed through artwork. Art therapy allows adolescents to express these experiences, to verbally share or not share the content of their art products, and to respond to any interpretation that the adult (therapist) might make about their creations.

This chapter discusses art therapy as a particularly effective modality with adolescent depression, a common complicating factor in this age group (Connor, 2002; Kendall, 2000). Traditional verbal therapies may fail to help adolescents with depression, because their resistance to therapy is so strong and their sense of disillusionment is so pervasive. However, if the therapist enters the adolescent's depressive world view by offering art as a means of communication, there is a good possibility of creating some alternative visions for these despondent youth. Art therapy provides a viable vehicle of treatment, a lens for viewing adolescents' perceptions through their own illustrations and narratives. Art making is less confrontive, less familiar, less judgmental, and without contamination from customary words that this age group often finds unacceptable.

OVERVIEW OF ADOLESCENT DEPRESSION

There is general agreement about the signs and behaviors that indicate adolescent depression (Bloch, 1995; Cyrtryn & McKnew, 1999; Goodyer, 2001; Kendall, 2000; Kopelwitz, Klass, & Kafantaris, 1993). Most agree that the classic indicators of depression in adults do not apply to teenagers. Adolescents are more likely to exhibit school problems, learning disabilities, social difficulties, and somatic symptoms (headaches, stomachaches) (Achenbach, 1991), and their depression is often central to a variety of emotional and behavioral disorders. Research has shown that the presence of depressed mood, whether based on the teenager's or the parents' reports, is the most significant single symptom separating adolescents referred to clinical treatment from those who are not (Achenbach, 1991).

Parry-Jones (1989) notes that "masked depression" takes the form of restless boredom, poor school performance, somatic symptoms, fatigue, promiscuity, and drug and alcohol abuse. Teenagers may also be angry or aggressive, as opposed to the lassitude of adult depression, and will generally act out feelings. Malmquist (1978) proposed that a large percentage of acting-out and delinquent behaviors are used to relieve depressive pain and self-deprecation. These acts demonstrate the anger that adolescents feel, and the resulting negative consequences are preferable to the experience of depression. In my clinical experience, I have observed that many adolescents substantiate the existence of depression after exploring reasons for acting-out behaviors. Because adolescents tend to act out their depression, there is an opportunity for an active therapy to be effective. Art is one action that can be used therapeutically and can be conformed to the needs of the adolescent client.

It is also important for the therapist to recognize the difference between normal and often exaggerated mood swings of adolescence and more serious and pervasive signs of chronic depression in this age group. Therapy will be more effective if the clinician understands the normal tasks of adolescence and the fluctuations that occur with the psychological and physiological changes of this age group (Parry-Jones, 1989). The greatest challenge to the therapist is to untangle all the various symptomatic behaviors of depression because some may be part of the teen's stage of maturation and others may be reactions to life circumstances, or even physical illness (Kendall, 2000).

Talk of suicide is, of course, always to be taken seriously. Waiting for absolute certainty that there is serious attempt at suicide is often too late. Any crisis that a depressed adolescent relates or expresses through art requires prompt intervention. Figure 17.1, a drawing by an adolescent, leaves nothing to the imagination. The drawing contains a grave that is isolated and barren, drawn in a manner that evokes a sense of bleakness and gloom. The adolescent has reinforced the underlying message through words written on the drawing: frustration, sorrow, miserable, depression, alone, help, and desire to die. An art expression such as this one is a powerful condensation of a verbal narrative of suicidal intent. For a therapist or any helping professional not to take the message of this drawing seriously would be a mistake.

ISSUES CONTRIBUTING TO ADOLESCENT DEPRESSION

The following sections address some of the major issues that induce or exacerbate depression in adolescents and how art therapy can be used to engage them in productive therapeutic exchange.

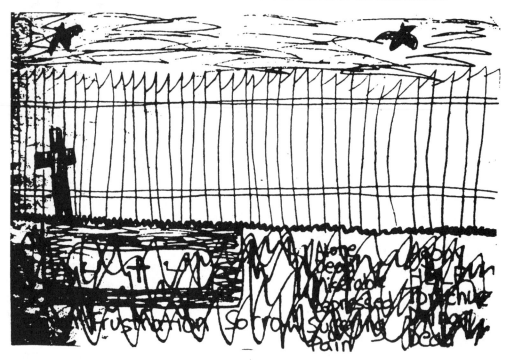

FIGURE 17.1. Example of drawing revealing depression by adolescent.

Peer Group Rejection

Acceptance or rejection by the peer group activates manifestations of adolescent depression. As adolescents turn away from parents in the struggle to individuate, they turn to their peers as a substitute for guidance and support. Unfortunately, the narcissism of this age leaves adolescents constantly seeking the approval of the group, and rejection by peers is a major source of depression.

For example, an attractive blonde Caucasian girl was shunned by her peers at the middle school she attended. Her parents were American, but the girl had been raised in Mexico City and considered herself to be a Mexican. She had proficiency in English, but it was actually her second language. Because of this cultural confusion, she did not respond to her peers at her new school in California; they decided she was "uppity" and called her a liar.

The girl struggled with this issue in an adolescent therapy group. She made a poignant drawing of a broken egg depicting her depression and loss of her friends in Mexico. The drawing helped her to convey her desperation to other group members and encourage them to give her the support she needed.

Societal and Familial Stress

Adolescents may be exposed to a variety of external stresses, including socioeconomic factors, living in dangerous neighborhood, or discrimination because of race or color. The perils of drug and alcohol abuse, violent victimization, and delinquency are widespread, cutting across family demographics, including those with stability, middle-class advantages, and parental love (Sandmier, 1996). Adolescents also face stresses within their own families, including physical or verbal abuse, neglect, poverty, divorce, and parental unemployment. Both societal and familial stressors can create a depressive environment, and under these circumstances, adolescents' depression is appropriate and should not be pathologized except when there is real pathology in the system (Hiscox, 1993).

Riley and Malchiodi (1994) note that societal stress such as street violence or riots have been the subject of adolescent art expression. For example, during the riots in Watts, a subsection of Los Angeles, adolescents frequently made images of being "jailed." They did not depict the violence they witnessed as much as they did the confinement to their homes which they experienced for days in order to be protected from the riots on the streets. This jail image has surfaced subsequently in other situations in which adolescents have been forced to remain in their homes or away from their schools because their parents were fearful of violence or harm to their children.

Despite the focus on the peer group, family relationships are still an important source of stability for adolescents, and stress within the family can have serious consequences at this time of transition and change (Gotlib & Hammen, 2002). The following example is one of the most poignant cases of the emotional stress and depression evoked by a parent's behavior toward his stepson.

Eddie was a 14-year-old teen in the adolescent group. He rarely spoke and had a depressed affect. He was tall for his age, fair, and did not have a strong muscular build. He was facile in art and joined in the art tasks but initially refrained from discussion. When the group was asked to picture "how other peers saw them," he drew a pajama clad asexual figure dancing behind bars with the word "Queen" written as the title (Figure 17.2). Eddie did not share the meaning behind the drawing. However, from that meeting on he felt free to draw violent pictures of hanging and burning his parents and pouring boiling oil on them as he tried to escape to join his dead grandparents.

Gradually, Eddie's story emerged. His stepfather was convinced, on the basis of his physical appearance, that Eddie was gay. He taunted Eddie unmercifully and, perhaps, even convinced Eddie that it was true. Eddie recited many stories about how his stepfather's treatment of him bordered on abuse.

Another group member made the proper therapeutic move. Sally was tough, sexually active, and often at risk of being raped and overdosing on drugs because of her behavior. She had a special place in group as the "experienced girl." When Eddie told of being ridiculed because he was gay, the group was enraged. Sally looked directly at Eddie and said, "Screw him (stepfather), I would F——you any day!!" The group cheered, Eddie smiled, and he stopped being afraid of what his stepfather said to him. His manhood had been confirmed!

Solutions such as these give a therapist pause. I am certain that few other statements would have made that great a difference to that boy. The stepfather was brought into the clinic and clearly informed that he was emotionally abusive and it must stop. The family was followed closely, and it appeared that the home situation greatly improved when the mother recognized how destructive this kind of taunting could be.

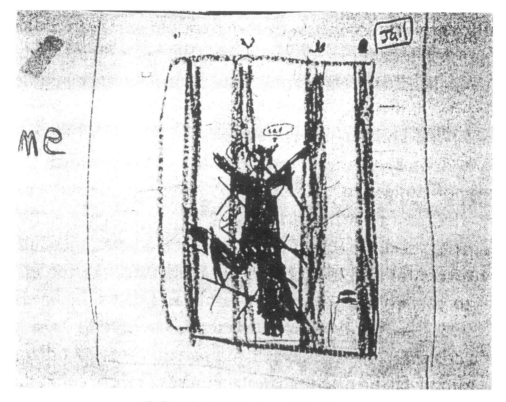

FIGURE 17.2. "A Queen behind bars."

It is interesting to think about the process that gave Eddie the tools he needed to disregard a negative projection that questioned his gender identification. He practiced making a verbal statement through his explicit art products that revealed his anger and his confusion. The art gave him courage to verbalize his abusive situation and his peer group (particularly a girl) repudiated the negative image.

All these steps were necessary to give Eddie the psychological equipment that he needed to refute the assault on his identity. The art expressions were also the key to unblock revelation of the trauma he was experiencing. The art he used was violent and aggressive and gave permission for him to silently disclose his misery. He was not psychologically capable of expressing these violent feelings until he was able to control them. The art acted as a form of gradual release until the time came that words were not so frightening. The conclusion of this process was a privilege to observe.

GENDER AND SEXUAL ISSUES

Adolescence is a period not only of emotional and cognitive change but also of puberty, the physical, gender-defining development. Who has not met the 12-year-old who is gangling toward 6 feet and still is family dependent and immature? Next to him or her in the classroom is the class genius who is readying for college and still has no facial hair to be seen. These discrepancies between the body and the mind can be enormously painful for the teen to endure.

In addition, there is the overriding concern about sex. Hormones come to the forefront before the physical signs are noticeable. The early adolescent is raging with fantasies and not yet ready to put them into action. During a teen's early adolescence, parents are shocked by transformation in attitude when their son or daughter has not yet physically shown signs of change (Nolen-Hoeksema, 2002).

Using gender-appropriate intervention in treatment is one way to engage adolescents in art therapy. In one group I had difficulty interesting the girls in any type of media or task. The girls were from a low economic group and had little or no exposure to any form of cultural imagery other than their own. They all were having difficulties at school and were angry with their parents but denied any sense of failure or unhappiness. Culturally, they were encouraged to look to an early marriage as their only goal, and the girls had all been sexually active by the age of 12 to 14 years. These girls (see Riley, 2001) were hopelessly disengaged from the therapy and used the hour to improve their makeup.

After a long period of frustration I decided to follow the group's lead. I helped them to draw an "ideal" girl's face, someone who was successful and happy. Following each teen's instructions, I drew a "beautiful" girl's face. The girls colored in and enhanced the drawings with their own cosmetics as a medium. As they decorated these idealized faces and talked through these "made-up" mouths, the girls acknowledged they were having some feelings and questions about the rules of their culture. They shared that they were angry and depressed at their status as second-rate citizens and handmaidens to more powerful males. The paper faces that were covered with lipstick, eye shadow, and foundation found a voice.

ADDRESSING RESISTANCE

The previous case is a good example of how to address resistance in art therapy with adolescents. The general complaint of therapists working with adolescents is that they are resistant. It is true that most teenagers are not interested in cooperating with a system they regard as useless. However, if therapy provides them with an expressive vehicle that they enjoy and control, there can be positive outcomes, even with adolescents who are depressed (Selekman, 1993).

In art therapy with adolescents, individual or group, therapists must make every effort to control their desire to ask questions or interpret the art. Teens are ready and waiting for this mistake and will feel they are justified in withdrawing whatever trust they may have invested in therapy. The following techniques are suggestions for working with resistance in adolescent clients:

- Ask teens to represent how they would handle a particular or current situation if they were in control. Drawing directives such as "How would you handle the situation? Or, "picture how a "successful" adults would problem solve and what would they do differently?" These questions engage adolescents' urge to be critical and the therapist has also shown interest and respect for their opinions.

• Use subject matter that is once removed from their immediate lives. This allows them to speak through drawings in a safe manner. For example, adolescents enjoy pontificating about the weaknesses of parents but would be less inclined to make an art expression about their own parents.

• Use art as the central focus of the session. In most situations we build rapport with another person by a positive attitude and the confirmation of trust by eye contact. This is not successful with teens. They often avoid looking in the eyes of the adult and prefer to keep their distance. However, both adult and youth can gaze at an art product that is created by the teen. By averting the gaze from eye to eye to eye to art, a midplace has been created where the therapist can speculate and "talk" to the art product, and the teen can respond (once removed) through the art. If the conversation is focused on the art and the teen is in control, the possibility of discussion increases.

• Offer the opportunity to express ambivalence. Present directives that address both sides of an issue, such as "How do your parents punish you?" and "How do you punish them?" or "What privileges do men have? and "What privileges do women have?" Through a "polarity drawing" (i.e., depicting opposites or contrasting viewpoints), the adolescent can demonstrate ambivalence as well as insights.

• Use the art of the street, graffiti, to therapeutic advantage. The techniques of art making familiar to adolescents can establish rapport when other subjects would set up defiance. For example, the technique and design quality of a large wall painting can be a starting place. Another sort of graffiti, tagging (the most basic form of graffiti, a writer's signature or logo with marker or spray paint), can also be used as a starting point; it may represent to a teen a way to be seen, recognized, or acknowledged. The conversation between therapist and adolescent can start around the desire to "make a mark" in our society. Respect instead of criticism of street art can provide a bridge to difficult to reach teenagers.

• Let the teen decide on the direction the art will take. As shown in the previous example, focusing on teens' interests can encourage participation in the art therapy group.

In every case of adolescent art therapy it is essential for the therapist to move into the teen's world as much as possible and then find a metaphor, a theme, or an art project that is individualized to meet their developmental need. This may entail giving up goals self-created by the therapist and searching for the adolescent goals on which to build a productive and relevant relationship.

CONCLUSION

Art therapy with adolescents with depression can be successful modality of treatment because the client does the following:

- *Controls communication.* The adolescent can draw whatever he or she wishes and share verbally what he or she chooses. Nonverbal communication is more comfortable than attempting to put ambivalent feelings into words.
- *Feels respected.* The therapist honors the content and meaning of the adolescent's art, reinforcing a sense of respect within the client.
- *Has an opportunity to feel omnipotent.* The adolescent can project idealistic viewpoints, intellectualize experiences, or criticize other adults or peers in a safe environment.
- *Externalizes problems.* Creating a tangible product provides the opportunity for the adolescent to take a fresh view of problems at a distance. They can experiment with changes to the problem through changing the art image before they risk making a change in reality.

Art therapy is a modality that suits adolescents' psychological needs and stage of development. With adolescents who are depressed, art therapy offers a unique way to communicate complex feelings in an active manner. Activity, in and of itself, is an antidepressant, at the same time stimulating the adolescent to take a step toward finding a solution. Art products allow the therapist to see the individual stressors that the adolescent is experiencing but may be too overwhelmed to manage. Letting adolescents express themselves creatively offers a greater possibility for understanding depression, its causes, and ways to reduce or eliminate it.

REFERENCES

Achenbach, T. (1991). *Manual for the Child Behavior Checklist.* Burlington: University of Vermont Press.

Allen, J. (1988). Serial drawing: A Jungian approach with children. In C. Schaefer (Ed.), *Innovative interventions in child and adolescent therapy* (pp. 98–132). New York: Wiley.

Bloch, H. (1995). *Adolescent development, psychopathology, and treatment.* New York: International Universities Press.

Connor, D. F. (2002). *Aggression and antisocial behavior in children and adolescents: Research and treatment.* New York: Guilford Press.

Cyrtryn, I., & McKnew, D. (1999). *Growing up sad.* New York: Norton.

Gotlib, I. H., & Hammen, C. L. (Eds.). (2002). *Handbook of depression.* New York: Guilford Press.

Goodyer, I. (2001). *The depressed child and adolescent.* Cambridge: Cambridge University Press.

Hiscox, A. (1993). Clinical art therapy with adolescents of color. In E. Virshup (Ed.), *California art therapy trends* (pp. 17–26). Chicago: Magnolia Street.

Kendall, P. C. (Ed.). (2000). *Child and adolescent therapy: Cognitive-behavioral procedures.* (2nd ed.). New York: Guilford Press.

Kopelwitz, H., Klass, E., & Kafantaris, V. (1993). *Depression in children and adolescents.* Switzerland: Harwood Academic.

Malmquist, C. (1978). *Handbook of adolescence.* New York: Jason Aronson.

Nolen-Hoeksema, S. (2002). Gender differences in depression. In I. H. Gotlib & C. L. Hammen (Eds.), *Handbook of depression* (pp. 492–509). New York Guilford Press.

Parry-Jones, W. (1989). Depression in adolescence. In K. Herbst & E. S. Paykel (Eds.), *Depression: An integrated approach* (pp. 111–123) Oxford: Heinemann.

Riley, S. (2001) *Group process made visible*. Philadelphia: Brunner/Routledge.

Riley, S., & Malchiodi, C. (1994). *Integrative approaches to family art therapy*. Chicago: Magnolia Street.

Sandmier, M. (1996). More than love. *The Family Therapy Networker*, pp. 20–22.

Selekman, M. (1993). *Pathways to change: Brief therapy solutions with difficult adolescents*. New York: Guilford Press.

CHAPTER 18

Working with Adolescents' Violent Imagery

Joan Phillips

Adolescence has always been recognized as a time of turmoil and testing of boundaries. While violent imagery occurs in the art of clients of all ages, adolescents are the most likely age group to portray images of violence, death, dismemberment, horror, and terror. Despite the influence of movies, television, and video games, their images are disturbing and frequently are seen as warning signs of pathology, disturbance, or impending violent action. Perhaps we sense the impulsive nature of adolescents and fear the universal impulse to violence.

This chapter addresses why both normal adolescents and those with emotional or behavioral problems create violent imagery, sources and types of violent imagery, and ways therapists can respond to these images. The term "violent imagery" is defined as art that depicts a violent intention or act, or aftermath of violence whether it be a fantasy or reality based. These images include body art, clothing, graffiti, cartoons, magazines, and Internet sites as well as drawings, paintings, and sculptures (Klingman, Shovlev, & Pearlman, 2000). The goal is to provide clinicians with an understanding of adolescents' art expressions in order to reduce impulsive interpretations and offer a more comprehensive understanding that leads to more effective work with this population. It also provides some guidelines on how to assess when violent imagery may be a cause for concern.

NORMAL ADOLESCENT DEVELOPMENT AND VIOLENT IMAGERY

Historically, the main psychological task of adolescence is the successful development of one's identity and transition into the adult world of productivity (Erikson, 1968).

It is commonly agreed that adolescence is a time of separation from parents, peer group influences, concern about appearance, and introspection (American Academy of Child and Adolescent Psychiatry, 1999).

Risk taking naturally goes with this territory, and for some adolescents making violent images is part of the risk-taking behavior of this age group. Violent imagery and horror evoke a level of emotional surrender and provide a way to embody deep fears and desires that must be sublimated in order for an individual to function as an adult in our society. Peer relationships become important during adolescence and some teens can gain acceptance through their mastery of the violent genre in art. For adolescents with limited interpersonal or social skills, such art can be their entree into interaction with peers. Violent imagery can represent a form of identification and initiation and can be generically part of psychological development, or more specifically related to membership in a particular peer group or subculture, such as a gang. In the latter, there may be specific visual imagery, usually kept quite secret, which represents the values and activities and individuals of the group. When an adolescent is reluctant to discuss artwork or interpret this "language" to the therapist, it may indicate involvement in such a "taboo" group. Becoming informed about these subcultures can assist the therapist confronted with these images.

Popular culture is important to teens and also influences their art expressions. In every generation and culture there are seminal works that inform the imagination, fantasy life, and fears of those reaching into adulthood. Perennial interest exists in Stanley Kubrik's *A Clockwork Orange*, the movies and books of Stephen King, and even Edgar Allen Poe's work. More recent films that have entered into the collective thinking of a generation are *The Crow* and *The Matrix*. Though these trends of popular culture are ever changing, they all have a common denominator of violence. Knowledge of and openness to the popular culture are assets in working with youth who appropriate the imagery, narratives, and metaphors from these sources. This is not to say that those working with violent imagery must steep themselves in heavy metal music or gothic pastimes. Nonetheless, some cursory awareness of trends of popular culture is useful and, at the minimum, helps in establishing rapport.

The art world has also influenced adolescents' expression of violent imagery. Horror and violence have long existed as a genre in art (Diamond, 1996). Adolescents are often drawn to the archetypal and enduring images of horror in paintings, film, and literature of the past. Psychologically, adolescents are vulnerable to such imagery as it addresses their growing existential awareness and their questions about their future. Seeing violent imagery elicits a visceral reaction, which is often why it is rejected by adults and embraced by adolescents. Adolescents are actively seeking a visceral understanding of the world and are highly critical of the "hypocritical" or detached thinking they see in adult behavior.

MEANING AND IMPLICATIONS OF VIOLENT IMAGES

There is relatively little specific research on the meaning and implications of adolescents' violent imagery. Silver (1995) conducted a study using the Silver Drawing Test (see Appendix I, this volume, for more information) with delinquent adolescents and noted that incarcerated juveniles often drew angry, aggressive drawings targeted at male authority figures. A pilot study examining the human-figure drawings of male prisoners notes some significant features but also cautions regarding possible influences from media such as television. It is observed that the drawings are reminiscent of "the figures of felons and criminals people usually see in the movies, which raises the question of cultural symbols of evil and violent appearance in human figure drawings. Do people identify with these symbols and draw themselves accordingly?" (Lev-Weisel & Hershkovitz, 2000, p. 175)

Because both normal adolescents and those at risk for violent behavior create violent images at one time or another, it has been difficult to determine whether violent imagery may be a predictor of violent behavior. There is anecdotal evidence that violent adolescents create violent art, and some therapists link violent imagery to early or current traumas, perpetuated by dysfunctional systems and families (Graham, 1994; Malchiodi, 1997). There may be representations of actual things the child has experienced and, in addition, "feelings of wanting to attack or of being attacked" may be evident in the artwork of children from violent homes (Malchiodi, 1997, p. 37). Flynn and Stirtzinger (2001) explore many of the aggressive and hostile themes that can appear in adolescent art in a full case study of a regressed adolescent.

A form of violent imagery often encountered is the secretive doodle or drawing not done in therapy or the classroom but rather confiscated or found during a search of a student suspected of inappropriate or antisocial acts. These artworks are usually on notebook paper, in pencil, and done with some skill. They often depict a gruesome, gory, bloody scene and may include words that threaten others by name or by group (e.g., "die you preppies!"). Although these artworks elicit concern and usually some form of punishment (suspension from school and/or therapy), they by no means are a causal link between an adolescent's thoughts and actions. Most if not all adolescents engage in fantasies of retribution, harm, and ill will toward those they feel have treated them unfairly. Many normal adolescents create imaginary "hit" lists or drawings of people they would like to see suffer yet do not carry through their fantasies.

WHEN TO BE CONCERNED

Researchers and clinicians agree that multiple factors place children and adolescents at risk for violent behavior (Bloomquist & Schnell, 2002; Connor, 2002). Home and family dysfunction, presence of a diagnosable conduct or other mental disorder, and the presence of specific and clear threats are all significant factors linked to adolescent violence. Art expression as an indicator of violence is particularly relevant with at-risk adolescents. However, all art products—especially those that depict violence—should be evaluated in context. For example McGann (1999) describes a client who presented a series of specifically threatening and graphically violent drawings. The client directed her aggression toward a specific staff member whom she felt had treated her unfairly. The client also had a history of taking a knife to school and threatening to kill a teacher. "These explicit threats are not always, or even often, the warning signs we get. It takes no special training to connect drawings of guns and express threats with possible homicide. The greater challenge is in reading the subtler messages" (McGann, 1999, p. 54). In this particular case, in addition to graphically violent drawings, there was a history of violent behavior and verbal threats that contributed to the therapist's deductions about the adolescent's art expressions.

Haessler (1987) notes that shocking symbols, dangerous situations, and violence toward self or others depicted in art may be nonverbal requests for intervention. An adolescent female with whom I worked in an inpatient art therapy group depicted a bloody knife piercing a head that was emblazoned with the title "I hurt and no one cares!!!" She was not openly voicing any suicidal thoughts, but her image was clearly stating some ideas, if not intention. Based on this drawing, a search was made of her room and several hidden razor blades were found. She had verbally denied any suicidal ideation, but the strength of her visual communication led me to collaborate with the staff in a more concerted effort to ascertain her true intentions and feelings.

As in the example, violent images may be related to feelings of depression or thoughts of suicide; they also may represent powerful feelings or emotional disorders. The therapist must address and explore these possibilities in the process of understanding the adolescents and their artwork. The danger of working with violent imagery lies in interpreting it one dimensionally and only responding to what is perceived as a threat or an inappropriate statement rather than delving into its complexity. Clearly, more research needs to be done before we can fully understand the types of violent imagery created by adolescents.

DISTINGUISHING BETWEEN SUBLIMATION, FANTASY, AND REHEARSAL

It is widely believed that art expression can provide an opportunity for sublimation, a process that is thought to be involved when art functions as a means of discharging tension or psychic disequilibirum. Normal adolescents often successfully displace anger through art; for others, allowing repetitive violent expression without some reflection or direction poses inherent risks.

Based on these risks, it is important to monitor and assess the level of involvement and aggression in the artwork of severely disturbed adolescents. At every opportunity, the therapist must encourage sublimation so the work in art therapy "does not perpetuate or instigate uncontrollable impulses, or unacceptable actions" (McGann, 1999, p. 53). It is also important to differentiate between rehearsal of violent impulses and sublimation of them in adolescent imagery. Art can be a forum where the adolescent plans and/or rehearses violence (Kramer, 1993) and violent images may depict something the adolescent is considering putting into action. As mentioned, this can be difficult to judge and requires excellent rapport and strong clinical skills and experience in the therapist. In particular, an awareness of the source of the imagery can help differentiate between rehearsal and sublimation. Sublimation is typically an unconscious process whereas rehearsal has an element of conscious awareness and planning.

When violent imagery is created to represent a fantasy, it is helpful to look more closely. Often, this imagery is consciously developed and may be influenced by comic books, video games, or other popular media. In conversation with the adolescent artist, one must determine whether the fantasy mimics popular culture or whether it is internally generated and original. Although the latter can sometimes be of more concern, due to its possible connection to delusional thinking, it is not an automatically a sign of trouble. Again, a more global look at thought processes and general mental functioning of the adolescent will help in determining the degree of pathology that fantasies may represent. Careful clinical interviewing will help sort out these issues, and determining the source of the imagery may be more important than the content of the imagery itself. When such art is accompanied by verbal threats to specific people, with access to weapons and the stated intent to carry out such threats, it is important to intervene.

RESPONDING TO AND WORKING WITH VIOLENT IMAGERY

The first step for any therapist confronted with violent imagery is to examine personal tolerance for such images. Not everyone can stomach or deal with the blatant messages of hate, pain, and evil that some adolescents depict. Rather than dismiss these images as only for "shock value," one must look further into the contexts and life experiences that motivate such art. Therapists must be willing to look at the darker side of life in working adolescents who depict violent imagery and explore the personal relationship they have to the violence. Exploring their own fantasies, fears, and imagery is a necessity in sorting out adolescents' meanings for their art expressions.

The key factor in assessing the meaning of violent imagery is context, rather than focusing on a single work of art with swift intervention, punishment, or censorship. The larger context informs intervention and the meaning that can be ascribed to the artwork. In addition to the larger context, "we must consider the progression in artworks, family dynamics, and treatment processes in order to assess our clients effectively" (McGann, 1999, p. 61). This family and clinical context is critical in being able to design interventions that will actually work.

In working with adolescents who create violent imagery there are guidelines that may help in effectively tapping the creative and healing potential while avoiding the possibilities of reinforcing or dismissing violent content. The aforementioned contextual background is an important piece in developing effective means of working with violent imagery. Do not get caught up in the content and forget the other contextual issues—the individual adolescent and his or her family, history, and behavior.

Based on a review of the art therapy literature, as well as my own clinical experience, I have come to rely on the following guidelines:

1. *Avoid reacting to violent imagery with disgust, fear, or extreme shock.* Immediate responses such as these almost always generate one of two outcomes in working with the adolescent who created the imagery. Either they begin to create volumes of the same sort of work in order to elicit that disgust repeatedly (possibly

reinforcing their own inner negative self-esteem) or the adolescent writes the therapist off completely as unable to comprehend him or her or be open to his or her expression or lifestyle. In either case, the adolescent has the accurate view of the situation. One can acknowledge the shocking or disgusting nature of an artwork without closing the door to other responses or reactions. Even just to say "at first I felt pretty nauseated by your image in that art, but now I would like you to help me understand it" is a good start in opening up a therapeutic dialogue. In addition, it is possible to affirm the value of expression without affirming the content that seems explicit at first glance. "I am glad you are showing me your art even though the themes in it are pretty disturbing to me." Almost every adolescent therapy group goes through a stage of profane and violent imagery as a part of testing the therapist or the setting.

2. *Allow, support, and, at times, even encourage the expression of strong affect—which can include anger, aggression, or violence—in adolescent art.* Adolescence can be a time of tumultuous emotion, which requires some form of expression to be tolerable. Music, poetry, drama, art, and other creative efforts may all serve as life rafts to the teen navigating the stormy waters of adolescence. "Creative work acts to realign the balance of what feels unjust, out of balance, and threatening to one's orienting framework. Violence is motivated by the same need" (Kapitan, 1997, p. 256). Haessler (1987), in discussing her work with adolescents, states: "In no way do I discourage the expression of affect in art. To the contrary, the art my patients produce is full of strong emotions and powerful images, and it sometimes contains frightening material-storms, agonized faces, graveyards, knives" (p. 12). Use of art therapy could be seen as the treatment of choice for the adolescent creating violent imagery: "Art therapy, a treatment modality that utilizes art expression as its core, has a unique role in the amelioration of violence and its effects. The very nature of image making makes it a powerful means of eliciting and dissociating painful and frightening images from the self" (Malchiodi, 1997, p. 5).

Figure 18.1, a doll, transformed by its owner's use of masking tape, red paint, nail polish, and glue, embodies powerful feelings of self-hatred. Fearing that the adolescent was using drugs, the mother found the doll during a search of her daughter's room, and this was the reason for the daughter's referral to treatment. After 8 months of outpatient art therapy, the final sessions were used, at the client's choice, to "clean up" the doll, using nail polish remover, scrub brushes, cotton swabs, and other cleaning solvents. She and I collaborated on this process, deciding how and what to use in order to "clean the doll," and her actions reflected the changes that had occurred in this adolescent's self image.

3. *Explore the meaning of the work with the adolescent.* A respectful dialogue must be entered into with the maker of the art about the meaning of the creation. Asking the artmaker to tell you about the work, why he or she chose that image or topic, why now in particular, and what it means are all appropriate questions. However, some makers of violent imagery are distanced from their own work and can only respond with a shrug or "I don't know" when attempts to engage them in such a dialogue are pursued. For these people, Speltz (1990) suggests asking, "If someone were to walk in here and see your picture, what message do you think they might

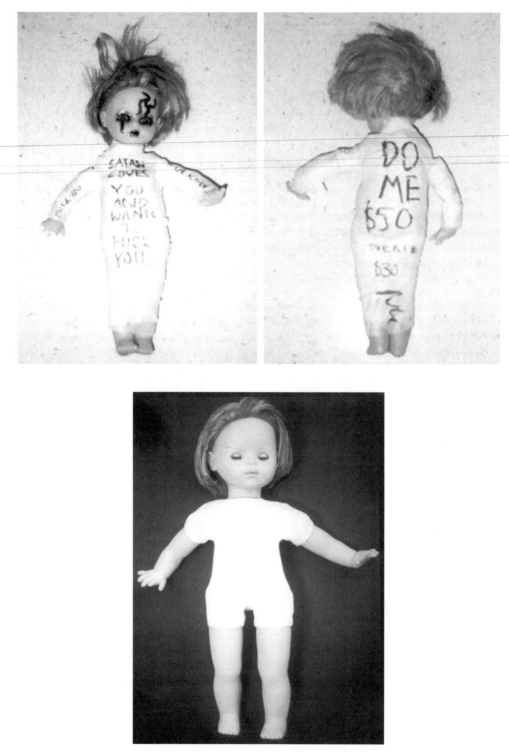

FIGURE 18.1. Left: Frontal view of doll; right: back view of doll; center: doll after being cleaned and restored.

get?" (p. 154). This type of question helps the artmaker stay in his or her position of distance yet entertain thoughts about the meaning to others, if not for themselves. This exploration of meaning can take place verbally, or by using one's own artwork in response to theirs. I call the latter "visual feedback." In response to a drawing depicting a violent death as fantasized by a client, I might draw a family crying and grieving for the victim shown in the art. Many times I find such visual feedback to be more effective in confronting and exploring meaning than a verbal response. Moon (1999) describes in fuller detail a similar process, which he calls "responsive artmaking."

It is appropriate to refer for further evaluation if there is evidence of problems, such as mental disorder. Violent imagery alone does not necessarily indicate a problem. If the artwork contains specific threats to named individuals, or if there is a history of involvement with the police, fire setting, or animal cruelty, these would be indicators of a need for much closer understanding of both the adolescent and the violent images.

4. *Develop and encourage creative expression overall, not just a focus on the violent content.* Even when the violent imagery is what brought an adolescent to treatment, the focus should not be solely on that issue. This may mean making suggestions for other forms of expression or use of media, using the skills or methods shown in the violent imagery as the starting point, for example, "You draw so well in this drawing, let's look at some of the work of M. C. Escher and see if you feel inspired." One could also share the work of artists throughout history who have expressed violent feelings, emotions, and acts through their art (Goya, Bosch, Picasso, Bacon, and many others). Do not assume that traditional art classes meet the developmental expressive needs of the adolescent. These are likely settings in which some degree of censorship must prevail and focus will be on skill building and technique, not on emotional expression. Skill is important but does not provide the therapeutic benefit that a more focused use of art by a clinician can; they are different experiences and not interchangeable although both are highly useful to the adolescent.

5. *Value the skill evidenced even when not valuing the content of the art and communicate this very clearly and consistently.* Speltz (1990), in discussing her work with Satanic imagery, emphasizes that it is often useful to dissociate the work and the person making it from the Satanism as a general concept (p. 153). There must be support for divergent views and ideas; art therapy must be an experimental ground, a safe haven for expression and trying out even repugnant ideas safely.

6. *Look for creative alternatives for expression of the violent imagery and/or associated feelings.* In addition to being a means of sublimation and catharsis, arts programs that address social problems and disenfranchised groups can provide the meaning and sense of justice that is sometimes denied adolescents in their everyday world. After not being scared off by the violent world an adolescent sometimes presents, it is ultimately the challenge to work with the larger existential issues the adolescent is facing. Does life make sense? What is the meaning of life? The clinician should help adolescents use this creativity in more positive venues and with more frequency.

CENSORSHIP ISSUES

No discussion of violent imagery is complete without considering the issue of censorship. As defined previously, violent imagery is designed to evoke a response and thus it is the very nature of these images to invite censorship or limits. Yet it is also true that art tasks can elicit much from the adolescent that verbal interactions will never garner: "Teenagers are willing to draw and create art as freely as they resist talking to an adult" (Riley, 1999, p. 37). So how do we negotiate these murky waters when the images seem to call for limits but also clearly have expressive and healing potential? It is important to remember that art and drawings are not "right" or "wrong"; what is done with them is what matters. The therapist should allow full expression with the only limits set being generated by the clinician's work setting or role.

An awareness of the setting and any inherent limits of it are essential in developing a consistent yet therapeutic approach to censorship issues. Clearly, there are different parameters for an art teacher, a probation officer, or a family therapist, and the exhibition of the artwork will also be key. Is the art for public consumption or created as a private communication within a confidential setting such as therapy (Graham, 1994; Haesler, 1987)? Nothing will do more to undermine work with adolescents creating violent imagery than being mired in a conflicted set of rules, expectations, and ideas about what is allowed, appropriate, or even desirable for creation.

In general, the more therapeutic the intent and setting, the less censorship is warranted. Basic therapeutic boundaries of no harm to self or others or the environment apply but do not solve each censorship dilemma. What if an art group member feels maligned, threatened, or demeaned by another's violent imagery? What if the therapist feels threatened? There are no black-and-white rules, but forethought can solve many of these dilemmas.

The therapist should avoid the temptation to confront the artist and instead confront the art; talk to *it*, ask *it* questions. This uses a basic principle of art therapy: Projection brings safety but still allows content to be addressed. For example, in an inpatient psychiatric art therapy group one patient created Nazi symbols. Rather than censoring, I engaged him in an intellectual dialogue about what those symbols represent to others and the feelings they were used to evoke historically. His own meaning emerged in this discussion as his sense that others hated him and he wanted to be "first" to hate. The Nazi symbol was just a quick way for him to open up this territory. The symbol served to protect him but also embodied his self-hatred, which had heretofore not been addressed in therapy.

CONCLUSION

Working with violent imagery evokes strong feelings in both therapist and client and challenges the therapist to balance caution with openness. A thorough understanding of the context and types of imagery forms the foundation for developing clinical techniques that will be effective. Without definitive research on adolescent artwork or violent imagery, one must use general clinical art therapy skills in combination with specific techniques related to the violent images and, in doing so, work toward fuller and healthier expression and living for the adolescents with which we work.

REFERENCES

American Academy of Child and Adolescent Psychiatry. (1999). *Normal adolescent development* [On-line]. Available: http://education. indiana.edu/cas/adol/development.html.

Bloomquist, M., & Schnell, S. (2002). *Helping children with aggression and conduct problems.* New York: Guilford Press.

Connor, D. (2002). *Aggression and antisocial behavior in children and adolescents: Research and treatment.* New York: Guilford Press.

Diamond, S. A. (1996). *Anger, madness, and the daimonic: The psychological genesis of violence, evil, and creativity.* Albany: State University of New York Press.

Erikson, E. (1968). *Identity, youth, and crisis.* New York: Norton.

Flynn, C., & Stirtzinger, R. (2001). Understanding a regressed adolescent boy through story writing and Winnicott's intermediate area. *The Arts in Psychotherapy, 28*(5), 299–309.

Graham, J. (1994). The art of emotionally disturbed adolescents: designing a drawing program to address violent imagery. *American Journal of Art Therapy, 34*(4), 115–121.

Haessler, M. (1987). Censorship or intervention: "But you said we could draw whatever we wanted!" *American Journal of Art Therapy, 26*(1), 11–20.

Kapitan, L. (1997). Making or breaking: art therapy in the shifting tides of a violent culture. *Art Therapy: Journal of the American Art Therapy Association, 14*(4), 255–260.

Klingman, A., Shovlev, R., & Pearlman, A. (2000). Graffiti: A creative means of youth coping with collective trauma. *The Arts in Psychotherapy, 27*(5), 299–307.

Kramer, E. (1993) *Art as therapy with children* (2nd ed.). Chicago: Magnolia Street.

Lev-Wiesel, R., & Hershkovitz, D. (2000). Detecting violent aggressive behavior among male prisoners through the Machover Draw-a-Person test. *The Arts in Psychotherapy, 27*(3), 171–177.

Malchiodi, C. (1997). *Breaking the silence: Art therapy with children from violent homes* (2nd ed.). New York: Brunner/Mazel.

McGann, E. (1999). Art therapy as assessment and intervention in adolescent homicide. *American Journal of Art Therapy, 38*(2), 51–62.

Moon, B. (1999). The tears make me paint: The role of responsive artmaking in adolescent art therapy. *Art Therapy: Journal of the American Art Therapy Association, 16*(2), 78–82.

Riley, S. (1999). *Contemporary art therapy with adolescents.* London: Jessica Kingsley.

Silver, R. (1995). Identifying and assessing self-images in drawings by delinquent adolescents. *The Arts in Psychotherapy, 22*(4), 339–352.

Speltz, A. (1990). Treating adolescent Satanism in art therapy. *The Arts in Psychotherapy, 17,* 147–155.

PART IV

Clinical Applications with Adults

Many therapists unfamiliar with art therapy believe that it is only useful with children who naturally embrace play and creative expression. While art therapy is a particularly effective modality with children as demonstrated in the previous section, it is also a method widely applied to work with adult populations. A major part of art therapy's foundations derives from the early work of psychiatrists and artists in the mid-20th century with people hospitalized for psychiatric disorders. Later, art therapist Margaret Naumburg (1950, 1953, 1966) published some of the first literature on art therapy with adults, illustrating her "dynamically oriented" approach to treatment. Since that time, art therapy with adults continues to use the psychoanalytic theories that Naumburg favored as well as more contemporary approaches to intervention.

Most of the reasons art therapy is effective with children and adolescents apply to work with adults: It serves as a form of nonverbal communication; it allows expression of feelings, thoughts, and world views; and it provides an opportunity to explore problems, strengths, and possibilities for change. The creative process of art making can be as life enhancing throughout the adult lifespan, well into old age (American Art Therapy Association, 1996). Landgarten (1981) explains another of the unique benefits of art therapy with adults: "Clients who are extremely resistant to treatment and refuse to talk about themselves or their problems tend to activate countertransference in the therapist . . . art psychotherapists have less difficulty with this type of person, for the client engaged in the art task is communicating on the symbolic level. It is this factor which often enables the therapist to remain interested in the silent or defended client" (p. 185). Art tasks are also a way for adult clients, especially those who are resistant to talking, to become invested in therapy.

Adults may be reluctant to use art materials in therapy for other reasons, perceiving art making to be "child's play" rather than real therapy. In my experience, most can be encouraged to try creative activities when they are explained by the therapist as another form of communication and an optional way to work on problems.

239

An emphasis on understanding that drawings, paintings, and collages do not necessarily have to have esthetic value to be therapeutic is often helpful for many adults to hear, especially those who are new to art therapy as a form of treatment. For some adults, it also helpful to provide a layperson's explanation of how art therapy works, describing in simple terms how our brains respond to and create images and how this can be beneficial in treatment.

Art therapy has been used with a variety of adult populations as well as with a wide range of problems including mood and personality disorders, medical illnesses, disabilities, addictions, family crises and domestic violence, loss and bereavement, and emotional trauma. Chapters in Part II ("Clinical Approaches to Art Therapy") demonstrate some of many applications of art therapy in work with adults. Case examples in the chapters on psychoanalytic, cognitive-behavioral, solution-focused and narrative, and humanistic approaches are good examples of the range of art therapy in the treatment of problems brought to therapy by adults. Additional chapters in Part V ("Clinical Applications with Groups, Families, and Couples") explain how art therapy is applied to adult art therapy groups, medical art therapy with adults, and adult family and marital issues.

This section describes additional clinical applications, covering several of the most popular applications of adult art therapy in greater detail. Gladding and Newsome open this section with an overview of the use of art in counseling (Chapter 19). The authors observe that there has recently been renewed interest in the use of art tasks in counseling with a wide range of adult clients. Because counselors and other therapists have come to realize the value of expressive modalities in therapy, their chapter provides a practical outline of just how art activities (drawing, collage, photography, and other media) can enhance a counseling session. Advice is also given on ethical issues associated with using art in counseling and the authors emphasize that therapists should determine the limits of their abilities to use art in counseling and seek additional training as needed. However, they also wisely advocate that counselors and other therapists should be able to bring art tasks into treatment, prompt a client to draw when talking becomes difficult; and use expressive, creative tasks to help individuals in therapy clarify and resolve issues, conflicts, and problems.

Art therapy is often used in conjunction with other expressive modalities such as movement, creative writing, and music therapies. Chapter 20 illustrates how sandplay is a useful form of art therapy because it uses visual imagery in the form of figures in the sand. Traditionally, therapists associate children with sandplay therapy, but as Steinhardt shows it is a method applicable to work with adults. Her work reflects a Jungian approach to treatment (see Chapter 4), one which involves understanding client-created symbols and allowing these symbols to emerge spontaneously in a nondirective manner.

Chapter 21, by Spaniol, addresses art therapy with adults with serious mental illness. Historically, art therapy has been used for many years with a variety of adult psychiatric populations with such disorders as schizophrenia, psychosis, depression, and dissociative disorders. The author brings a more contemporary art therapy model to light in this chapter, emphasizing the therapist's comfort and understanding of three concepts when working with this population: authenticity, creativity, and recovery. The concepts of authenticity and creativity echo the humanistic values discussed in Chapter 5, underscoring the importance of the individual's experience of therapy and the value in the role of creative expression in everyone's life despite illness or disability. Spaniol's values highlight the therapeutic value of acknowledging people with mental illness as creative individuals as well as art's capacity to normalize psychotherapy. In working with those with mental illness, therapists can capitalize on the personally empowering qualities of artistic expression that normalize the treatment setting and encourage the person to be an active participant in his or her therapy.

Art therapy has been applied for many years to work with substance abuse with individuals, families, and groups. In fact, art therapy has a long tradition of use in the treatment of substance abuse, dating back to the 1950s when art therapist Elinor Ulman worked in alcohol rehabilitation (Rubin, 1998). Wilson, in Chapter 22, offers her experience in applying art therapy to addictions treatment with individuals within a group setting. She provides suggestions for specific art activities to address safety, the nature of addictions, denial and shame, and the process of recovery. The author integrates art therapy within the popular 12-Step program widely embraced by individuals with addictions.

Chapter 23 demonstrates that older adults are a population that also can benefit from art therapy. It is now known that art expression can reveal neurological deficits that result from stroke, Alzheimer's, or dementia, assisting the therapist in understanding the older individual's physical and mental functioning. Recently, neuroscience has demonstrated that a great deal can be learned from offering drawing tasks to older adults with neurological disabilities (Ramachandran & Blakeslee, 1998) and visual tasks can be a method of both assessment and treatment (Wald, 1999). Creative activities with this age group may be used to address psychosocial issues or simply as an expressive mode of communication that stimulates attention span, decreases depression, and alleviates stress or boredom in those who are unable to engage in physical activities.

Landgarten (1981) observed that art therapy with adults facilitates communication in therapy and helps them to "listen with their eyes" (p. 4). It can be particularly useful as an adjunct to traditional talk therapy but also as a way to encourage adult clients to view problems in new ways and to tangibly create solutions to those problems. Incorporating art expression in therapy with adults offers the therapist a versatile modality that enhances and deepens treatment and provides an empowering and meaningful addition to the therapeutic exchange.

REFERENCES

American Art Therapy Association. (1996). *Mission statement*. Mundelein, IL: Author.
Landgarten, H. (1981). *Clinical art therapy*. New York: Brunner/Mazel.
Naumburg, M. (1950). *Schizophrenic art*. New York: Grune & Stratton.

Naumburg, M. (1953). *Psychoneurotic art*. New York: Grune & Stratton.

Naumburg, M. (1966). *Dynamically oriented art therapy*. New York: Grune & Stratton.

Ramachandran, V. S., & Blakeslee, S. (1998). *Phantoms of the brain*. New York: Quill.

Rubin, J. (1998). *Art therapy: An introduction*. Philadelphia: Brunner/Mazel.

Wald, J. (1999). The role of art therapy in post-stroke rehabilitation. In C. A. Malchiodi (Ed.), *Medical art therapy with adults* (pp. 25–42). London: Jessica Kingsley.

CHAPTER 19

Art in Counseling

Samuel T. Gladding
Debbie W. Newsome

This chapter focuses on ways mental health professionals, including professional counselors, can assist adult clients by integrating visual arts into the counseling process. This chapter provides a rationale for using art in counseling with adults and describes specific ways mental health workers can use art-based interventions to facilitate the counseling process.

BENEFITS OF THE USE OF ART WITH ADULT CLIENTS

Mental health professionals are more likely to integrate art activities in their work with children than their work with adults. The greater incidence of use with children may reflect a view that art activities are childlike, having little relevance to other age groups (Stewart & Brosh, 1997). Mental health workers also may refrain from using art in counseling adults because many adults feel inadequate about their skills or embarrassed over expressing themselves artistically (Gladding, 1998).

Nevertheless, there are many documented benefits of employing art as a part of a treatment plan with adult clients. Although these benefits have been described throughout this text, the following list summarizes specific advantages of art in counseling with adults:

- Taps the unconscious and helps individuals express covert conflicts, bringing into awareness thoughts and feelings that were previously hidden (Liebmann, 1990).
- Acts as a metaphor for the conflicts, emotions, and situations experienced by clients (Ulak & Cummings, 1997).

- Assists people in picturing themselves or their situations in a concrete, objectified manner (Rubin, 2001).
- Acts as a bridge between the counselor and the client, especially when the subject matter is too embarrassing or difficult to talk about, such as family violence and abuse (Brooke, 1995; Liebmann, 1990; Trowbridge, 1995).
- Creates a visible trail, provides a tangible record, and allows clients and counselors to review a series of past sessions and note development and change (Ganim, 2000; Liebmann, 1990).
- Inspires and helps people become more connected with the transcendent and growth sides of their personalities (Mills & Crowley, 1986).
- Provides a process that is energy enhancing (Kahn, 1999); art gets clients "doing" rather than thinking and therefore can be more activating than verbal counseling (France & Allen, 1997).
- Can easily be combined with other expressive arts such as music, movement, creative writing, and imagery (McNiff, 1997; see Chapter 7, this volume, for more information).

THE COUNSELING PROCESS AND ART

Counselors working with adult clients can use various forms of visual arts to facilitate different stages of the counseling process. The key to successfully employing art in counseling is to understand the goals of each stage of the process and then carefully select art directives that are consistent with the process and needs of the client (Kahn, 1999). Counselors must ask themselves questions such as, "What needs to be expressed through art during this stage?" and "What art activity will help the client move through this stage of the counseling process?" With some clients, art may facilitate the establishment of rapport. With others, it may help with the exploration of the client's world, issues, and concerns. In other situations, art may best be used to establish therapeutic goals and interventions. Counselors may select art directives to confront inconsistencies in thoughts and behaviors, develop and narrow options, move a client to action, or help with termination of the therapeutic relationship.

Although much of art therapy is grounded in psychodynamic theory, numerous methods have evolved that can be integrated into different theoretical approaches to counseling (Kahn, 1999). For example, a person-centered counselor may encourage clients to use art for self-actualization through self-expression and integration of perceptions of self and the environment (Cochran, 1996). A cognitively oriented counselor may ask a client to explore irrational thoughts by drawing cartoon strips. A solution-focused counselor may find it helpful to ask the client to reflect on a time when things were going well and to draw what he or she was doing at that time. A counselor following a constructivist approach might encourage a client to draw a life map representing important things that have happened over time, using different colors and symbols to represent positive and negative events.

PRACTICE OF THE USE OF VISUAL ARTS IN COUNSELING

In setting up situations for using the visual arts in counseling, the best-quality art materials should be purchased so that clients who might otherwise be intimidated by the use of these media will become more relaxed and creative (Makin, 1994; Nadeau, 1984). Other conditions important to visual art counseling sessions are enough space, quiet, freedom of movement, encouragement, and time. It is essential for those who assist to be patient, too. Just as great art takes time, so does psychosocial change. It may take several sessions before clients actually begin to enjoy and benefit from visual art experiences and even longer to integrate art into their lives in a productive way.

As with all interventions, it is important for the counselor to establish a relationship with the client based on genuineness, empathy, and positive regard. Counselors can ensure a reluctant client that the experience is not about artistic ability but, instead, is an opportunity for self-exploration using a different medium than words. If a client continues to resist, it should be remembered that art interventions are not appropriate for all clients, and refusal to engage in an artistic experience needs to be respected (Ulak & Cummings, 1997).

The field offers a number of possibilities for clients who are willing to engage in visual art experiences: interventions involving sketching, drawing, or painting; interventions using counselor-made drawings; and interventions using photography.

Sketching, Drawing, and Painting

The selection of which artistic intervention to use should be based on the clients' issues and their preferred modes of self-expression. The many types of activities that involve sketching, drawing, and painting are limited only by the counselor's and client's imagination. Five are described next.

Lines of Feeling

At times, people cannot find words to express their emotions, although they may have a strong sense of what those feelings are. To help with awareness and expression, the counselor asks the client to draw lines representing his or her emotions using various art media (e.g., markers, colored pencils, paints, and crayons). The lines vary in length and shape, but often jagged, rough lines in red or orange are used to signify anger or discontent, and smooth, flowing pastel-colored lines are used to represent peacefulness (Gladding, 1997, 1998).

Depending on the stage of counseling and the particular issues presented, the approach counselors take with this activity can vary. One approach is to ask clients to draw using only lines to represent feelings at the present moment. Clients then are asked to explain the lines and to draw what they hope the lines will become in the future. An alternative approach is to ask clients to reflect on specific past, present, and future events that relate to the issues with which they are struggling. Using lines, clients draw out feelings associated with the events, thereby providing an avenue for exploring thoughts, feelings, and behaviors.

Road Maps

The road map and its numerous variations (e.g., the life map and the lifeline) can be used to help people review significant periods in their lives and anticipate the future. Such activities help clients explore patterns, expand self-expression, and plan their lives more effectively (Gladding, 1998; Kahn, 1999; Miller, 1993). They also can serve as forms of qualitative assessment that stimulate counseling interaction (Goldman, 1990).

The road map provides an opportunity for counselors to help clients plan for the future by looking back on where they have been and thinking about where they are going. Clients are asked to paint or draw their life paths and career influences in the same manner that they map out directions to a specific destination (Gladding, 1998; Liebmann, 1986). In this procedure, clients are encouraged to sketch in significant events and experiences along the way. The counselor may introduce the activity by saying, "I want you to represent your life as a road map. Some roads are straight and wide; others are narrow and winding. Some are bumpy, and others are smooth. There may be some road blocks or detours. It is possible that the road of your life has been many of these." These directions give clients free reign to evaluate the factors that have been most influential and then symbolize them in a form that allows them to see the past, present, and future simultaneously. After completing the drawing, clients are encouraged to talk about the map and the events depicted on it. What events were expected? Which ones were unexpected? What people were associated with these events? What feelings are remembered? These and other questions encourage self-exploration while providing the counselor with a picture of clients' contextual development.

In a variation of the road map, clients begin by drawing the current road they are on. Then they asked to draw three paths branching off the main road: the high road, the expected road, and the low road. Along each path, clients draw or paint symbols to represent an ideal future, an anticipated future, and the worst possible scenario. After the paths have been drawn, clients are encouraged to explore possible action steps that need to be accomplished to stay on the preferred path. This activity can be particularly helpful for clients facing career decisions and other major life choices.

Another method designed to stimulate client reflection and counseling interaction is the "lifeline" (Goldman, 1990; Miller, 1993). The lifeline is a relatively simple and straightforward strategy designed to assist individuals with the reality of their lives. A line is drawn horizontally across a piece of paper, representing the "average" level. Above the line, clients chronologically plot symbols of positive, happy, or rewarding experiences. Below the line, they draw negative, unhappy, or painful experiences. The distance above or below the line represents the relative impact of the positive or negative feeling. The completed lifeline can be used to process values, moods, needs, sense of self, factors affecting development, and implications for resolving current issues (Goldman, 1990).

The Bridge

For clients dealing with difficult life situations, visual representations of the situation and possible solutions can be empowering (Gladding, 1997; Mills & Crowley, 1986). To begin the activity, clients divide a piece of paper into three panels or sections. On the first panel, clients are invited to draw a picture of a problem or concern they are currently facing. After drawing the particular situation, they are asked to draw on the third panel a picture of what things would look like if the problem were solved. Between these two scenes clients draw symbols of obstacles blocking their movement toward the "solution." Clients then are asked to draw a bridge over the obstacles, providing a connection between the problem and problem solved. The counselor encourages client inclusion of symbols or word phrases on the bridge that represent varied solutions for circumventing the obstacles and living life more effectively. A variation of this activity requires the client to draw a picture of him- or herself before a particular crisis (divorce, traumatic experience, hospitalization), a picture of him- or herself in the present, and a picture of how he or she would like things to look in the future. The sequential drawings can serve as a springboard for discussing coping skills and new patterns of behavior.

Comic Strips and Cartoons

Liebmann (1990) found that using comic strips facilitated communication and helped get clients involved in the counseling process. In her work with offenders in the context of a probation office, she designed this method to help them look at problem behaviors and alternatives. Liebmann introduces the concept of the comic strip as a way of learning more about their perceptions of the offense. Often the client needs prompting, and the cartoon strip becomes a dialogue, with the counselor encouraging the client to draw out as much information and as many stages as possible. After the comic strip is completed, the counselor and client look at it together. This process provides an opportunity for offenders to distance themselves from what happened. It may prompt them to see themselves as actors in the center of the story rather than mere victims of circumstance, thereby marking the first step on the road to taking responsibility for their choices, actions, and consequences.

Comic strips also can be used to help clients explore irrational thoughts. For example, a woman may seek counseling because of feelings of anxiety associated with job expectations. Closer evaluation reveals that she has dealt with perfectionistic tendencies most of her life. In counseling, she can be asked to draw a comic strip of herself at work and the thoughts that accompany her anxious feelings. After talking about what she has drawn, she can be encouraged to rewrite the script, exchanging irrational thoughts and fears for more healthy, realistic messages.

Published cartoons, with or without words or captions, can be used in counseling as well as client-drawn strips (O'Brien, Johnson, & Miller, 1978). Cartoons can serve as stimulus material to summarize the nature and foibles of people and their world. The counselor can use cartoons as an intervention within the counseling session, for homework, and for encouraging discussions of self-selected materials and dialogue completion. Within counseling, published anthologies of cartoons can be shared to illustrate particular concerns and help the client reconceptualize the problem and its implications, as illustrated in the following example:

> One man concerned about his deteriorating marriage was shown a *New Yorker* illustration portraying a tough, karate-attired couple advancing belligerently toward the office of a marriage counselor. This husband, when shown the cartoon, paused, looked at it carefully, and said, "That's us all right. Mary and I bring to everything, even counseling, that aggressive, I've got-to-win attitude." He saw himself in a new way; his defensiveness and unproductive hostility were revealed and could be dealt with in subsequent counseling. (O'Brien et al., 1978, p. 55)

Using cartoons and comic strips in counseling can defuse tension with humor and help clients become involved in the counseling process in an unthreatening manner. There are some precautions to take, however. The nature of the material used should be considered carefully, especially in sensitive problem areas. It is important for clients not to feel that their concerns are being treated superficially.

Images

The process of creating images to represent inner experiences was inspired by Jung (1965), who drew, painted, and sculpted representations of dreams and fantasy experiences. Based on the psychological value he personally discovered from exploring the images, Jung later encouraged his patients to make visual images of their own inner experiences (Edwards, 1987). The use of images in counseling is not limited to therapists trained in Jungian psychology. Counselors of various theoretical orientations can provide clients with opportunities to create images to facilitate the release of emotional or traumatic experiences that might otherwise be repressed.

France and Allen (1997) employed a Gestalt approach to image making with a disruptive adolescent client to help enhance his awareness of feelings and reintegrate conflicting forces into a more healthy self. The approach consists of four steps: warm-up, action, sharing, and dialoguing. In the warm-up stage, clients talk about specific concerns or dilemmas and their thoughts and feelings about those concerns. In the action stage, clients are invited to create an image representing the concern. After the image has been created, clients share what they have drawn with the counselor. This step is followed by dialoguing, with the counselor asking specific questions to help clients explore possibilities related to the image. The counselor might ask questions such as the following: "What is the image telling you?" "What are you aware of right now?" "What is the energy of the image?" "What is missing?" Or, the counselor may encourage clients to select specific objects in the picture and role-play those objects. At times, it is beneficial for the counselor to play the role of one of the images (Coan, 2000). Image-making experiences of this nature help put the dilemma into perspective, provide opportunity for insight, and reveal additional possibilities and choices for living.

Counselor-Made Drawings

Another way counselors can combine art with therapy is by making their own impromptu sketches during counseling sessions. These drawings delineate issues brought forth by the client in order to promote dialogue and objectify concerns. The sketches provide opportunities for situations to be exposed and then explored in a nonthreatening manner (Edens, Newsome, & Witherspoon, 1996). According to Cudney (1975), pictures drawn by counselors in sessions can help in understanding and objectifying counseling issues, increasing openness to oneself, promoting counselor–client conversations, clarifying problems, and reaching nonverbal clients.

Sketches can pave the way for discussion when the counselor's perception of the issue differs from that of the client. For instance, if a client states that a problem is so large it cannot be overcome and yet solid evidence indicates the contrary, the counselor might draw two pictures. Each would be of a mountain with the first mountain much higher and steeper than the other. The counselor then might indicate that he or she hears the client describing the problem in terms of the first mountain but that the counselor perceives the difficulty as more similar to the second, more gently sloping mountain. Challenges of this nature may help clients reevaluate how they are presenting situations and then modify their outlooks accordingly (Gladding, 1998).

Another way to use counselor-made drawings in sessions is by sketching out the problem, sometimes using only doodles, as the client describes a particular situation or set of relationships (Trimble, 1975). These doodles or sketches help clarify the situation and illustrate complex relationships. It is difficult if not impossible to communicate all the interconnections of a complicated problem concerning relationships or career by relying entirely on words. By graphically representing the problem, all parts of the puzzle are revealed at once, including feelings and nuances of relationships. The complexity of the problem as it unfolds on paper can be seen as a whole, not just a series of fragmented parts, which can help clarify the problem for both the counselor and the client.

Counselor-made drawings often take the form of characterizations. For example, a quick sketch of what "stressed" looks like can generate dialogue concerning a client's lifestyle. If a client talks about feeling "weighted down" with burdens, the counselor can characterize the burdens in a drawing, thus encouraging the client to explore the issue further. It is important for the sketches to be impromptu, individualized, and confidential (Edens et al., 1996). These and other implementations of counselor-made drawings have the potential to provide counselors with a unique way to enter fully into a client's world.

Photography

"Photographs are footprints of our minds, mirrors of our lives, reflections from our hearts, frozen memories we can hold in silent stillness in our hands—forever, if we wish. They document not only where we may have been but also point the way to where we might perhaps be going, whether we know it yet or not" (Weiser, 1993, p. 1). According to Weiser, photography, or "phototherapy," is a way to capture and express feelings and ideas in a visual–symbolic form across the lifespan. It works "particularly well for people who find other visual arts too demanding or too risky to try" (Weiser, 1993, p. 13). Phototherapy can personalize the counseling process while promoting self-awareness and increasing sensitivity. It can help assess client concerns, build the counselor–client relationship, facilitate communication, and measure progress and change throughout the counseling process (Amerikaner, Schauble, & Ziller, 1980; Gladding, 1998; Krauss, 1981).

Typically, photographs used in counseling focus on relationships. Photographs may include pictures taken of the client, pictures taken by the client, pictures taken as self-portraits, and biographical pictures of groups of friends and family, which may or may not include the client. When photography is used in counseling, processing the project is emphasized, giving clients opportunities to examine their emotional and cognitive responses to the experience (Weiser, 1993).

One example of using photography in counseling involves asking clients to take several photos that represent who they are and who they want to become. After taking the pictures, clients are asked to order the photographs from most self-descriptive to least self-descriptive then write captions for each picture (Amerikaner et al., 1980; Ziller, Vera, & Camacho de Santoyo, 1981). The photographs provide the counselor with a vision of the client's world, and at the same time provide the client with an opportunity to reflect, set goals, and envision the future.

Older adults represent a population with whom the use of phototherapy may be especially beneficial. Old photographs can provide an excellent way to facilitate the life-review process that is so important to fostering a sense of ego integrity (Myers, 1989; Weiser, 1993). The procedure used in introducing this activity can vary depending on the counseling setting. For example, counselors employed in older adult day-care centers can ask members of the center to bring in photographs of their lives. On the other hand, counselors employed in inpatient facilities where clients do not have ready access to their personal possessions may have to be more active and find some representative photographs. Regardless, the goal is to accentuate the positive and help clients reflect on early recollections while reframing negatives to promote the building of self-esteem (Gladding, 1998).

To help clients examine situations from different perspectives, I (S.G.) have devised an exercise called Mailbox. In this exercise, a client is instructed to photograph a mailbox from as many angles as possible and then bring the photographs, mounted on poster board, to the next session. When the assignment is completed the counselor and client discuss the task and examine the pictures. It soon becomes obvious that a familiar object can be seen in a multitude of ways. Likewise, problems with which the client is dealing can be viewed from more than one perspective. By discussing the experience, the client may discover ways to modify or completely change his or her approach to resolving those problems (Gladding, 1997).

LIMITATIONS AND ETHICAL CONSIDERATIONS

A number of considerations need to be taken into account when making decisions about when and how to use art in counseling with adults. If applied in a whimsical way, art can be "distracting at best and dangerous at worst" (Kottler, 1993, p. 252). Approaches become unbalanced if counselors present activities without adequate reflection about their purposefulness or without allowing adequate time for processing (Gladding, 1997). Related to this point is the potential of using art in a mechanical, gimmicky, or otherwise nontherapeutic way. When used appropriately, the arts involve full use of one's imagination, enhancing clients' problem-solving skills and broadening their perspectives.

The use of arts in counseling may not be helpful to clients who are professional artists. According to Fleshman and Fryrear (1981), "For artists, the use of art in therapy may be counterproductive" (p. 6). One reason for this negative phenomenon is that artists support themselves through creative expression and to be asked to perform in a therapeutic environment may feel too much like work. Conceivably, this barrier can be overcome if artists are asked to relate in creative ways that differ greatly from their professional specialty.

Hammond and Gantt (1998) addressed the issue of mental health professionals other than trained art therapists using art with clients. Ethical codes dictate that no mental health professional should practice beyond that which he or she was trained to do. However, Hammond and Gantt (1998) stated that "any well-trained counselor should be able to talk with a client about a piece of art brought into a session" (p. 275). Further, counselors should be able to prompt a client to draw or paint an image when talking becomes difficult, clarification is needed, or the client is blocked in describing something. However, it is important to avoid challenging ethical boundaries by interpreting the client's art to the client or making generalizations about the meaning of the art to others, such as an agency's treatment team. Counselors need to be conscientious in determining the limits of their ability to use art in therapy and recognize when consultation or referral to an art therapist is indicated (Olivera, 1997).

Other issues associated with the use of art in therapy include confidentiality, documentation, ownership, research and publication, and displays; many of these topics are addressed in Appendix II (this volume). As a rule of thumb, artwork should be given all due consideration and protection as that of any other form of speech (Hammond & Gantt, 1998). Ramifications include using caution when entering material into clients' records, taking photographs of the clients' artwork only after informed consent has been granted, and adequately disguising the identity of a client whose work is used in research and publication.

CONCLUSION

Counseling at its best employs an artistic quality that enables individuals to express themselves in a creative and unique manner. In this chapter the premises, practices, limitations, and ethical considerations of using the visual arts in counseling have been explored. The procedures presented here represent but a few of the many ways visual art can be employed effectively to help people both prevent and resolve problems. There are multiple considerations to keep in mind when employing the arts in therapeutic ways with adults, and those who use art must do so with caution and care.

Choice and change in counseling are the result of clients' consideration of aspects of life that heretofore have gone unnoticed. Art serves as both a catalyst and conduit for understanding oneself in a larger world context. It does so through stirring up feelings and opening up possibilities. Thus, through affect and awareness, the use of art in counseling creates possibilities and broadens horizons so that the world becomes ever new and the view of what can be, if worked on, becomes what is.

REFERENCES

Amerikaner, M., Schauble, P., & Ziller, R. (1980). Images: The use of photographs in personal counseling. *Personnel and Guidance Journal, 59,* 68–73.

Brooke, S. L. (1995). Art therapy: An approach to working with sexual abuse survivors. *The Arts in Psychotherapy, 22,* 447–466.

Coan, K. (2000, March). *Expressive arts in counseling.* Paper presented at the Wake Forest University Counselor Education Program Spring 2000 Seminar, Winston-Salem, NC.

Cochran, J. L. (1996). Using play and art therapy to help culturally diverse students overcome barriers to school success. *School Counselor, 43,* 287–298.

Cudney, M. R. (1975). *Eliminating self-defeating behaviors.* Kalamazoo, MI: Life Giving Enterprises.

Edens, M. B., Newsome, D. W., & Witherspoon, E. L. (1996, February*). Creative arts in counseling: Bridge to a client's world.* Poster session presented at the annual meeting of the North Carolina Counseling Association, Charlotte, NC.

Edwards, M. (1987). Jungian analytic art therapy. In J. A. Rubin (Ed.), *Approaches to art therapy: Theory and technique* (pp. 92–113). New York: Brunner/Mazel.

Fleshman, B., & Fryrear, J. L. (1981). *The arts in therapy.* Chicago: Nelson-Hall.

France, M. H., & Allen, E. G. (1997). Using art: A gestalt counselling strategy for working with disruptive clients. *Guidance and Counselling, 12*(4), 24–26.

Ganim, B. (2000). *Art and healing: Using expressive art to heal your body, mind, and spirit.* Three Rivers, MI: Three Rivers Press.

Gladding, S. T. (1997). The creative arts in groups. In H. Forester-Miller & J. A. Kottler (Eds.), *Issues and challenges for group practitioners* (pp. 81–99). Denver, CO: Love.

Gladding, S. T. (1998). *Counseling as an art: The creative arts in counseling* (2nd ed.). Alexandria, VA: American Counseling Association.

Goldman, L. (1990). Qualitative assessment. *The Counseling Psychologist, 18*(2), 205–213.

Hammond, L. C., & Gantt, L. (1998). Using art in counseling: Ethical considerations. *Journal of Counseling and Development, 76*(3), 271–276.

Jung, C. G. (1965). *Memories, dreams, reflections.* New York: Random House.

Kahn, B. B. (1999). Art therapy with adolescents: Making it work for school counselors. *Professional School Counseling, 2*(4), 291–298.

Kottler, J. A. (1993) *On being a therapist* (rev. ed.). San Francisco: Jossey-Bass.

Krauss, D. (1981). *On photography: Uses in psychotherapy.* Paper presented at the Annual Convention of the American Psychological Association, Los Angeles, CA. (ERIC Document Reproduction Service No. ED 209 628)

Liebmann, M. (1986). *Art therapy for groups.* Cambridge, MA: Brookline.

Liebmann, M. (1990). "It just happened": Looking at crime events. In M. Liebmann (Ed.), *Art therapy in practice* (pp. 133–155). Bristol, PA: Jessica Kingsley.

Makin, S. R. (1994). *A consumer's guide to art therapy.* Springfield, IL: Charles C Thomas.

McNiff, S. (1997). Art therapy: A spectrum of partnerships. *The Arts in Psychotherapy, 24,* 37–44.

Miller, M. J. (1993), The Lifeline: A qualitative method to promote group dynamics. *Journal for Specialists in Group Work, 18*(2), 51–54.

Mills, J. C., & Crowley, R. J. (1986). *Therapeutic metaphors for children and the child within.* New York: Brunner/Mazel.

Myers, J. E. (1989). *Infusing gerontological counseling in counselor preparation.* Alexandria, VA: American Counseling Association.

Nadeau, R. (1984). Using the visual arts to expand personal creativity. In B. Warren (Ed.), *Using the creative arts in therapy* (pp. 61–86). Cambridge, MA: Brookline.

O'Brien, C. R., Johnson, J., & Miller, B. (1978). Cartoons in counseling. *Personnel and Guidance Journal, 57,* 55–56.

Olivera, B. (1997, Winter). Responding to other disciplines using art therapy. *American Art Therapy Association Newsletter, 30,* 17.

Rubin, J. A. (2001). *Approaches to art therapy: Theory and techniques* (2nd ed.). New York: Psychology Press.

Stewart, T., & Brosh, H. (1997). The use of drawings in the management of adults who stammer. *Journal of Fluency Disorders, 22,* 35–50.

Trimble, W. B. S. (1975). Doodle counseling. *Social Work, 20*(2), 152–153.

Trowbridge, M. M. (1995). Graphic indicators of sexual abuse in children's drawings: A review of the literature. *The Arts in Psychotherapy, 22,* 485–494.

Ulak, B. J., & Cummings, A. L. (1997). Using clients' artistic expressions as metaphor in counselling: A pilot study. *Canadian Journal of Counselling, 31*(4), 305–316.

Weiser, J. (1993). *Phototherapy techniques.* San Francisco: Jossey-Bass.

Ziller, R. C., Vera, H., & Camacho de Santoyo, C. (1981). Federico: Understanding a child through autophotography. *Childhood Education, 57,* 271–275.

CHAPTER 20

Sandplay Therapy and Art Therapy with Adults

Lenore Steinhardt

Sandplay, the construction of an image with sand, water, and a large choice of minia-tures in a tray of prescribed dimensions, adds natural materials to art therapy and promotes access to certain deep internal states that may be less readily engaged with established art therapy materials. This visual, concrete experience may be new to many therapists, although it is now more frequently integrated into the expressive therapies (Carey, 1999; Case, 1987; Gray, 1983; Halliday, 1987; Lewis, 1988; McNally, 2001; Steinhardt, 1997, 1998, 2000; Toscani, 1998). The universal forms that result from play with sand and water can be categorized according to use of the sand surface, its penetration, and use of water. The different approaches to the use of sand reflect symbolic meanings and may be linked to stages in the therapeutic pro-cess. If clients are coping with similar issues, their sandplays may display similar sand forms and the same choice of miniature objects at times.

This chapter discusses the basic premises of sandplay from a Jungian perspective, approaches to constructing sand pictures, universal phenomena in sandplay, and the integration of sandplay into work with adult clients. The healing use of archetypal imagery in sandplay is illustrated with the work of a woman who experienced infer-tility.

JUNGIAN SANDPLAY

Sandplay originated in 1928 as a form of children's play therapy using sand and wa-ter and miniature objects to build a world (Bowyer, 1970; Lowenfeld, 1935). It was later given a Jungian perspective by Swiss child psychotherapist Dora Kalff (1980) and used individually with children and adults, often as an adjunct to verbal psycho-therapy (Ammann, 1991; Bradway & McCoard, 1997; Markell, 2002; Mitchell & Friedman, 1994; Ryce-Menuhin, 1992; Weinrib, 1983). Kalff included miniatures from various cultures in her collection and saw the relevance of Neumann's develop-mental theory to stages in the sandplay processes of children, and later of adults (Neumann, 1973/1988).

Jungian sandplay incorporates two shallow wood trays whose inner measure-ments are $19'' \times 28'' \times 3''$ or higher, standing at table height, and filled about halfway with fine white sea sand. In one tray the sand is dry; in the other it is moist. A client's choice of moist sand is believed to indicate readiness to access a deeper unconscious knowledge (M. Kalff, 1993). Both sandtrays' interior bottoms and sides are painted blue, to represent water or sky when the sand is moved aside (D. Kalff, 1980). Blue is considered to be a tranquilizing color that signals the human brain to bring calmness to the body and to slow the pulse rate (Luscher, 1969; Walker, 1991). Steinhardt (1997) prefers cerulean blue for the dry sandtray, where depth may be less important, and the deeper cobalt blue for the moist sandtray, where expression of deeper physi-cal and emotional depth may be desired.

Hundreds of miniature objects are available to the client on nearby shelves. These may be chosen or "found" and placed on the sand, a process resembling that of spontaneous play with sand or earth and found objects in childhood, a time when play and art making are nearly identical. This is similar to assembling a collage, inte-grating disparate items into a meaningful configuration. A completed sand picture may also be seen as a "bas relief" of protruding forms attached to a supportive foun-dation. The sandplay miniature collection contains both natural and manufactured objects, in categories ranging from people of all ages, occupations, and ethnic groups to film characters and gods, life forms of the sea, land and air, dwellings, food, types of vehicles, fences, bridges, and other figures. An object's identity, material, and color can activate in the sandplayer a sense of affinity to its universal, cultural, and per-sonal implications leading to a choice of relevant objects.

Sand, water, and the color blue evoke the experience of nature and recall the pri-meval ocean environment where life first originated. They are believed to provide ac-cess to specific metaphors for human growth and healing; for example, sand is made of stones and shells pulverized in ocean water, the primordial womb of life, perhaps evoking our deep inborn instincts. Sand and water are also thought to represent the limitless flow of creative imagination and access to the unconscious, whereas the sandtray provides a safe container for the client's image making (Weinrib, 1983).

Sand pictures cannot be kept and stored as artworks are. After joint observation by client and therapist the sand picture is photographed and dismantled out of sight of the client, who has left the session. Photographs are kept for review at termination of therapy, recording the client's healing process.

C. G. Jung's own healing process of symbolic play began after his break with Freud in 1912–1913. Jung worked daily on the banks of a lake, constructing a village with mud, water and stones, as he had done in childhood (Jung, 1961/1995). This process released streams of fantasies and helped clarify his thoughts. He later deliber-ately developed the dialogue between himself and the fantasy figures encountered, advocating his patients to do the same. He named this technique "active imagination." Storr (1983) writes:

> Jung encouraged his patients to enter a state of reverie in which judgement was suspended but consciousness preserved. They were then enjoined to note what fantasies occurred to them, and to let these fantasies go their own way without interference. Jung encouraged his patients to draw and paint their fantasies, finding that this technique both helped the patient to rediscover hidden parts of himself and also portrayed the psychological journey upon which he was embarked. (p. 21)

Sandplay came to be known as a form of concrete active imagination, the images taking shape as the sandplayer's hands move and create spontaneously (Ammann, 1991; Chodorow, 1997; Kawai, 2002; Weinrib, 1983).

APPROACHES TO CONSTRUCTING A SANDWORLD

In general, sandplay should be chosen voluntarily. Sand as a surface with a penetrable interior may become a metaphor for the body. Sand may arouse positive or negative tactile memories of the skin as the zone of communication between mother and child, or of favorable or forcible penetration of body apertures such as the mouth, vagina, and anus. If the skin shield has not been able to prevent abusive wounding and unwanted penetration (Anzieu, 1989), touching sand may be resisted due to a sense of the body as defenseless and vulnerable. In such cases sandplay may be contraindicated. For those who use sandplay, the three primary approaches are use of the sand surface, penetration of the surface, and the addition of water, each with its own symbolic significance (Steinhardt, 1998, 2000).

Surface

Early beach play often begins by packing loose sand into a mold and carefully overturning it to release a transformed "pie" into the world, like the birth of a new independent structure. Gathered sand becomes a mound, perhaps symbolic of a breast or womb, or a Tel, a layered tomb. Lines drawn on flat sand in the sandtray may become paths leading to the destinations of therapy, and activating the archetype of the hard and dangerous "way" (Neumann, 1963/1983, p. 8). Hands impressed in the sand may be spontaneously ornamented with shiny objects, resembling a "Hamsa," a Middle Eastern hand-shaped talisman embellished with fertility symbols such as fish, or a divine eye for protection against evil.

Penetration

Digging is the act of penetrating the sand's interior to create holes and tunnels, or to bury and unbury. A hole may become a well, a volcano, a cave, an oracle's residence, or a grave. Tunnels connect descent, an underground sojourn, and ascent into a new place, resembling a birth and transformation. Burial may refer to hiding, preserving, hibernating, or dying. Unburying may expose, reveal, exhume, or release into new life (Steinhardt, 1998, 2000). Entering the sand and emerging mirror the psyche's polarities, concealed or revealed, light and darkness, protected or vulnerable, death and rebirth.

Water

As a liquid water flows and changes shape, moving continuously, never stable or rigid, it symbolizes the "fluidity of life, as opposed to the rigidity of death" (Cooper, 1978, p. 188). Water may represent depth, the unconscious, the womb, flow and change, cleansing and purification, or turbulence and drowning. Human emotion may be expressed by the secretion of body fluids such as sweat, tears, urine, saliva, and blood. The particular aspect of water that a sandplayer needs to be in touch with may take the form of a well, pond, river, lake, or ocean. When real water is preferred to the sandtray's blue symbolic water, and used with control, sand and water form fragile spires that crown sandcastles. When control is relinquished, flooding may result, destroying all form and reducing mass to an undifferentiated mud. Whitmont (1990) states: "urges of violence and aggression are likely to be aroused by any stagnating or deadlocked life situation which calls for the need for regeneration, a new birth" (p. 18). Mud, then, represents not only chaos but the beginnings of new life and form.

UNIVERSAL PHENOMENA IN THE SANDTRAY

Specific sand forms or choice of miniatures do reoccur and may be identified with certain client populations or with stages undergone in the therapy process. For example, Bradway notes that at termination of therapy, turtles often appear in a client's final sand picture, perhaps symbolic of the client's new ability to negotiate life, just as turtles autonomously navigate the ocean after leaving the coast of their birth (Bradway & McCoard, 1997).

    C. G. Jung postulated the existence of a "myth producing level of mind which was common to all men." Jung wrote that the collective unconscious "as the ancestral heritage of possibilities of representation, is not individual but common to all men, and perhaps even to all animals, and is the true basis of the individual psyche" (Jung 1927/1931, pars 320). Jung recognized the forms of the objective psyche as "a collective a priori beneath the personal psyche existing as forms of instincts, that is, as archetypes" (Jung 1961,1995, p. 185). Edinger (1968) defines four inclusive categories of archetypal imagery:

    1. The Archetype of the Great Mother contains both the nourishing and devouring attributes of the feminine principal. Miniatures may represent the feminine range, from goddesses, queens, princesses, fairies, witches, to ordinary girls and women of all kinds. Neumann (1963/1983) writes:

The archetypal image symbol corresponds, then, in its impressiveness, significance, energetic charge, and numinosity, to the original importance of instinct for man's existence. . . . The representation of the instincts in consciousness, that is to say, their manifestation in images, is one of the essential conditions of consciousness in general, and the genesis of consciousness as a vital psychic organ is decisively bound up with the reflection of the unconscious psychic process in it. (p. 5)

One archetypal image frequently chosen by women concerned with achieving pregnancy is a metal Middle Eastern goddess holding her breasts. Her weight, secure stance, and turquoise color, potent against the evil eye, can evoke desire to receive her nurturing protection. A metal bare-breasted Cretan goddess holding a snake in each hand with a cat signifying wisdom perched on her head is popular in the role of invincible protector. In a second group, the fiery nature and determination of the crafty black witch of Oz are often feared, until she becomes a comfortable companion and example. Pinocchio's Blue Fairy, the gentle Chinese goddess Kwan Yin, and an American Statue of Liberty are archetypal feminine images that represent quiet compassion, dignity, and independence.

2. The Archetype of the Spiritual Father personifies the masculine principle of consciousness and spirit as opposed to matter. The union of opposites is necessary for all new life, and in the sandplay miniature collection, the full masculine range must be represented. One male archetypal image, a small metal African god holding a stick, is frequently chosen as a consort for the turquoise fertility goddess. Small metal soldiers, a golden Buddha, and a black totem have also increased the archetypal male presence at significant moments in the sandplays of women whose quest touched issues of identity, motherhood, and individuation.

3. The Archetype of Transformation includes themes of journey, descent, search for hidden treasure, death and rebirth, and hero or wonder child.

4. The Archetype of the Self, a symbol of totality and wholeness, is defined by Jung as being at once the center and the circumference of the psyche. It is the central organizing factor of the personality and includes both the collective unconscious, personal unconscious and consciousness of which the ego is the center (Edinger, 1968).

APPLE WORSHIP: A CASE EXAMPLE
OF THE SANDPLAY PROCESS

The following case example briefly presents the sandplay process of one young woman trying to get pregnant. Discussion of her work, illustrated with six of her sand pictures, exemplifies collective imagery concerned with fertility and may represent the imagery of other women with similar experiences (Steinhardt, 2000).

Sheila was considered a helping angel by family, friends, and those with whom she worked. After she had undergone medical fertility treatments, her one pregnancy had miscarried. A fertility treatment after her seventh sandplay was successful. She created six more sand pictures until her sixth month of pregnancy when she was confined to home rest until the birth. Her 13 sandplays were completed over 7½ months, each one helping to prepare the way for the next (Weinberg, 2002).

Sandplays 1, 2, and 3

A dialogue between opposites was apparent in Sheila's first three sandplays. In the first, a boat-like central sand shape points downwards to the right, a form she called "the mouth of the ocean." This image could have symbolized an entry to the unconscious and Sheila's therapeutic process, or an opening for fertilizing substances to enter her womb. In her second sand picture a triple spiral path moves counterclockwise from a shell in center to the lower right corner. Opposites are present in the spiral's high sand ridges studded with turquoise sea glass versus its gullies lined with a band of orange and red crepe. Four miniatures contrast masculine and feminine, and innocence with demonic power: a girl and boy are in the right corners and a witch and Indian chief in the left corners (Figure 20.1).

Sheila's third sandplay established fire and water as relevant opposites. Fire and water, and archetypal figures such as the turquoise goddess and metal African god, large apples, and other objects appeared in the sandplays of two other women with fertility problems just prior to conception (Steinhardt, 2000). In the center of the third sandplay is a palm tree shape made of two curving symmetrical incised blue lines. Its branches resemble two ovaries, each with a blue stone in its center. An imprinted hand filled with sea glass (a Hamsa) and other wet or blue elements represent water. A fire, two suns, stars, and red marbles represent fire. A rainbow, the merger of fire (as light) and water (as vapor), fills the upper right corner and will appear six more times.

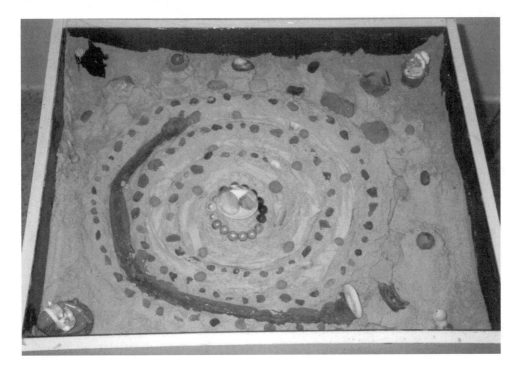

FIGURE 20.1. Sandplay 2.

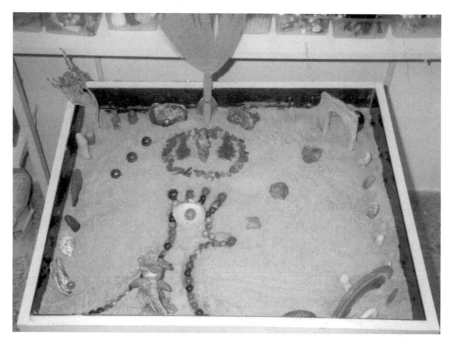

FIGURE 20.2. Sandplay 4.

Sandplay 4

Archetypal powers now enter as feminine and masculine opposites, the turquoise goddess in upper center, enclosed in a sea-glass circle, and the little African god unobtrusively standing in the upper left corner. They will appear together in five consecutive sandplays until, after successful conception, the god vanishes. Below the goddess, imprinted on the sand, is a large Hamsa, a hand and arm outlined by marbles reaching out from the bottom left. Fire and water (a shell) are present within, as well as a seed in the receptive feminine shell like a fetus in the womb (Eliade, 1991). Three blue stones lead from the hand to a portal in the upper right corner beyond which is a black egg. Another symbol of "egg" or "seed" is a path of three marbles on the upper left leading to a black shell with a pearl. Under the rainbow in the lower right corner, a little boy observes as he did here in the second sandworld. Awareness of the need to block intrusion is demonstrated by rows of stones and shells on the left and right edges of the scene (Figure 20.2).

Sandplays 5 and 6

The next two sand pictures are opposites, the fifth an angel's grave and the sixth a fruit-filled fertility rite to promote new growth. In the fifth sandplay the angel's funeral mound is reached through a black portal below. Above the grave stands the turquoise goddess with a watering can at her feet, the god outside to the mound's left and the black witch visibly on the right. "Seeds" in shells and a large metal fish are present. In the sixth sandworld the goddess is part of a group of four, including a fire, witch, and large apple, in the center of a large mandala cluttered with many other objects (Figure 20.3). The little god is behind and to the left of the goddess. Sheila wanted water to grow new things in the mandala and placed the watering can on the witch's arm. "Who will help the goddess to water? Her hands hold her breasts. The witch can help," she said. Fire and water are together in the center. Large fruits—apples and strawberries—newly appear inside the mandala, and as part of its circumference. Outside its boundaries, babies, children, and dwarfs represent the demands of others on her. The large metal fish waits again in the lower right. Sheila realized that she did not want to be an angel and had liked witches as a girl, but seemed to have forgotten their language.

Sandplay 7

This sandworld integrates the work done in the previous two. Sheila was saddened at first that spectators who had come for "apple worship" had also come to a funeral. An apple ringed by marbles, a fire just above it, and a watering can and open shell below are in the center of a mound enclosed by a circle of sea glass and nine evenly spaced objects. The reclining boy, goddess, metal fish, witch, twin kittens, black stone egg, little girl in a bucket, Chinese wise woman, and little god are closely unified in a rather ceremonial structure. And indeed Sheila put water in the can and

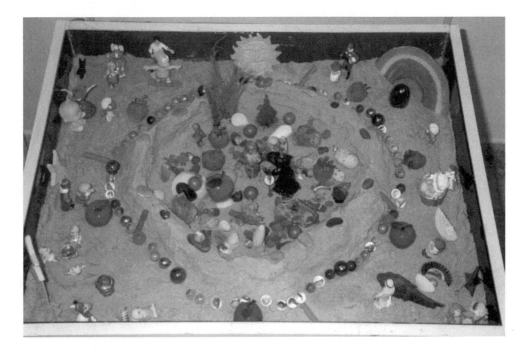

FIGURE 20.3. Sandplay 6.

dripped it into the shell "so something could grow on the grave." Above the circle are orange Garfield the cat and a rainbow behind him. Below, the black egg and twin kittens—new objects that also represent new life—and the baby in a bucket are closest to the black portal with a tiny owl on it and a mushroom on each side. A metal soldier guards beneath the gate as if an entry is imminent. This "guarding of the womb" by a male before fertilization, was present in two other women's sandplays. Four strawberries outside the mandala "square" the circle. According to Jung, the "squaring of the circle," the quaternity with the circle, could "even be called the archetype of wholeness" (Storr, 1983/1988, p. 236). A black totem introduces a new powerful male presence and a dinosaur hatches from an egg to the right above. A sun glows in the upper left. Sheila experienced this sandworld as her own domain, enjoying the mushrooms "after the rain," and the witch who speaks and is heard. The presence of black in four powerful objects may refer not only to the absence of light and death but to the void from which new life emerges (Kandinsky, 1977; Luscher, 1969; Walker, 1991). The fish, symbolizing fertility and the fruit of the unconscious (Cooper, 1978), puzzled Sheila. After a successful fertility treatment 9 days later, the fish never returned (Figure 20.4).

Sandplay 8

After 8 weeks of pregnancy, Sheila's sand picture shows a decisively protected inner womb, fortified with double sand walls, containing two blue marbles representing

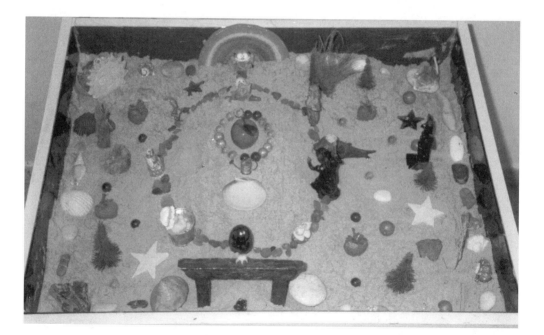

FIGURE 20.4. Sandplay 7.

her twin fetuses, covered by a palm branch. Six concentric circles, made of sand, glass, stones and nuts, shells, a blue moat, and a fence, separate the womb from the outside. Circular configurations may appear as symbols of wholeness and as a manifestation of the Self that "seems to guarantee the development and consolidation of the personality" (D. Kalff, 1980, p. 29). Inside the moat are four sentries facing outward: turquoise goddess at bottom, Cretan goddess above (just arrived on the sandplay shelves), little god facing left, and witch facing right. Sheila saw the trees as watching for approaching danger. The needy creatures facing outward at the sandtray's left and right edges, must look elsewhere for help. Sheila now related clearly to her archetypal guardians. The turquoise fertility goddess was full of feeling, connected to the earth, reminding her from where she came and to where she was going. The witch was a good old friend, a healthy part of her that she could now use. The Cretan goddess seemed aggressive and warlike, helping the witch, and saying, "Don't even think about messing around with me." The male god was protective but also had a therapeutic role—"hurting, wounded, helping others connect to their own wounds, he blocks shocks from the outside. His stick is like a lightening rod, he can absorb into himself sorrow, despair, loss, anxiety, mostly pain and frustration" (Figure 20.5).

Sandplays 9, 10, 11, and 12

Sheila's next two sandplays reflected her recurring anxiety about the success of her pregnancy. Even after the results of genetic blood tests were reassuring she remained

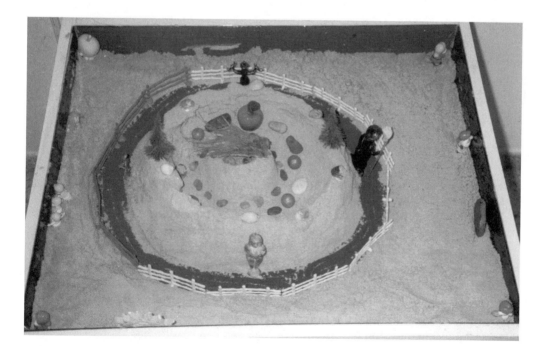

FIGURE 20.5. Sandplay 8.

uncertain. Yet the Cretan goddess, apples and sea glass, and trees and blue marbles seemed to bring back hope and she was able to access a victorious, flowering side of herself in her 10th sandplay, a large sandwoman crowned with trees like the Statue of Liberty in a blue-water semicircle and a rainbow and both goddesses above. The 11th and 12th sandplays are quietly guarded by the two goddesses facing each other and four trees. In the 11th, twin blue wombs each contain an open shell holding a nut. The 12th sandplay done in Sheila's fifth month of pregnancy shows a circle of smooth flat stones, the two goddesses and two blue stones, perhaps representing her twins, inside. Above, a sun and rainbow lie flat, as if to prescribe rest.

Sandplay 13

This final sandplay in Sheila's sixth month of pregnancy shows a mandala of sea glass reinforced by a sand ridge, containing a central turquoise stone with two shells with a red marble in each on either side. The squaring of this circle, portraying her sense of wholeness, manifests in the presence of the number four (Eastwood, 2002). Outside the circle are four archetypal figures and four hills with four stones on them. Inside are four trees, four nuts, two closed shells, seed pod and watering can, four together. The outer edges are guarded by the turquoise goddess in the rear facing us, the Cretan goddess facing outward in front, black witch facing left, and black totem facing right, perhaps replacing the male god (Figure 20.6).

Summary of Sessions

In this sandplay case example a series of symbolic steps were taken to engender conception and to provide a sense of protection for mother and fetus until birth. Differentiation of the opposites, masculine and feminine, fire and water, was initially achieved. Sheila's old role—her "angel" persona—was ceremoniously buried and upon the grave new growth was watered. Boundaries were strengthened to prevent the dependency of others on her. Differentiation of archetypal feminine roles gave rise to the turquoise goddess with her male god-consort presiding over conception, helped by the witch who brought water to the fire. Many seeds in shells, the black egg, the metal fish, a baby in a bucket, and the small boy were constant symbols of new life potential.

After her conception, uncertainty and doubt were transformed into a sense of protection by masculine and feminine guardians, the invincible Cretan goddess and the black totem. The last four sandplays prescribe rest and secure boundaries serving maturation of the fetus. A central mandala predominated in the three sandplays before conception and in the last two sandplays, which seem quiet and secure. Repetitive use of spontaneously chosen specific objects and introduction of new objects at appropriate moments seem to confirm the self-regulating power of the psyche in the service of healing and individuation.

Sheila became the helper not of others but of herself, allowing the sandplay process and spontaneous archetypal imagery to instill hope that she could clarify the boundaries and priorities in her life and be victorious in her own cause.

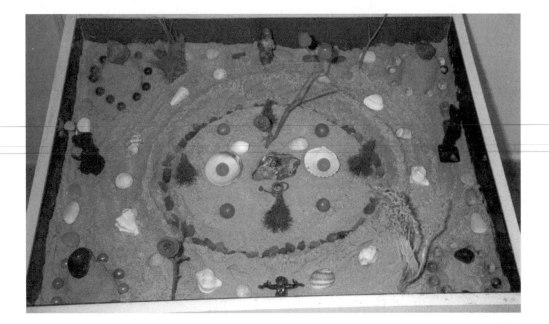

FIGURE 20.6. Sandplay 13.

CONCLUSION

Sandplay in the art therapy setting adds natural materials and their innate metaphoric potential for healing and growth, accessing deep instinctual layers of the psyche. Play with sand, water, and miniatures integrates creation of self-made forms from primordial materials and choice of already formed objects existing in the world. It is a way of balancing natural instinct and cultural knowledge. It joins those who use it in an unacknowledged communal ceremony of creating universal forms, as part of the life path. Sandplay clients often say "I have no idea what I have done or what it means," accompanied by a sense of physical "knowing" that the image must be this way and no other.

Weinrib (1983) states that "the primary thrust of sandplay is the reestablishment of access to the feminine elements of the psyche in both men and women" (p. 37). The case study presented demonstrated the feminine aspect of nurturance and fertility. Of the universal approaches to sandplay, Sheila used several—mounds, a spiral path, and imprinted hands, or Hamsas. She penetrated the sand to bury an angel, her persona. She used both real water for purification and blessing and blue symbolic water. The sandforms instinctively chosen reflected her goals, those that would help her. The miniatures she chose represented those qualities of herself that had to be done away with if she was to bring new life into the world, and archetypal images that brought her support, hope, and inspiration that her dream was possible. Sandplay was the vehicle of this process.

REFERENCES

Ammann, R. (1991). *Healing and transformation in sandplay.* LaSalle, IL: Open Court.

Anzieu, D. (1989). *The skin ego.* New Haven and London: Yale University Press.

Bowyer, L. R. (1970). *The Lowenfeld world technique.* Oxford: Pergamon Press.

Bradway, K., & McCoard, B. (1997). *Sandplay—silent workshop of the psyche.* London: Routledge.

Carey, L. (1999). *Sandplay therapy with children and families.* Northvale, NJ: Jason Aronson.

Case, C. (1987). A search for meaning: Loss and transition in art therapy with children. In T. Dalley, C. Case, J. Schaverien, F. Weir, D. Halliday, P. Nowell Hall, & D. Waller (Eds.), *Images of art therapy: New developments in theory and practice* (pp. 36–73). London: Tavistock.

Chodorow, J. (1997). *Jung on active imagination.* London: Routledge.

Cooper, J. C. (1978). *An illustrated encyclopaedia of traditional symbols.* London: Thames and Hudson.

Eastwood, P. S. (2002). The archetypal meaning of numbers in the sandplay process. In N. Baum & B. Weinberg (Eds.), *In the hands of creation: Sandplay images of birth and rebirth* (pp. 65–72). Toronto, Canada: Muki Baum Association.

Edinger, E. F. (1968). An outline of analytical psychology. *Quadrant, 1,* 1–1.

Eliade, M. (1991). *Images and symbols.* Princeton: Princeton University Press.

Gray, E. (1983). Review: Images of the self: The sandplay therapy process, by Weinrib, E. *American Journal of Art Therapy, 3*(1), 35–38.

Halliday, D. (1987). Peak experiences: The individuation of children. In T. Dalley, C. Case, J. Schaverien, F. Weir, D. Halliday, P. Nowell Hall, & D. Waller (Eds.), *Images of art therapy: New developments in theory and practice* (pp. 128–156). London: Tavistock.

Jung, C. G. (1927/1931). The structure of the psyche. The structure and dynamics of the psyche. *Collected works* (Vol. 8, p. 320). London: Routledge.

Jung, C. G. (1961/1995). *Memories, dreams, reflections.* London: Fontana Press. (An imprint of HarperCollins)

Kalff, D. M. (1980). *Sandplay.* Boston: Sigo Press.

Kalff, M. (1993). Twenty points to be considered in the interpretation of a sandplay. *Journal of Sandplay Therapy, 2,* 2.

Kandinsky, W. (1977). *Concerning the spiritual in art.* New York: Dover.

Kawai, H. (2002). Creation myths and sandplay therapy. In N. Baum & B. Weinberg (Eds.), *In the hands of creation: Sandplay images of birth and rebirth* (pp. 33–40). Toronto, Canada: Muki Baum Association.

Lewis, P. P. (1988). The transformative process within the imaginal realm. *The Arts in Psychotherapy, 15*(4), 309–316.

Lowenfeld, M. (1935). *Play in childhood.* London: Victor Gollancz Ltd. (Reprinted, 1976, New York: Wiley; 1991, London: Mac Keith Press)

Luscher, M. (1969). *The Luscher color test.* New York: Random House.

Markell, M. J. (2002). *Sand, water, silence—the embodiment of spirit: Explorations in matter and psyche.* London: Jessica Kingsley.

McNally, S. P. (2001). *Sandplay: A sourcebook for play therapists.* Campbell, CA: Universe.

Mitchell, R. R., & Friedman, H. S. (1994). *Sandplay, past, present and future.* London: Routledge.

Neumann, E. (1963/1983). *The great mother.* New York: Bollingen Foundation.

Neumann, E. (1973/1988). *The child.* London: H. Karnac.

Ryce-Menuhin, J. (1992). *Jungian sandplay: The wonderful therapy.* London: Routledge.

Steinhardt, L. (1997). Beyond blue: The implications of blue as the color of the inner surface of the sandtray in sandplay. *The Arts in Psychotherapy, 24*(5), 455–569.

Steinhardt, L. (1998). Sand, water and universal form in sandplay and art therapy. *Art Therapy: Journal of the American Art Therapy Association, 15*(4), 252–260.

Steinhardt, L. (2000). *Foundation and form in Jungian sandplay.* London: Jessica Kingsley.

Storr, A. (1983/1998). *The essential Jung.* London: Fontana.

Toscani, F. (1998). Sandrama: Psychodramatic sandtray with a trauma survivor. *The Arts in Psychotherapy, 25*(1), 1–29.

Walker, M. (1991). *The power of color.* New York: Avery.

Weinberg, B. (2002). Crossing thresholds of initiation: Images in sandplay. In N. Baum & B. Weinberg (Eds.), *In the hands of creation: Sandplay images of birth and rebirth* (pp. 99–116). Toronto, Canada: Muki Baum Association.

Weinrib, E. (1983). *Images of the self.* Boston: Sigo Press.

Whitmont, E. C. (1990). *Return of the goddess.* New York: Crossroad.

CHAPTER 21

Art Therapy with Adults with Severe Mental Illness

Susan Spaniol

Each year, the lives of about 5 million Americans and those close to them will be affected by a severe and persistent mental illness that interferes with their ability to think, to feel, to work, and to sustain meaningful relationships. These often disabling conditions include schizophrenia, a thought disorder that can cause delusions and hallucinations, and the more severe cases of depressive disorders, which include major depression and bipolar disorder (manic–depressive illness). More common than diabetes, cancer, or heart disease, these mental illnesses fill 21% of all hospital beds at any given time. The need for effective approaches to treating people with severe mental illness is often a matter of life and death; the lives of 1 in 10 persons diagnosed with schizophrenia and 1 in 5 with bipolar illness will end in suicide.

The prevalence and urgency of severe mental illness challenges therapists to develop hope-inspiring approaches for working with this population. However, therapists are often discouraged in their efforts to provide adequate treatment due to the realities of health care in the United States. Treatment is brief, often limited to one or two sessions within hospital settings, and a few months in day treatment. Individual art therapy is nearly obsolete, and people are often seen in large groups with various diagnoses, emotional states, and cognitive abilities, and at widely different stages of their recovery. Given the current constrictions of the mental health system, most group art therapy with people with mental illness is conducted along traditional lines, in prosaic rooms, with limited supplies.

Despite these troublesome realities, art therapy with people with severe mental illness can be deeply rewarding work. It can be intensely gratifying to build connections with and between people who have felt entirely alone, to provide hope to those who feel hopeless, and to guide them in using art's tools and processes to develop a sense of meaning and purpose. This chapter describes necessary conditions for working successfully with people with mental illness and how they can be applied in traditional mental health settings. It also suggests resources that can help people with mental illness extend their artistic engagement beyond the treatment setting.

There are three necessary conditions for therapists to be confident and competent working with people with severe mental illness: authenticity, creativity, and recovery. "Authenticity" describes the deeply human relationship between the therapist and clients, which becomes a model for clients' relationships with one another. "Creativity" relates to clients' engagement in the arts and the therapist's awareness of the special role that creativity can play in the lives of people with mental illness. "Recovery" represents the therapist's belief that people with mental illness can build lives of meaning and purpose despite their illnesses.

AUTHENTICITY

Therapeutic skills, theoretical knowledge, and proper technique are requisites to any successful treatment. In working with people with severe mental illness, the therapist's attitude is even more essential than what she says or does because authentic and sincere engagement with people, and the art materials themselves, are the basic curative elements in art therapy with this population.

The art therapeutic alliance should be a genuine relationship, not a technique for stimulating transference or a strategy for facilitating group participation. Therapists who are successful with this group of people are honest, warm, and active. Their primary role is as a fellow human being who does not perceive people as "mental patients," but as people with mental illness who once had dreams and hopes that were the same as theirs. They acknowledge their inability to find a "quick fix." They tolerate despair and offer hope in the face of their clients' hopelessness. They are willing to disclose aspects of their lives to make clients more comfortable; to use outside supports when necessary; and to address the consequences of major mental illness, such as poverty, stigma, discrimination, and self-doubt (Deegan, 1993, 1996).

By connecting with clients in a real and genuine fashion, therapists become models for how to connect with others. In successful art therapy groups, people with mental illness often develop empathy and compassion for one another, sometimes for the first time in their lives. Most people with mental illness long for intimacy because it makes them feel whole and intensely alive, yet many also feel too anxious, vulnerable, and exposed to try to connect with others (Davidson & Stayner, 1997). Group members learn that they, too, can relate to people in safe, creative ways to feel less alone and more complete. They begin to develop interpersonal confidence that they can carry with them beyond the art therapy group and into their lives.

CREATIVITY

For those working with people with severe mental illness, the role of creativity is heightened due to its special connection to mental illness. The notion that artistic creativity and mental illness are related has been embedded in our culture since classical antiquity. We can all name great visual artists who are now believed to have been mentally ill, such as Bosch, Durer, van Gogh, Nolde, and Pollock. In fact, empirical studies of possible connections between creativity and mental illness are providing strong support for a relationship between them, especially with the mood disorders of depression and manic depression (Jamison, 1993; Ludwig, 1995; Post, 1994; Schildkraut & Otero, 1996).

Although it is erroneous to believe that all people with mental illness are creative, it can be useful to consider the transformative role the arts have played in the lives of many people with mental illness. Although it may be a high price to pay, some people with mental illness consider artistic creativity to be a compensatory benefit of their illness. For those who build art making into their lives, the positive social identity of "artist" often furnishes an empowering alternative to the negative stereotype of the "mental patient." Since the 1990s, growing numbers of people with mental illness have recognized that art can effect social change. Around the country, groups of people are promoting the use of the arts outside treatment settings to challenge social stigma and build a sense of community (Bluebird, 1996, 2000). Therapists who understand the growing role of the arts in the self-help movement will be more empathically attuned to their clients and better able to help them extend their artistic involvement beyond clinical art therapy groups.

RECOVERY

Therapists who are successful with people with severe mental illness focus on their hopeful long-term prognoses rather than their pessimistic medical diagnoses. They know that despite the grave and damaging effects of severe and persistent mental illness, the concept of chronicity is not considered accurate. The term "recovery" has been used to include the deeply human experience of transcending afflictions which anyone might experience, such as illness, loss, and trauma. For people with mental illness, it suggests growing beyond the limits of the illness to build a meaningful life, even when the illness persists. Recovery is a developmental process of self-discovery and transformation that empowers people with mental illness to develop lives of dignity and purpose.

High rates of recovery for mood disorders have long been acknowledged. What is less familiar is the optimistic outcome for schizophrenia. The classic study by Harding (Harding, Brooks, Ashikaga, Strauss, & Breier, 1987) of people deinstitutionalized from the back wards of Vermont's State Hospital found that 62 to 68% showed no signs of schizophrenia at all several decades after their first admission. Nine other long-term studies of people hospitalized for schizophrenia (McGuire,

2000), conducted worldwide, reveal a recovery rate of 50% or higher over time. Given these results, the possibility of recovery is more hopeful than ever.

Researchers are discovering that a key to successful treatment of severe mental illness is understanding its impact and course from the viewpoint of the person experiencing it (Anthony, 1993; Baxter & Diehl, 1998; Davidson & Strauss, 1992; Deegan, 1993, 1996; Spaniol, Gagne, & Koehler, 1999; Young & Ensing, 1999). They propose a concept of recovery that challenges the traditional medical model of treatment because it addresses the impact of mental illness rather than its symptoms, and focuses on human potential rather than disease. Therapists who are most successful with people with mental illness recognize that the majority will grow beyond the limits of their illness. Therapists can offer hope for the future because they hold a vision of what is possible.

During recent years, researchers have been differentiating various phases of the recovery process (Baxter & Diehl, 1998; Spaniol et al., 1999; Young & Ensing, 1999). While each client's journey of recovery is unique, studies describe a similar path leading from a sense of being overwhelmed by the disability, to struggling with the disability, to living with the disability, to living beyond the disability. With the onset of the illness that characterizes the first phase, people feel powerless and desperate for some sense of control over their lives. During the second phase, people begin to accept that they have a mental illness and need information and strategies for coping with their disability. During the third stage, when people can better manage their mental illness, they often focus attention on strengthening their sense of selfhood and regaining valued social and vocational roles. Finally, those who reach the fourth stage and grow beyond their illness can begin to develop contributing lives that express their talents and abilities. Knowledge of these phases can greatly assist therapists in creating treatment plans grounded in the wellness-oriented vision of recovery.

HOSPITALIZATION

Phase 1: Overcoming Crises

During the first phase of recovery from mental illness, people are often hospitalized in a state of severe crises. Due to the brevity of treatment, emphasis is on stabilization and discharge planning rather than psychotherapy. Most therapists find themselves running groups on hospital wards where members meet once or twice and barely know each other. These groups are usually tightly structured, address common themes, and use easy-to-control materials. Despite these limitations, hospital art therapy groups are especially important because they are often patients' only psychotherapeutic group as well as their first contact with the use of art for healing.

Therapists leading hospital groups are challenged to provide meaningful art experiences in a single session (Riley, 2001). They can follow the brief therapy model and meet the hospital's goal-oriented expectations by framing the art process as a metaphor for life. Themes should be simple and directed toward the here-and-now of patients' lives rather than dredging the past. Therapists can ask clients to identify a specific concern or goal when they introduce themselves at the beginning of groups. Emergent themes might include the experience of their hospitalization, issues in the milieu, or hopes for the future.

More important than the choice of theme, however, is identifying how the process of art therapy parallels life. Most people become hospitalized when they are unable to tolerate strong feelings. They have become immobilized by depression, terrified by delusions, or overcome by anger. Art therapy group leaders can introduce art making as an action-based activity that provides skills for managing difficult emotions.

Before people begin making art, the leader can explain that the art experience will be a three-step process of expressing, integrating, and containing their feelings and thoughts. When the works are complete, the therapist points out that members have expressed strong feelings in a safe way and are ready to integrate them by sharing them with others. At the end of the group, the therapist acknowledges members' courage in expressing and sharing and points out that they will be able to integrate their learning and resume their functioning within the milieu. She can also suggest that people experiment with drawing as a strategy for coping with distressing feelings after they are discharged.

DAY TREATMENT

Assessment

Group psychotherapy for people with mental illness usually takes place in day treatment centers, where people are often in the early phases of their recovery. Although the pace of admission has become so rapid that art therapists rarely do intake assessments, they often use assessments to help them place people in suitable groups. A particularly useful instrument is the Drawing from Imagination subtest of the Silver Drawing Test of Cognition and Emotion (SDT) (Silver, 1996), which consists of a set of 15 stimulus cards showing people, animals, and things.

People are asked to select two stimulus drawings, imagine something happening between them, draw a picture of what they imagine, and then tell a story about what is happening. The protocol suggests using a pencil and 8½″ × 11″ piece of paper, but a creative chromatic adaptation uses oil crayons and 12″ × 18″ paper (Sandburg, Silver, & Vilstrup, 1984). An advantage of this test is that it is a gentle introduction to the creative process that can be presented as a problem-solving task.

How a person selects, combines, and integrates the pictures provides information about his or her cognitive functioning; how the person describes his or her pictures and the stories the person tells suggest the person's level of creativity and use of fantasy. People who demonstrate concrete cognitive functioning and a limited ability to fantasize are well suited to psychoeducational art therapy groups. Those with richer fantasy lives and the ability to express and contain them in images are ready for psychosocial groups that help them strengthen their sense of selfhood.

Phase 2: Developing Coping Strategies

One of the greatest losses accompanying severe mental illness is loss of a sense of control. With schizophrenia, reality may seem to slip away as people lose the ability to distinguish between external and internal experiences; with depression, energy and hope may erode as people are overtaken by despair and emotional pain; with bipolar disorder, the ability to focus is overcome by escalating agitation. Clinicians using a psychoeducational focus inform their clients about their conditions and give them methods of management. While verbal instruction is helpful, concretizing learning in artwork helps clients define their feelings and rehearse solutions.

It is useful to frame clients' symptoms as stress because stress is a common human experience. Clients can be taught that stress can stimulate or exacerbate the symptoms of mental illness, such as hallucinations, agitation, or a sense of hopelessness. They should also recognize that stress can be stimulated by environmental events, such as stigma and discrimination. Art therapy directives can be designed to frame symptoms of illness as messengers that carry clues about sources of stress and resources for managing them. For example, art therapy treatment can be organized around the following sequence of questions:

1. *What are your symptoms of stress?* By creating a visual analog for stressful feelings, people learn to identify and recognize their individual experiences of stress. Consistent with a psychoeducational approach, it is useful to use art therapy directives that are concrete rather than vague. To "get a picture" of how a person experiences stress, the clinician can ask the client to "Draw a picture of how you experience stress, using color, line, and form," or "Draw a picture of your stress as a weather condition." The expressive range of this exercise can be broadened by using unusual and evocative art materials such as collage or three-dimensional assemblage.

2. *What makes you feel stressed?* It is important for people to recognize situations that are potentially stressful. One way to accomplish this is by asking people to depict situations that trigger stress. Another way is to suggest that they use art materials in a way that evokes a stressful situation (e.g., using dissonant colors or unpleasant forms).

3. *What are some effective strategies for dealing with your symptoms of stress?* Here, again, the focus can be the content or the process of creating artwork. People can be encouraged to visualize a peaceful, stress-reducing scene, to draw or paint it, and then to display it where it can reawaken feelings of serenity and competency. Clients can also learn to use art activity as a form of stress reduction that evokes the relaxation response (Malchiodi, 1999). For example, painting to music with a wide brush and water colors on wet paper can be soothing if the activity is carefully framed as a relaxation technique. Modified contour drawing can also be a meditative practice because it trains people to focus their attention outside themselves (Edwards, 1979; Franck, 1973). To create a contour drawing, a person observes an object (natural objects are recommended) for a period of time and then—very, very slowly—draws the outlines he or she sees as though creeping ever so slowly along the edges, noticing each change and twist of the contour, peeking only to adjust the relation-

ships in the drawing. Through the use of art for stress reduction, clients learn strategies for controlling their symptoms and become ready to focus on developing a fuller sense of self.

Phase 3: Strengthening Selfhood

Research interviews with people with persistent psychiatric disorders indicate that a critical requirement for recovery is "rediscovering and reconstructing an enduring sense of the self as an active and responsible agent" (Davidson & Strauss, 1992, p. 131). Results of these interviews suggest that the task of developing a sense of self as an active agent in one's life is the key to improvement in the course of persistent mental illness. The study concludes that steps for developing a sense of self include "taking stock" of oneself, discovering a more active self, and putting that self into action.

Visual art as a therapeutic modality is especially useful for strengthening a fragile sense of selfhood. Not only do art activities build identity, but their concrete products can also furnish a form of self-identification. Nucho (1987) and DiMaria (1982) have described the "Self-System," which consists of interrelated components of the self. These components are (1) abilities and endowments, (2) relationships, (3) work performance, and (4) values and ideals.

By using these areas as treatment planning foci, therapists can monitor their groups so they address all facets of the lives of group members. The content of this system is especially appropriate to the recovery vision because it focuses on people's strengths and aspirations rather than their pathology and deficits.

I have modified the Self-System somewhat over the years. The four components of this modified system are (1) Self-Definition: Who are you?, (2) Self-in-Relation: What are your intimate and distant relationships?, (3) Self-Achievement: What are your accomplishments and what would you like to accomplish?, and (4) Self-Value: What gives your life meaning and purpose? These components can become the basis for building a sense of selfhood as well as strengthening and modifying aspects of the self. Based on these components, clinicians can select art therapy activities that develop particular aspects of their clients' selfhood. As Nucho (1987) indicates, change in one component shifts the entire system, creating conditions for growth.

The Self-System can be visualized as a series of four concentric circles. The first, central circle represents the client's current view of their core self. Like DiMaria's (1982) and Nucho's (1987) model, it includes people's physical endowments and functioning. In addition, it also includes their private, internal self—the part of the person that declares, "I am." In psychological terms, it includes the part of self known as the "subconscious" or "unconscious"; in archetypal terms, as the "psyche"; and, in religious terms, the "soul." Examples of directives include a visual self-symbol, drawing a tree and giving it a voice, a time line or road of life of specific memories, or how your best friend would portray you.

The therapist may want to use the same directive periodically to get an idea of whether or how a group member's self-image has shifted over time. The tree drawing in Figure 21.1 is inscribed with the message, "I am strong but empty at times. Am waiting for Spring." The tree in Figure 21.2, done by the same person at a later time, is identified by the word "peacefulness," suggesting a growing sense of well-being.

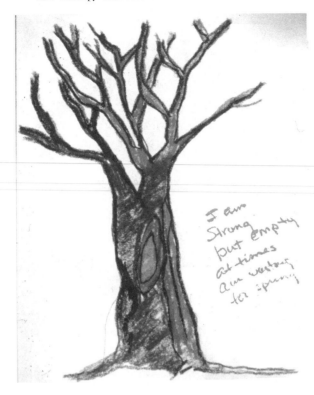

FIGURE 21.1. Tree drawing with message, "I am strong but empty at times. Am waiting for Spring."

The second concentric circle represents the social self—a person's place and space in relationship to others. Self-definition is based largely on how people are with others—their intimate, dyadic relationships, and their social roles and memberships in various groups. Life begins with the intimate relationship between mother and child, and future personality develops in the context of others. All people define themselves through membership in national, religious, and/or ethnic groups, as well as various cultural subgroups, such as gender and age. Examining one's social self helps people establish their uniqueness by understanding their relatedness to others. Examples of directives include a diagram of your support system and your place in that system, a picture of an ideal relationship and a difficult relationship, and your best friend. The person who drew Figure 21.3 depicted the importance of relationships in her life by portraying herself seated next to a friend at her residence, watching television, listening to music, and waiting for the phone to ring.

The third circle represents the achieving self. This component describes the self as an effective agent in the world. It is a broad category related to a person's roles and activities based on his or her strengths and abilities. Roles may be social as well as vocational. For clients who discover or rediscover their artistic interest and skill, making art can furnish a positive self-identity as an artist—a sense of self as a person who contributes to society by expressing the joys as well as the sorrows of being human (Spaniol, 1995). Examples of directives include "the proudest moment of my

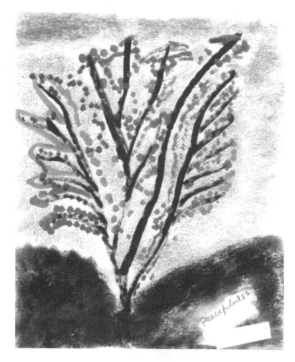

FIGURE 21.2. Tree image and word, "peacefulness," suggesting a growing sense of well-being.

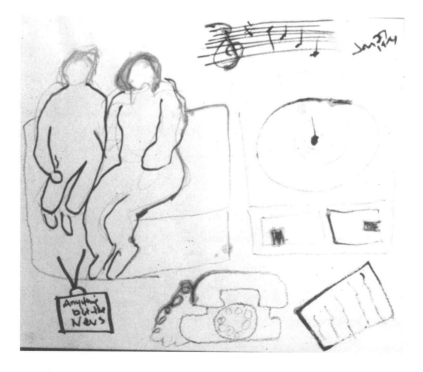

FIGURE 21.3. Image depicting the importance of relationships.

life," "the various roles you play," "a bridge between your present and your future," and "a portrait of yourself as an artist."

The fourth and last circle represents the valuing self. It is the meaning-making aspect of selfhood based on beliefs and values. Although it derives from people's interactions with the external world, it is an internal process of building one's preferences, hopes, and dreams, as well as identifying dislikes, fears, and regrets. It is a way of developing a sense of purpose that allows people with serious mental illness to "get on with their lives" as they grow beyond the limits of their psychiatric disorder. Examples of directives include "something important to you," "the person you most admire," "an image of your inner guide," and "a crystal ball showing where you would like to see yourself in 5, 10, or 25 years."

STUDIO SETTINGS

Creative Transformation

Thus far, this chapter has focused mainly on content-based art therapy directives because they provide structure and containment that help people strengthen their sense of self. But art is a way of transforming the self, as well as a way of knowing the self (Allen, 1995). When a person grasps internal images, wrestles with them, and concretizes them in two- or three-dimensional form, art becomes a "way of knowing." The process of grappling with the media can become a metaphor for the struggle to wrestle a new identity from strengths remaining from the former self and from newly developed capabilities.

Most therapists working in day treatment offer open studio sessions where clients can master the unique properties of various art media, giving physical existence to shapes and forms. The field of psychiatric rehabilitation is also beginning to recognize the role of the arts in enriching the lives of people with mental illness. Therapists are finding employment in clubhouses, which provide vocational support, and social clubs, which provide opportunities for companionship.

With the studio focus to art therapy, therapists become facilitators and collaborators rather than treaters. Instead of selecting materials because they provide containment, they offer artist-quality materials that provide dignity and respect. These media might include acrylic paints and canvases, printing processes such as monotypes, and sculptural materials that require persistence over time. Therapists using a studio approach educate people about the use and potential of the media available so they can make informed choices. They avoid suggesting themes, providing only enough guidance to prevent excessive anxiety.

When art tasks are complete, the facilitator demonstrates curiosity about the artwork produced instead of allowing long silences, asking probing questions, or interpreting. Therapists can assist people to find words to describe their artwork by asking them for concrete descriptions of what they see. Betensky (1995), Nucho (1987), and B. Moon (1990) have described variations of this method of questioning. These variations are familiar to therapists as examples of the phenomenological approach to interpretation of artworks. Betensky guides clients simply by repeating the key phrase, "What do you see?" Nucho describes a structured dialog that includes an inventory of shapes and objects in the artwork, and Moon begins by encouraging artists to list the colors and shapes of things before naming objects. Phenomenological approaches are useful for people with schizophrenia and depression because they are concrete and reality based, grounding imagination in the world outside the artist's thoughts and feelings. They are also supportive because they respect the client's reality, encouraging the client to talk about his or her art in his or her own words, syntax, and personal style.

Advocacy through Art

Therapists should be aware that a growing number of people with severe mental illness are using the arts as self-help tools and as vehicles for social change. The person who painted Figure 21.4 considers herself a professional artist who attends an art studio for ex-patients in Western Massachusetts. This painting is both a powerful visual image and a strong statement about the lack of privacy in state institutions.

Many self-help groups use visual art for personal growth and transformation (Spaniol, 2000). A.R.T.S. Anonymous (Artists Recovering Through the Twelve Steps) was founded in 1985 as a self-help organization that now has over 100 chapters worldwide for people who want to fulfill their creative potential. National Artists for Mental Health (NAMH) is a New York-based organization run by people with men-

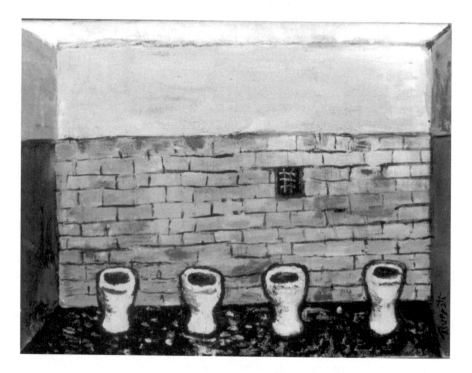

FIGURE 21.4. Painting by artist with mental illness.

tal illness to promote self-help activities that use of the creative arts. Its annual "Art of Healing" conference brings together consumers and interested professionals from across the country. The Center for Mental Health Services of the U.S. Government has sponsored annual Alternatives conferences, which have spawned a quarterly journal called *The Altered State* and a self-help manual for and by people with mental illness called *Reaching Across With the Arts* (Bluebird, 2000). These groups signal a decisive shift from the illness paradigm to a wellness orientation (Spaniol & Bluebird, 2002). They should remind therapists to explore the culture created by people with mental illness in order to empower themselves as clinicians and support their clients' transformation and growth.

Picturing Hope

Clinicians working with people with severe mental illness are often desperate to feel competent as healers. Clients with severe mental illness are often desperate to feel competent as a human beings. Both practitioners and clients are often desperate for interventions that provide a sense of hope and dignity to people with mental illness.

Through the therapeutic use of art, people with mental illness can develop and strengthen their connections to themselves, to others, to their environment, and to a greater purpose and meaning (Farrelly-Hansen, 2001). By projecting their internal lives into their artworks, they can connect with their emotions, developing a deeper sense of empathy and compassion for themselves (C. Moon, 2002). By identifying relationships of value and exploring ways to deepen them, they can take steps toward overcoming the subjective experience of loneliness. By using art to explore their values, they can gain a profound sense of meaning and connect with something beyond themselves. Finally, by immersing themselves in the creative process, people with mental illness can feel more fully whole, more fully human, and more fully the unique individuals they truly are (Spaniol, 2001).

REFERENCES

Allen, P. (1995). *Art is a way of knowing*. Boston: Shambhala.

Anthony, W. (1993). Recovery from mental illness: The guiding vision of the mental health service system in the 1990s. *Psychosocial Rehabilitation Journal, 16*(4), 11–23.

Baxter, E., & Diehl, S. (1998). Emotional stages: Consumers and family members recovering from the trauma of mental illness. *Psychiatric Rehabilitation Journal, 21*(4), 349–355.

Betensky M. (1995). *What do you see?: Phenomenology of therapeutic art expression*. London and Bristol, PA: Jessica Kingsley.

Bluebird, G. (1996). View from the arts: Arts as equal partners for social change. *Resources, 8*(2), 19–20.

Bluebird, G. (2000). *Reaching across with the arts: A self-help manual for mental health consumers*. Washington, DC: Center for Mental Health Services.

Davidson, L., & Stayner, D. (1997). Loss, loneliness, and the desire for love: Perspectives on the social lives of people with schizophrenia. *Psychiatric Rehabilitation Journal, 20*(3), 3–12.

Davidson, L., & Strauss, J. (1992). Sense of self in recovery from severe mental illness. *British Journal of Medical Psychology, 65*, 131–145.

Deegan, P. (1993). Recovering our sense of value after being labeled. *Journal of Psychosocial Nursing, 31,* 7–14.

Deegan, P. (1996). Recovery as a journey of the heart. *Psychiatric Rehabilitation Journal, 19,* 91–97.

DiMaria, A. (Ed.). (1982). *Art therapy: Still growing.* Mundelein, IL: American Art Therapy Association.

Edwards, B. (1979). *Drawing on the right side of the brain: A course in enhancing creativity and artistic confidence.* Boston: Houghton Mifflin.

Farrelly-Hansen, M. (Ed.). (2001). *Spirituality and art therapy.* London and Philadelphia: Jessica Kingsley.

Franck. F. (1973). *The Zen of seeing.* New York: Knopf.

Harding, C., Brooks, G., Ashikaga, T., Strauss, J., & Breier, A. (1987). The Vermont Longitudinal study of persons with severe mental illness, I: Methodology, study sample, and overall status 32 years later. *American Journal of Psychiatry, 144*(6), 718–735.

Jamison, K. (1993). *Touched with fire.* New York: Free Press.

Ludwig, A. (1995). *The price of greatness: Resolving the creativity and madness controversy.* New York: Guilford Press.

Malchiodi, C. (1999). Art therapy, arts medicine, and arts in healthcare: A vision for collaboration in the next millennium. *International Journal of Arts Medicine, 6*(2), 13–16.

McGuire, P. (2000). New hope for people with schizophrenia. *Monitor on Psychology, 33,* 24–28.

Moon, B. (1990). *Existential art therapy: The canvas mirror.* Springfield, IL: Charles C Thomas.

Moon, C. (2002). *Studio art therapy.* London and Philadelphia: Jessica Kingsley.

Nucho, A. (1987). *The psychocybernetic model of art therapy.* Springfield, IL: Charles C Thomas.

Post, F. (1994). Creativity and psychopathology: A study of 291 world-famous men. *British Journal of Psychiatry, 165,* 22–34.

Riley, S. (2001). Groups in psychiatric hospitals and day treatment programs: Art as an entree into unfamiliar realities. In S. Riley (Ed.), *Group process made visible* (pp. 193–208). Philadelphia: Routledge.

Sandburg, L., Silver, R., & Vilstrup, K. (1984). The Stimulus Drawing Technique with adult psychiatric patients, stroke patients, and adolescents in art therapy. *Art Therapy: Journal of the American Art Therapy Association, 1,* 132–140.

Schildkraut, J., & Otero, A. (Eds.). (1996). *Depression and the spiritual in modern art: Homage to Miro.* New York: Wiley.

Silver, R. (1996). *Silver drawing test of cognition and emotion* (3rd ed.). New York: Albin Press.

Spaniol, L., Gagne, C., & Koehler, M. (1999). Recovery from serious mental illness: What it is and how to support people in their recovery. In R. Marinelli & A. Dell Orto (Eds.), *The psychological and social impact of disability* (4th ed., pp. 409–422). New York: Springer.

Spaniol, S. (1995). Art is all the feelings trapped inside: An interview with Marilyn McKeon. *Art Therapy: Journal of the American Art Therapy Association, 12,* 227–230.

Spaniol, S. (2000). Guest editorial: "The withering of the expert": Recovery through art. *Art Therapy: Journal of the American Art Therapy Association, 17*(2), 78–79.

Spaniol, S. (2001). Art and mental illness: Where is the link? *The Arts in Psychotherapy, 28,* 221–231.

Spaniol, S., & Bluebird, G. (2002). Report: Creative partnerships—People with psychiatric disabilities and art therapists in dialogue. *The Arts in Psychotherapy, 29,* 107–114.

Young, S. L., & Ensing, D. S. (1999). Exploring recovery from the perspective of people with psychiatric disabilities. *Psychiatric Rehabilitation Journal, 22*(3), 219–231.

CHAPTER 22

Art Therapy in Addictions Treatment: Creativity and Shame Reduction

Marie Wilson

An alcoholic or chemically addicted person has a pathological relationship with a mood-altering substance. The addicted individual's relationship with the substance becomes primary and, with continued use, affects the person's psychological adjustment, economic functioning, and social and family relationships (Kinney & Leaton, 1995). The relationship between person and substance progresses to the point at which alcohol or the addictive substance is necessary to feel normal. This leads to isolation because the primary relationship is with a substance not with other people. Distortions in thinking, especially denial, become part of how the addict keeps painful feelings and associations related to substance abuse at a distance.

"Addiction" is a term traditionally associated with compulsive and out-of-control use of alcohol or drugs. The term, however, is now used to describe other compulsive behaviors such as gambling, overeating, or sex when these behaviors are also uncontrolled. Compulsivity is the loss of the ability to choose whether or not to stop or to continue a particular behavior. The continuation of behaviors and patterns that have resulted in adverse consequences such as arrests, divorce, loss of health, employment, or freedom clearly define behavior that is compulsive and out of control. Such behavior is called addiction.

In the United States, the predominant model for understanding alcoholism and other addictive illness is the view that these disorders are diseases (Thombs, 1999). This view is particularly popular within the treatment community and within the self-help fellowships such as Alcoholics Anonymous. The disease model provides the individual with a conceptual framework for understanding behaviors that he or she does not understand and cannot control and helps affirm the personal worth of the addict. It places value on who the addict is as a person and decreases some of the shame of being out of control.

Art therapy has been adapted to the specific needs of addiction treatment over the last two decades. Allen (1985) delineated the need for therapists to integrate art therapy into the overall treatment of alcoholism through highly structured groups on an alcoholism unit. Julliard (1994) and Feen-Calligan (1995, 1999) designed art therapy sessions based on concepts embraced by Alcoholics Anonymous and the 12 Steps, particularly the concepts of powerlessness and Higher Power. Chickerneo (1993) asserted that the visibility of art helped clients with addictions clarify spiritual beliefs. Moore (1983) addressed the uniqueness of the art product as tangible documentation and used it to assist in the recognition and reduction of distortions such as denial and Dickman, Dunn, and Wolf (1996) researched the use of images as predictors of relapse in chemically dependent adults. Therapists have also offered clinical observations on art therapy with chemically addicted, sexually abused women (Spring, 1985), with adolescent substance abusers (Cox & Price, 1990), and with sex addicted individuals (Wilson, 1998, 1999).

SHAME AND ADDICTION

Shame is an issue at the core of all addiction and a concept frequently addressed in addiction treatment programs. Terms such as "shame based" are used by addiction professionals to describe the feelings of worthlessness, powerlessness, and personal failure often experienced by the addicted person. Bradshaw (1988) says that shame is often preverbal in origin, making it difficult to define in words. Kaufman (1989) states, "It is a total experience that forbids communication with words . . . " (p. 119).

Other authors describe shame as intangible and elusive, yet complex and complicated. This is often the experience for the addicted person as well, making shame a particularly difficult issue to identify, especially in early treatment. The process of shame reduction, however, is crucial to the recovery process since it can be masked in many ways and interrupt the treatment process if not properly identified and addressed. It can take the form of silence, limit testing, anger, noncompliance, confusion, and projection, as well as other disruptions in thinking, especially denial (Wurmser, 1981).

SHAME THEORIES

Traditional psychoanalytic theory views shame as tension between the id, the ego, and the superego. Erikson (1950) included the concept of shame in the second stage (autonomy vs. shame) of his developmental model. This stage is described as a time when the child exercises control and develops self-esteem or becomes helpless and loses self-control.

In the 1970s and 1980s, shame became a focus of growing interest and research among theorists and clinical practitioners. Lewis (1971) described shame as a primitive and irrational state and connected it with the specific defense of "hiding or running away" (p. 38). Wurmser (1981) examined how issues of power are often tied to self-esteem and "to be powerless is to be shamed" (p. 220). These viewpoints provided a conceptual framework for a theory of shame compatible with current treatment philosophy in addictions literature.

Strongly connected to the experience of shame is the mechanism of denial, which is considered a primary symptom of chemical dependence. Denial is the inability to correctly perceive an unacceptable or painful reality. Denial protects the ego of the addicted individual from the threat of inadequacy (Thombs, 1999), and is used to manage the shame. Powerlessness is also a concept strongly associated with addiction. Step 1 of the 12 Steps of Alcoholics Anonymous begins with the need for addicted individuals to admit their powerlessness over the substance or behavior of which they have become addicted (Alcoholics Anonymous World Services, 1952). The addicted person's struggle to avoid recognition of their powerlessness over their addiction is also their struggle to avoid feelings of shame.

More recently, writers in addiction literature have examined shame as the foundation of all addictive behaviors. Carnes (1991) believes that shame is at the core of all addiction and that shame-based persons are particularly vulnerable to addictive illness. Bradshaw (1988), a recovering alcoholic himself, defines shame as toxic, dehumanizing, and terrifying to face and differentiates between healthy shame which is similar to remorse and in response to "what I did" and toxic shame which is about core beliefs and "what I am."

CREATIVITY AND SHAME REDUCTION

Although concepts of shame are not directly addressed in the literature, the self-affirming and life-giving nature of the creative process in humanistic theory is inherently shame reducing and corrective. May (1975) viewed the creative process with the highest regard and believed that creative individuals were on the path of self-actualization.

Addictive use of substances or behaviors becomes a conditioned response to stress and pain. Addicts feel powerless to break their conditioned response and the recovery process, like the creative process, offers individuals with addictions choices that the addiction does not. Arieti (1976) believed that creativity helps humans establish a bond between themselves and the world and enlarges the universe in an enriching and expansive way. Theories that embrace concepts of emotional health, self-actualization, enrichment, and expansiveness are compatible with treatment concepts outlined in addiction treatment and the recovery process. Zinker (1977) embraced creativity as life affirming and a celebration of life. He equaled creativity to the expression of each person's Godliness. The concept of spirituality and Higher Power are an integral part of 12-Step philosophy.

ART THERAPY AND SHAME REDUCTION

Art therapy seems particularly well suited for the expression and processing of deeper forms of psychic pain such as shame. McNiff (1986) stated that the arts, accustomed to speaking the language of the soul, have more immediate access to emotional conflicts and psychological pain. Moon (1994) described the artistic process as meta-verbal, or beyond words, suggesting that the images that artists create come from some place deep within them. Experiences that are difficult to articulate with words or are preverbal in origin lend themselves to expression more naturally through creative medium.

Art therapy provides an optimal arena for addressing early recovery issues related to honesty, accountability and change in both residential and outpatient addiction treatment programs. Education about addiction, confrontation of denial, and introduction to 12-Step philosophy are considered the basics of early intervention. In addition, art therapy is particularly well suited for the exploration and integration of shame within the context of the traditional addiction treatment model. I have included a set of five basic guidelines for therapists that follow specific identifiable tasks involved with recovery from addiction and shame reduction (Carnes & Rening, 1994).

Task 1: Establishing Safety with Self and Group

Establishing safety and containment within the therapeutic framework is essential to the process of treatment. Little else can happen until these basics are accomplished. Judging oneself as shameful builds a wall that successfully keeps others out. If a person sees no value in him- or herself, then it follows that others won't either. Most addicted individuals have issues of trust and any disclosure about themselves in a group involves both trust and risk taking. Initially, experimentation with art materials requires risk also. Many are fearful of being judged or looking foolish and often struggle with the need for perfectionism and control. These issues are reflections of shameful feelings.

Clients may feel more comfortable with the introduction of group norms and expectations at the beginning of each session. Asking older clients to mentor newer clients by describing the purpose of the group and their experience with art therapy helps create connections between members. Having all clients take a vow of confidentiality sets the tone for serious work and will help newer clients feel safer. Using treatment terms that are familiar to the client and compatible with addiction philosophy is recommended so that art therapy will be viewed as a continuation of the treatment process. In initial sessions, art therapy can assist with shame reduction by:

1. *Helping develop a language for the self.* Addicted clients can begin to explore the use of art as a language for their thoughts and feelings. Until clients are more accustomed to using art materials, it is best to offer materials that are easy to use and require minimal clean-up. This author prefers to limit the use of magazines for collage since most addicts are accustomed to looking towards external sources for an-

swers. Given adequate time and support, addicts can begin to access inner resources of wisdom and knowledge and images will begin to reflect their personal style.

2. *Providing safety and containment for raw and unprocessed feelings.* Unresolved emotional issues that have been kept submerged by the addiction now come to the surface. Feelings that have been numbed, avoided and denied by compulsive and out of control behaviors begin to surface in early treatment. Johnson (1990) stated that "often, the first creations of a recovering addict are disclosures of extreme shame, anguish, and rage" (p. 300). Art materials allow for ventilation and transformation of aggressive and violent emotions previously dealt with by compulsive and out-of-control behaviors.

3. *Learning self-reliance.* Addiction gives few choices. In the art room, clients are given the opportunity for choice. Art making provides a sense of mastery and control over media and outcome, unlike the unmanageability of the addiction.

Art directives

- Introduce yourself in a picture.
- Draw a picture about what circumstances brought you to treatment.
- Draw how you feel about being here.

Task 2: Understanding the Nature of Addictive Illness

The hardest challenge for some addicts is acknowledging that they have a problem since addiction cripples their ability to know what is real (Carnes, 2001). Therefore, education is an important aspect of addiction treatment since knowledge is empowering for the addicted individual. Giving addicts ways to describe their experience gives them tools for mastery and objectivity. Learning about the disease concept of addiction and that they are not to blame for having an addiction assists with shame reduction. There is power in naming the addiction for what it is and addicts are relieved to have words to describe their experiences. The art therapy session provides an excellent environment for both didactic and experiential learning. Use of creative modalities enhances the learning experience, allowing for a shift in the energy of the group and providing a tangible outcome. Using art materials to depict their own individual experiences of the concepts they are learning helps addicts personalize the experience and be accountable for their actions.

1. *Labeling the addiction.* Art is instrumental in helping addicted persons visualize their illness, providing both objectivity and distance from the chaos of their inner experiences. Images assist with reality orientation and many times addicts view, fully, for the first time, the negative consequences of their addiction.

Art directives

- Draw your addiction.
- Draw what happens to you when you are "under the influence" of mood altering substances or behaviors.

- Group exercise—draw the outline of someone's body on a large sheet of paper and have the group fill in the effects of substances on the body (Feen-Calligan, 1999).

2. *Unmanageability and powerlessness.* An understanding of the first step of a 12-Step fellowship sets the stage for the beginning of the recovery process. Twelve-Step work, which related originally to the 12 Steps of Alcoholics Anonymous (AA), currently is used successfully in numerous self-help fellowships, worldwide (Gamblers Anonymous, Narcotics Anonymous, Overeaters Anonymous, Sex Addicts Anonymous, etc.). Each step is fashioned around a particular task and each works in connection with the next. Although the exact wording of each task may vary from group to group, philosophically, the message remains the same. This first step requires an admission of powerlessness over living life in the extremes. An essential part of early recovery is the task of having addicts list evidence that documents both powerlessness and unmanageability in their lives as a result of addiction. Creating artwork around basic 12-Step concepts helps addicts visualize themselves working their recovery program and assists with integration of the recovery model.

Art directives

- Draw the unmanageability of your addiction (see Figure 22.1).
- Draw how being powerless feels to you.
- Draw the effects of unmanageability and powerlessness on your family.

Task 3: Breaking through Denial

Denial masks shame. Most clients who seek help for addiction are in considerable denial about the extent and severity of their problems. Most fail to recognize the enormous impact that their addiction has had on their lives and on the lives of those closest to them. Ignoring the problem, blaming others, and minimizing the severity of their behaviors are all part of their defensive repertoire. Adverse consequences that occur as a result of their addiction are overlooked or justified in an attempt to hide from a truth that is painful. Art therapy can break down defenses more quickly and less traumatically than verbal tactics. Creative modalities tend to bypass intellectual controls such as denial and speed up the therapy process. In addition, the artwork may reveal primary defenses when addicts continue to rationalize or minimize that they have a problem (Moore, 1983).

In the early stage of treatment, the emphasis should be on helping clients understand the role of denial in the maintenance of their addiction. Until they understand how hidden all addiction can be and still thrive, addicts will continue to see it as a rare illness, affecting other people but never themselves.

Art directives

- Draw a fantasy versus reality picture that compares and contrasts what the ad-

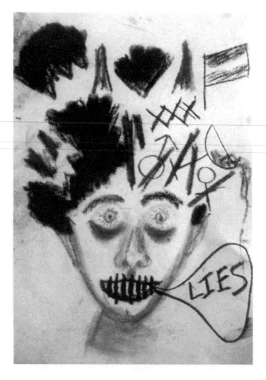

FIGURE 22.1. One client depicts the unmanageability of his addiction to alcohol and sex with a picture of his exploding head. His mouth is sutured shut as he tries desperately to speak the truth, but all that comes out is "lies."

diction promised you and what the reality of the experience actually was (see Figure 22.2).

- Draw a picture that depicts all that you have lost as a result of your addiction.
- Draw the consequences of the addiction, both external and internal.

1. *Forms of denial.* Educate clients as to the many forms of denial such as rationalizing, minimizing, intellectualizing, compartmentalizing, blaming, and the like.

Art directives

- Illustrate three (or more) forms of denial that you have used.
- *Self bag/box.* Use a bag or box to depict the inside and the outside of yourself (the outside represents what you let people see and the inside what you are afraid to let them see) (see Figure 22.3).

2. *Becoming aware of situations that trigger acting out.* It is essential in the beginning stages of treatment to educate clients about the situations in their lives that trigger acting out. The therapist should help them problem solve around ways

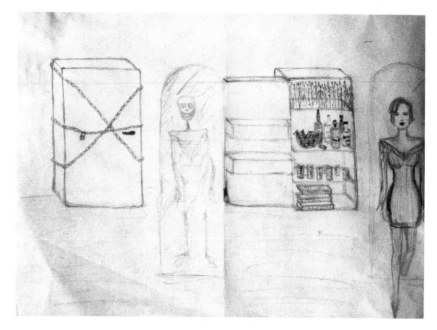

FIGURE 22.2. A female client drew this picture to illustrate the illusion versus the reality of her addiction to sex, alcohol, spending, cocaine, and nicotine. On the right side of the paper she drew an open refrigerator filled with all of her addictions. It is filled with people, bottles of alcohol, a bowl filled with money, cans of Coke to represent cocaine, and cartons of cigarettes. The mirror to the right of the refrigerator holds the image of herself as young, sexy, and beautiful. This represents the illusion that the addiction perpetuated. On the left side of the paper is a chained refrigerator. In that mirror she only sees the reflection of a skeleton. This represents the reality of how she really felt about herself.

to avoid the people, places, and things that electrify impulses. Clients can complete a checklist of triggers and spend time with the therapist reviewing the list.

Art directives

- Draw your checklist of triggers including emotional triggers.
- Draw a picture about when you are most vulnerable to addiction.
- Draw yourself with the tools of recovery to help you deal with triggers.

Task 4: Surrendering to the Process of Recovery

The transformation from active addiction to recovery is a process that requires an act of surrender. For the addict, the essence of surrender is accepting limitations since limits teach us about our humanness. Addiction is a denial of those limitations and accepting our humanness is part of shame reduction. The purpose of treatment is not to push the addict into deescalation but, rather, to bring about a profound shift of beliefs and behavior in which the addiction loses its power. This shift requires a radical change in the addict's view of the world.

1. *Support involvement in a 12-Step community and sponsorship.* In early treatment, it is essential for addicts to be with other recovering people and begin to build supportive relationships outside of treatment. The treatment center and the 12-Step community serves as a standard reality test for the addict entering recovery. When addicts do not possess inner resources, they can "borrow" some hope and strength from the 12 Steps and fellowship with other recovering people. A sponsor is an individual with some recovery time who mentors a newcomer in 12-Step work and basic recovery concepts.

Art directives

- Draw a picture about all the benefits of attending 12-Step meetings.
- Draw yourself surrounded by people who nurture you.
- Draw the qualities that you want to look for in a sponsor.
- Use a cartoon format to walk yourself through approaching someone at a meeting to be your sponsor.

2. *Help addicts structure a belief in a Higher Power of their choice.* The tremendous success of AA and other 12-Step programs may rest on the fact that they are so open ended with regard to spirituality and do not promote a specific belief system. Structuring one's belief begins with visualization. Many addicts begin with a portrayal of Higher Power being outside them and some distance away. As recovery progresses, the connection to Higher Power becomes closer, as a more intimate relationship with self and God emerges.

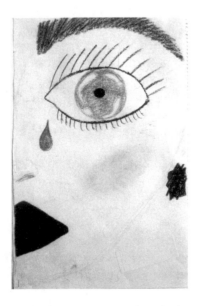

FIGURE 22.3. One female client used this picture to describe how she only shows a part of herself to other people and that no one ever sees all of her. Compartmentalization is a form of denial frequently used by sex addicts to keep shameful thoughts and feelings away from consciousness.

Art directives

- Draw your relationship to a Higher Power.
- Use a cartoon strip format to dialogue with your Higher Power.
- Draw a picture about forgiveness.

Task 5: Understanding the Origins of Shame

When clients in early recovery begin to feel safe enough to drop the facade of "looking good" they may become bombarded by feelings of shame and remorse over past behaviors and finally facing reality for the first time. Addicts who were raised in dysfunctional or abusive families of origin or are adult children of alcoholics carry the additional burden of traumatic experiences that have not been processed or integrated into conscious awareness. Often these families did not provide the structure, predictability, or nurturing necessary for teaching self-regulatory or problem-solving skills. Children who come from addicted families experience profound losses. Some addicted individuals experienced physical, emotional, or sexual abuse or neglect. From the age of onset of the addiction, the addict learned that mood-altering behaviors and/or substances took away feelings that caused discomfort or anxiety and came to rely on these as ways to cope.

There is a high comorbidity for addiction and posttraumatic stress disorder. Literature on the subject recognizes the use of addictive substances and compulsive behaviors for self-regulation of traumatic memory (Herman, 1992; van der Kolk, McFarlane, & Weisaeth, 1996). Although traumatic experiences are repressed and memories forgotten, the pain continues to accumulate. Trauma specialists such as Herman (1992) address the need for reconstruction of the trauma narrative with creation of new understanding and meaning.

Traumatic memories lend themselves more easily to images than to words. Art provides both safety and distance from the content of the experience through use of metaphor and symbolism yet also allows opportunity for full expression of traumatic experiences. Art gives preverbal trauma a voice while facilitating the exploration of deeper levels of emotional memory and experience. The unspeakable can be spoken while still maintaining safety and support in treatment. van der Kolk et al. (1996) said, "Prone to action, and deficient in words, these patients can often express their internal states more articulately in physical movements or in pictures than in words. Utilizing drawings and psychodrama may help them develop language that is essential for effective communication and for the symbolic transformation that can occur in psychotherapy" (p. 196).

1. *Addressing family-of-origin messages.* Addicted clients may either minimize their abuse or deny the long-term implications. Exercises that help them recognize the connection between childhood abuse and patterns of addiction are useful. The realization that they too were once victims helps with shame reduction. Behaviors that were established in childhood in the form of survival roles frequently become the self-defeating behaviors that create problems for early recovery.

Art directives

- Draw a family portrait.
- Draw the outline of a house. Outside the house, draw the image that the family portrayed to others. Inside the house, draw the way the family really functioned.
- Draw a picture about what you never got as a child and still long for today (see Figure 22.4).

2. *Breaking through addicts' myths and rules such as their perfectionism and need for control or their fear of change.* The creative forum gives permission for adult addicts to play in healthy, structured ways. Clients can explore and create without fear of reprisal. They are allowed to make mistakes and take risks. The simple act of building up and tearing down may be an activity never experienced by a client who was fearful that his or her every move was either under the scrutiny of critical parents or never tried because mistakes were not allowed (Rubin, 1984). Creativity gives adult addicts permission to play without serious regression or significant loss of control, thereby nurturing the child within and providing opportunity to accomplish as adults what they could not do as children (Wilson, 1998).

3. *Self-affirmation and empowerment.* The addict must let go of damaging and dysfunctional messages carried from childhood. By receiving affirming messages from others, addicts learn to construct a new, positive sense of themselves, eventually learning how to affirm themselves from within.

For many, healing the inner child is synonymous with recovery. Recovery literature abounds with books that use art exercises to help individuals get in touch with their inner child. It is no accident that the inner child expresses its feelings and needs more easily through art because children turn to these forms of expression when they cannot articulate their needs. Part of the repair work at this stage is for clients to learn to nurture their inner child so that childlike qualities so essential to growth can be reclaimed (Carnes, 1991).

Art directives

- Have clients each make an outline of their bodies. Have them fill the inside with positive affirmations and images.
- Have clients work together to build a road to recovery.
- Ask clients to create images of their inner child being attended to by their adult part.
- Have clients make a fabric doll or puppet of their inner child and create an environment of safety.

CONCLUSION

The process of surrender to a new lifestyle that does not include compulsive use of chemicals or behaviors is gradual and requires commitment. Addiction professionals

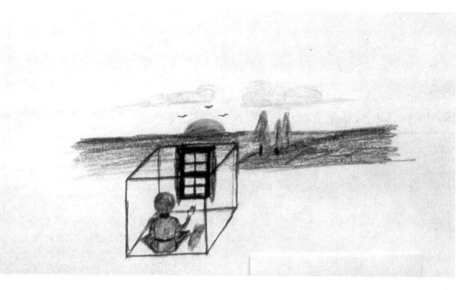

FIGURE 22.4. A sex- and drug-addicted client drew this picture to represent what he never got as a child and what he still longed for today. He felt isolated and lonely as a child and what he longed for was connection to other people.

have the task of teaching basic recovery concepts and skills while also addressing shame responses in a manner that is supportive yet holds the addict accountable. Art therapy can play an instrumental role in these treatment services and can be used in either a primary or adjunctive capacity.

Addicts must learn to recognize and identify their own shame response. By learning to label their shame, they can then separate reality from their feelings of shame, and in doing so, decrease cognitive distortions. Traditional cognitive approaches to shame reduction may allow intellectualization. Understanding alone is not sufficient to reduce shame since shame must be felt and reprocessed in order to reduce its impact on shaping perceptions and experiences. As shame is reduced, the individual begins to feel fewer urges to return to shameful, addictive patterns (Adams & Robinson, 2001).

Since the creative arts are accustomed to speaking the language of the soul, they have more immediate access to deeper forms of psychological pain such as shame. Often preverbal in origin, shameful feelings flow more easily via imagery and symbolism. The creative process itself is self-affirming, life giving and inherently shame reducing and corrective.

REFERENCES

Adams, K., & Robinson, D. (2001). Shame reduction, affect regulation, and sexual boundary development: Essential building blocks in sexual addiction treatment. *Sexual Addiction and Compulsivity*, 8(1), 23–45.

Alcoholics Anonymous World Services. (1952). *Twelve steps and twelve traditions*. New York: Author.

Allen, P. (1985). Integrating art therapy into an alcoholism treatment program. *American Journal of Art Therapy, 24,* 10–12.

Arieti, S. (1976). *Creativity: The magic synthesis.* New York: Basic Books.

Bradshaw, J. (1988). *Healing the shame that binds you.* Deerfield Beach, FL: Health Communications.

Carnes, P. (1991). *Don't call it love: Recovery from sexual addiction.* New York: Bantam Books.

Carnes, P. (2001). *Facing the shadow: Starting sexual and relationship recovery.* Wickenburg, AZ: Gentle Path Press.

Carnes, P., & Rening, L. (1994). *The 27 tasks for changing out-of-control, compulsive, and inappropriate sexual behavior.* Plymouth, MN: Positive Living Press.

Chickerneo, N. B. (1993). *Portraits of spirituality in recovery: The use of art in recovery from codependency and/or chemical dependency.* Springfield, IL: Charles C Thomas.

Cox, K., & Price, K. (1990). Breaking through: Incident drawings with adolescent substance abusers. *The Arts in Psychotherapy, 24,* 10–12.

Dickman, S., Dunn, J, & Wolf, A. (1996). The use of art therapy as a predictor of relapse in chemical dependency treatment. *Art Therapy: Journal of the American Art Therapy Association, 13*(4), 232–237.

Erikson, E. H. (1950). *Childhood and society.* New York: Norton.

Feen-Calligan, H. (1995). The use of art therapy in treatment programs to promote spiritual recovery from addiction. *Art Therapy: Journal of the American Art Therapy Association, 12*(1), 46–50.

Feen-Calligan, H. (1999). Enlightenment in chemical dependency treatment programs: A grounded theory. In C. Malchiodi (Ed.), *Medical art therapy with adults* (pp. 137–161). London: Jessica Kingsley.

Herman, J. (1992). *Trauma and recovery.* New York: Basic Books.

Johnson, L. (1990). Creative therapies in the treatment of addictions: The art of transforming shame. *The Arts in Psychotherapy, 17,* 299–308.

Julliard, K. (1994). Increasing chemically dependent patients' belief in step one through expressive therapy. *American Journal of Art Therapy, 33,* 110–119.

Kaufman, G. (1989). *The psychology of shame: Theory and treatment of shame-based syndromes.* New York: Springer.

Kinney, J., & Leaton, G. (1995). *Loosening the grip: A handbook of alcohol information.* St. Louis, MO: Mosby-Year Book.

Lewis, H. B. (1971). *Shame and guilt in neurosis.* New York: International Universities Press.

May, R. (1975). *The courage to create.* New York: Norton.

McNiff, S. (1986). *Educating the creative arts therapist.* Springfield, IL: Charles C Thomas.

Moon, B. (1994). *Introduction to art therapy.* Springfield, IL: Charles C Thomas.

Moore, R. (1983). Art therapy with substance abusers: A review of the literature. *The Arts in Psychotherapy, 10,* 251–260.

Rubin, J. (1984). *The art of art therapy.* New York: Brunner/Mazel.

Spring, D. (1985). Sexually abused, chemically dependent women. *American Journal of Art Therapy, 24,* 13–21.

Thombs, D. L. (1999). *Introduction to addictive behaviors* (2nd ed.). New York: Guilford Press.

van der Kolk, B. A., McFarlane, A. C., & Weisaeth, L. (1996). *Traumatic stress: The effects of overwhelming experience on mind, body, and society.* New York: Guilford Press.

Wilson, M. (1998). Portrait of a sex addict. *Sexual Addiction and Compulsivity, 5*(4), 231–250.

Wilson, M. (1999). Art therapy with the invisible sex addict. *Art Therapy: Journal of the American Art Therapy Association, 16*(1), 7–16.

Wurmser, L. (1981). *The mask of shame.* Baltimore, MD: Johns Hopkins University Press.

Zinker, J. (1977). *Creative process in gestalt therapy.* New York: Vintage Books.

CHAPTER 23

Clinical Art Therapy with Older Adults

Judith Wald

I'm growing old
Growing older, growing, maturing,
Phooey!
I'm growing old.

I don't like it.
Not one bit.
I'm all alone.
I'm unhappy.

I'm slower.
Sometimes I can't walk.
I have to learn to cry.
Nobody wants to die.

Yet . . .
I'm older than my mother ever was
I don't have to do the things
I had to do when I was young

I'm lucky.
I have a husband
I have children
I did a good job.

Now I'm painting
Reading.
Getting out.
Having a delicious time.

But, I'm growing old.
I'm growing old.

—GROUP POEM WRITTEN BY CLIENTS AT A GERIATRIC
DAY TREATMENT PROGRAM

I usually begin workshops for professionals with an experiential: "Draw a picture of an elderly person." This statement serves to introduce issues of personal and societal attitudes toward the older adult. How does one perceive an "elder"? As vigorous, decrepit, with a smile or a frown? Is this a grandparent, a special older person in one's life, a client one has encountered? Do one's own fears about the aging process surface? Can you work with this population and handle the countertransferential issues that emerge? What are the goals of art therapy treatment and what can a therapist expect in working with older adults?

Everyone, of any age, needs to believe there is something to live for, to experience pleasure in living. By understanding and acknowledging age-related changes and losses that the elderly suffer, therapists can help them to maintain hope despite physical, psychological, and/or cognitive losses. This chapter reviews these specifics with older physically disabled, psychiatric, and dementia populations, as well as how to motivate these populations to activity by building on the positive and on their strengths through art therapy.

CHANGES RELATED TO AGE IN THE OLDER ADULT

The older adult must cope with major life losses, physical decline, sexual changes, changes in dependency status, role as receiver, and reduction in social contacts by developing new leisure activities, learning new skills, and making new friends. According to Blau and Berezin (1975), one is expected to sustain mild feelings of depression, anxiety, and grief, and one needs to reduce somewhat one's aspirations. They define the difference between normal and pathological aging as "the ability to handle both external losses and narcissistically perceived internal and external changes without becoming seriously disturbed" (p. 226).

Changes related to aging fall into two general categories: physical–biological and psychosocial losses and crises.

Physical–Biological

Physical changes occur to the hair, which thins and grays; visual and hearing acuity declines; skin wrinkles; muscles and bones weaken; joints become inflamed; and sexuality changes with menopause and impotence. These minor narcissistic injuries can cause more discomfort and anxiety than more apparent major external traumatic events yet elicit less sympathy (Blau & Berezin, 1975). Normal changes also occur in all systems and organs, and physical disabilities can result from injury and illness to any organ.

Cognitive impairment, memory loss, reduced rate of response, and organic bodily ills can play a causal role in mental illness in the elderly. Common psychiatric disorders among the elderly include mood disorders of major depression, bipolar disorder, dysthymic disorder; psychotic disorders of schizophrenia and paranoia; and neurotic disorders of anxiety disorder, somatoform disorder, dissociative disorder (which may involve psychotic features), sexual and gender disorders, and personality disorders. Cognitive disorders, including Alzheimer's disease and other dementias, delirium, and amnestic disorder, as well as physical illnesses, are often complicated by paranoia, depression, or psychosis.

Psychosocial Losses and Crises

In our culture that favors beauty and youth, one's job status may be lowered in favor of promoting a younger less experienced colleague, leading to loss of self-esteem. Whether retirement is forced or self-chosen, it requires an adjustment. Loss of income may result in loss of independence and increased financial concerns. Loss of social contacts through work; death of peers, relatives, and spouse; and fear of crime and vulnerability, compounded with isolation and inactivity, lead to stress. Mental illness in the elderly is usually caused by stress—economical, social, and psychological.

Historically, families provided for their relatives, and aging was accepted as part of the life cycle, not an illness. Kerr (1999) notes, "Where once our elders were revered for their wisdom and encouraged to inspire the intergenerational family constellation, now our aged are often viewed as burdensome and subordinate" (p. 38). Now group homes and institutions substitute for families. Usually the decision to enter an institution is made by another, against one's will, which gives older individuals the message that they are no longer capable of self-care. It is not surprising that losses of family role, work role, close relatives, familiar people, and places and things lead to depression, withdrawal, and regression—all natural responses to losses and crises (Weiss, 1984).

Finally, many defense mechanisms may surface in behavior in an attempt to handle anxiety and protect the ego in reaction to the changes brought on by aging. The stubborn, inflexible elder is really trying to maintain his or her independence and integrity, and to protect against a crisis or a threat. Lack of understanding and treatment of these and other defenses can result in personality changes, paranoia, depression, anxiety, and psychiatric illnesses.

THE CREATIVE PROCESS IN LATER LIFE

Arieti (1976) writes that creative work establishes a "bond between the world and human existence" (p. 4), between the individual and the creative product. He says that everyone can be creative, and that creativity lifts morale, liberating one from conditional responses toward making new choices, and "dispels or decreases neuroses" (p. 10). Butler feels that longevity and creativity are associated, noting examples of artists Michelangelo, Titian, Tintoretto, Hals, Picassso, Grandma Moses, and O'Keefe. Butler also noted the positive combination of aging and creativity: a broader vision of life and easy associative powers (cited in Arieti, 1976). Gardner (1976) studied the question of whether we need the whole brain to create, noting artistic changes and adaptations following brain lesions.

The creative process of art expression can rekindle new energy and reawaken potential in the older adult. Art therapy can serve a role in increasing and sharpening cognitive and perceptual skills, in stimulating the senses, and in regenerating social interaction. While the therapist usually plays a supportive role, psychotherapy may be in order as a client attempts to resolve problems through life review (Butler, Lewis, & Sunderland, 1998). Fenton (2000) described three elderly women with schizophrenia who used the creative process to rework unresolved issues of motherhood. Zeiger (1976) recommends that "the sensitive use of art activities can stimulate the recall of forgotten or repressed material and thereby further the personality reorganization of the life review process" (p. 50).

ART-BASED ASSESSMENT

In work with older adults, art-based assessments help determine assets and deficits in cognition, interpersonal skills, task performance, physical–manipulative ability, sensory–perceptual ability, and psychological status. Art-based assessments for the physically disabled, elaborated by Wald (1999) specifically for stroke clients, are:

1. Copy a geometric shape, to test for brain damage, spatial concepts, and ability to concentrate and to follow directions.
2. Draw a clock, to test for concept retention, execution, and neglect.
3. Draw a self-portrait, to test for conceptualization, body-image, affect, and psychological state.
4. Use Silver Drawing Test (Silver, 2000) to test cognition, sensory–perceptual and manipulative skills, and emotional outlook.
5. Choose colors to represent how one is feeling and to evaluate affect and mood.
6. Create a free-choice painting to evaluate ability to abstract, conceptualize, imagine, and express ideas and feelings.

To test for organicity, predominant signs in the art work include perseveration, fragmentation, misproportion, concreteness, and incomplete shapes. This can occur in both psychotic disorders and dementia. Dementia is characterized by problems of memory, especially short-term memory; possible personality changes; problems in abstract thinking and intellectual functioning and behavior, confusion, disorientation, self-care, and appearance; and gradual deterioration of cognitive functions (language, perception, memory) and motor skills. "One of the main characteristics of the Alzheimer's disease [client] is difficulty in integrating and organizing information; the art therapist can use a variety of art tasks to ascertain more comprehensive information about the [client's] visual perception and ability to process sensory input, translate it, and organize ideas into a graphic modality" (Wald, 1989, p. 206). As Alzheimer's disease and other dementias are progressive disorders, the degree of deficits and stage of dementia can be observed in each art therapy session rather than by a formal assessment. Ability to follow directions, reality orientation, omissions, and ability to notice mistakes can be evaluated in drawings of another person, portraits following the leader's step-by-step directions. Perceptual, organizational, and manipulative skills can be checked in a watercolor painting of a vase of flowers. Intellectual ability and retention are tested by asking the client to title a picture, sign his or her name, and recall what he or she drew (Wald, 1983, 1986b, 1989). Psychotic ideation appearing in dementia can be identified by merging of symbols in the client's artwork (Wald, 1984, 1986a, 1993).

For the older psychiatric client, level of depression, suicidality, psychosis, memory strengths, and cognitive impairments are also continually evaluated in art works. The House–Tree–Person Test (Buck, 1981) can be used informally as art themes, with the underlying purpose of evaluation. Social skills and isolation can be evaluated in a group mural. Comparisons of artwork are made from session to session to observe improvements and declines in psychiatric status (see Figure 23.3, which appears on page 304).

TREATMENT CONSIDERATIONS

Assessments help guide treatment considerations. Zweig (1994), presenting an overview on psychotherapy with older adults, described three types of older clients:

1. The aging group, who were dealing with developmental, retirement, and realignment issues with their spouses and children, and losses, were found to be the best candidates for psychological insight, with resulting gains in self-concept and social functioning.
2. The crisis group, who needed to adapt to external losses such as the death of a spouse, benefited from supportive therapy.
3. The frail and debilitated, characterized by mild organicity or chronic illness, were helped by limited supportive therapy with small environmental changes in day programs.

Lang and Heaney (1993) listed three levels of support for inpatient geriatric services as follows: Clients returning to community living require minimal support; the therapist aims to facilitate increased client independence, empowerment, and self-esteem. Moderate support is needed for older adult clients with partial symptom resolution, such as mild cognitive impairment and depression, but are still alert and oriented; the therapist takes an increased role in organizing art activities in which the client can feel successful and productive. Maximum support is required for clients who are very regressed due to major depression, schizophrenia, and/or moderate or severe cognitive impairment, dementia. These clients benefit from reality orientation and require supervision regarding safety, decision making, problem solving, and frequent support, cueing, encouragement, sensory stimulation, and simple step tasks.

Choice of art media merits careful consideration of individual problems and losses specific to the client's personality, illness, and life. For clients with physical dexterity deficits, such as shaking and lack of fine/gross motor control, media that require less control and can even assist with control include paint and clay. A paintbrush handle covered by a sponge improves control for a physically ataxic or apraxic client. Taping paper to the table prevents frustration in a stroke client who has lost control of one hand. Objects need to be placed in the intact visual field for clients with visual deficits; a dark marker used on a light paper decreases figure/ground confusion. The therapist can place drops of water on watercolor blocks and squeeze acrylic and tube watercolor on a palette to suit the preferences of a client with a disability (Wald, 1999). Separate paintbrushes can be placed in tempera jars to prevent confusion due to visual or cognitive deficits. Pasting of collage materials requires assistance for the cognitively impaired and physically challenged client. Collage shapes should be precut for those who can no longer use scissors, and scissors and other sharp items need to be accounted for at the end of the session when working with potentially suicidal clients. Nontoxic materials must always be used, especially with a confused client.

The fluidity of watercolor stimulates the expression of emotions and imagination, and soft music played in the background can provide relaxation for the anxious client. Acrylic paints are more tactile and mistakes can be corrected; used on canvas they give the feeling of being an artist. Poster paint is bright and colorful and provides sensory stimulation; its application on large paper or mural paper can encourage movement in a withdrawn, depressed, or controlled client. Oil crayons and magic markers are also bright but require good manipulative skill. Clay may be too regressive for a low-functioning client but provides good tactile stimulation and can be used to make a useful object (Wald, 1986b, 1989). The therapist should be sure to provide good-quality art materials, which help promote respect and dignity, and quality background music from the client's era. Lectures on art history and art demonstrations also elevate the level of the group, especially for resistant clients who regard art making as a child's activity (Wald, 1984).

ART THERAPY GOALS

The therapist can build on strengths and motivate toward activity through creative therapies, demonstrating creative solutions to old and new problems. Kerr (1999) proposes that the therapist take a more positive attitude: "We often approach the problems of aging for the commendable purpose of correcting them rather than finding a workable social and theoretical perspective to describe what is healthy and adaptive during this remarkable stage" (p. 37). Based on the perspectives of Erickson and Jung, she recommends "advocating the creative process of generactivity [that] encourages respect for the wisdom of older adults" (p. 38). General art therapy goals (Wald, 1983, 1986b, 1989) applicable to all geriatric populations include the following:

1. Provide art activities within a framework in which the client can succeed. In other words, gear the activity and art materials to the level of the group, minimizing deficits and maximizing strengths.
2. Allow the release of pent-up emotions and expression of underlying psychosis, problems, and organicity. This will arise in art, verbalizations, and writings.

3. Preserve a sense of pride and dignity as productive adults by making a visual, tangible product.
4. Encourage reminiscence and life review to help resolve and integrate unresolved conflicts and to take pride in one's past. Reminiscence and life review can be encouraged through themes of memories of childhood, school, work, trips, family, special events, holidays, and hobbies.
5. Provide a visual focus for reality orientation, particularly for clients with psychotic disorders or dementia.
6. Provide a nonverbal, visual means of communication for clients whose language skills are compromised, especially the dementia or stroke clients.
7. Bring clients out of personal isolation and despair by encouraging socialization and group support in creative therapy groups.
8. Allow clients to make their own choices, to be original, to feel a sense of self-worth and integrity.
9. Improve self-esteem by giving the artistically skilled an opportunity to gain recognition.

Additional goals especially, but not exclusively, for clients with physical disabilities, are:

10. Make the client aware of individual problems.
11. Teach compensatory techniques to deal with deficits.
12. Improve functional, manipulative ability.
13. Assist the client to mourn, grieve, and accept change in body image.
14. Support efforts to work through his emotional reaction to losses and limitations.
15. Assist finding inner strengths and old and new resources and "coping mechanisms" (Wald, 1999, p. 36). Keep in mind that "by virtue of their years, [older adults] possess a "wisdom of survival" (Callanan, 1994, p. 1).

STIMULATING THE DEPRESSED, UNMOTIVATED, RESISTANT, OR CONFUSED CLIENT

There are some specific ways to stimulate older adults who are having difficulties engaging in art making. Crosson (1976) suggests having a client choose a favorite color, then make a mark with it; this may evolve into a picture. Suggesting an easy form such as a circle can serve as a stimulus. I have drawn a wiggly or jagged line on a paper, and asked a client to turn it into a design or picture. A simple still life setup, looking at art books and magazines for ideas, pasting part of a scene on a blank paper, and asking the client to complete the scene with art materials all serve as stimuli.

Crosson (1976) found that placing a depressed, resistant client next to an active motivated one encouraged artistic engagement. Landgarten (1983) suggested fostering the therapeutic alliance with a depressed client through a dual drawing created by the client and the therapist together, either by taking turns or by working simultaneously, the therapist responding as needed. All levels of clients are assured success by following the therapist's demonstration of a wet-on-wet watercolor sunset, painting broad bands of horizontal colors that softly blend together; it may be suggested to add the sea, a beach, and so on.

And let us not forget that we, too, experience fear, panic, and helplessness when faced with the blank canvas. It is so important to create a peaceful, relaxed, nonthreatening atmosphere, conducive to creativity. Once we begin and relax, one line and form and color lead to another, take over, let us play and imagine and free associate, and absorb us in concentration. While absorbed in the art process, one is distracted from psychological needs and physical pain and able to release emotions in the art object. Gently placing a hand on a resistant or inhibited person's hand and helping to move the brush, suggesting a change in color, and painting to the rhythm of background music helps to engage the most regressed, obstinate client.

CASE EXAMPLES

The following brief vignettes illustrate some typical examples of older adults in art therapy treatment.

Case 1

When I began working in one day treatment program, I noticed one client who continued to make slow "progress" with a tile tray project given to him by an occupational therapist. He struggled to pick up the small tiles and often pasted them upside down, not able to distinguish between the colorful shiny side and the colorless dull side, due to double vision. Sid was suffering from Parkinson's disease. He drooled and appeared sluggish and depressed. He barely spoke due to his slurred speech.

One day I decided to introduce a new media, watercolor. I set up a vase of flowers. He asked me to squirt out specific colors for his palette, not the exact colors of the flowers. Asking him why he chose these colors, he came to life, explaining that purple is needed to complement and contrast with yellow. It turned out that he had worked as an art teacher! Using a big handled brush to help with his grasp, he created a beautiful watercolor. His double vision worked in his favor, as the painting looked like an Impressionist-style rendition—vivid, spontaneous, alive (Figure 23.1). That was the end of the tile project. We continued in the same method, he telling me what colors to place on his palette and why—and I indeed got a good refresher color course from this former art teacher. From then on care was taken to match media to his specific physical disabilities and artistic skills; paints and brushes require less control and visual acuity. He produced many beautiful "Impressionistic" watercolors, which led to an exhibit in the halls of the program, resulting in physicians and therapists requesting his paintings for their office walls. Sid regained his role as an artist and teacher and, above all, his self-esteem and joy in life.

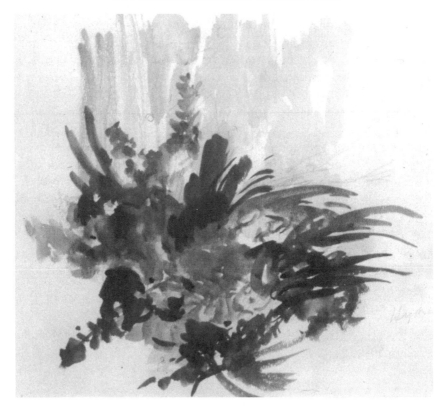

FIGURE 23.1. A client with Parkinson's disease depicts his adaptation to his limitations.

Case 2

Mel, a man with dementia and psychosis secondary to dementia, had became bellig-erent and difficult to control. A former prolific architect, he had also painted fine wa-tercolors. Though his artwork had became notably regressed and repetitive due to the progressive dementing illness, he loved art therapy. Mel retained his sense of work order and discipline by always putting on an apron and sitting close to the art therapist in the "best student's chair," and he was able to draw for long periods. His best work was rendered in pencil, the medium of the architect; now it served to chan-nel his impulsivity and compulsivity into concentration and productivity. Maximum support in a structured day treatment program lowered his anxiety; art therapy gave him a visual focus for reality orientation and a safe outlet for psychotic ideation. The many compliments he got from staff and other clients placed him in a special role and increased his self-esteem (see Wald, 1993, for further analysis of this client).

Case 3

John was a physically frail elderly gentleman who was still able to live with his family but was becoming increasingly depressed and confused from lack of socialization and activity. Referred to a painting group in a day program, he patiently focused his failing eyesight through trifocal lenses, to paint scenes of his former outdoor adventures, mountain climbing in the Colorado Rockies and Mt. Rainier. His paintings led to stimulating conversations with other clients as they reminisced about their travels and adventures, and, subsequently, his mood improved. His daughters were so surprised and proud of the accurate detailed renderings of Mt. Rainier that soon his whole family asked him to paint each of them a "Mt. Rainier" (Figure 23.2). With minimal support, John recovered his self-esteem through his paintings, increased his socializing, felt empowered by his past accomplishments, and was able to remain relatively independent.

Case 4

Art therapy can help remove language barriers and give older immigrants who can barely communicate verbally an opportunity to express themselves. An Italian woman with bipolar disorder had difficulty communicating her thoughts and emotions verbally due to the language barrier. We would overhear Maria shouting angrily at her son on the telephone in a Sicilian dialect. In the art room she could express her range of emotions graphically in colorful floral drawings; when she felt calm and in

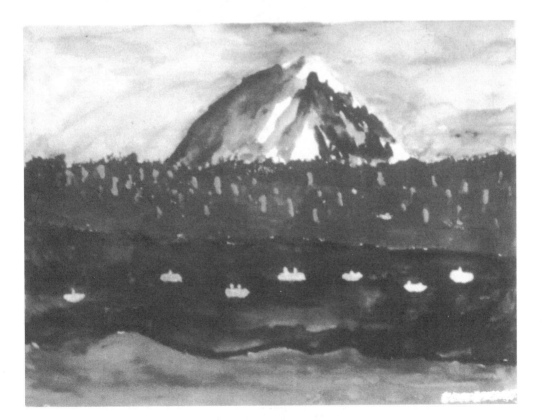

FIGURE 23.2. Reminiscing about a favorite place: Mt. Rainier.

control, the flowers were even and symmetrically balanced, and when she was angry and confused, these flowers became jagged and disorganized (see Figure 23.3). She also shared her background in Sicily with us in drawings of donkeys pulling carts, herself standing at the doorway of her house to greet her husband returning from work. Details of lacy curtains in the windows and the husband's fedora hat enhanced the story of her former life in a different culture. When Maria got psychotic, the steps of the house, her husband, the donkey, and the flowers all merged in confusion.

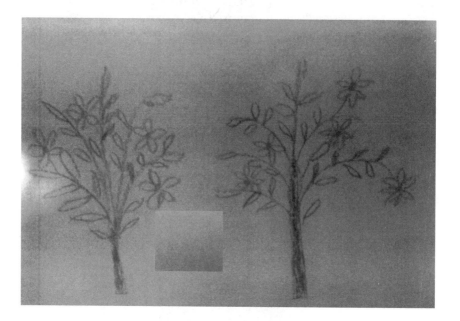

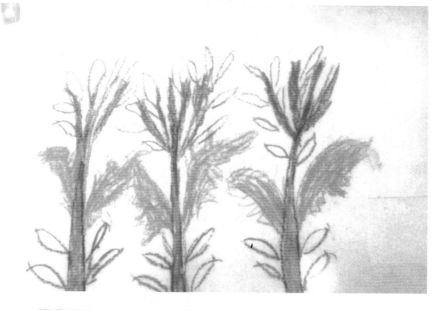

FIGURE 23.3. Drawings by a woman with bipolar disorder.

Maria's artwork provided graphic clinical indications of the need to monitor her antipsychotic medications. The structure and support of the day treatment program and a group home kept this elderly woman with chronic bipolar disorder out of the hospital.

GROUP ART THERAPY

As loss of friends, family, and social network result in isolation and despair, which in turn can lead to the aforementioned confusion and maladaptive defense mechanisms, group art therapy can serve as a primary catalyst to social rekindling. With all populations, murals bring people together; each client contributes artistically at his or her own level and is encouraged to make contact with others by observing their contributions and listening to their ideas. A lower-functioning or resistant client can contribute ideas, words, and lettering and can help color in another's outline (Wald, 1989).

Group clay projects also work well with all geriatric populations, as each person can work at his or her own level of comfort and ability. Themes my art therapy groups have come up with include a band, a baseball game, meatballs and spaghetti, and people sitting on a bench. Individual abstract clay shapes can be combined into a chiming mobile.

Most art therapists working in geriatric programs are required to lead other groups besides art. This can serve an integrative function by combining art with gardening, cooking, music, dance, and writing. For example, planting seeds, watering them, and watching them grow into flowering plants can be nurturing and reparative. The colors and aroma provide sensory stimulation, evoking memories of past enjoyment of gardening. Drawing and painting their own plants gives them a sense of pride and reality focus. Finally, the flowers can be combined into a large spring mural, a symbolic visit to a botanical garden.

Combining creative writing with art therapy can be done in a group "Once upon a time" story, wherein each client adds a phrase and illustrations. This has resulted in story booklets in which expression of dreams, fears, hopes, and worries were creatively expressed and worked through with group support. This project also helps build cognitive skills and reality orientation.

Through a group, long-term project combining reminiscence, writing, drawing, cooking, and eating, therapists can learn about each client's family and cultural background. I asked each client to tell me about a favorite food from his or her childhood, or something he or she liked to cook. The whole group listened as I "interviewed" each client, asking about the recipe and memories about making and eating it. I wrote up summaries of the interviews, each with the recipe and personal memories; the group members would, if they could, copy them over neatly and carefully and then decorate or illustrate their own page. Then each Monday, one client would take charge or help with the cooking of his/her recipe, and we would all enjoy eating it! This resulted in a booklet titled *Cooking Down Memory Lane* by the Monday Lunch Bunch. We licked our fingers eating Betsy's fried chicken which her mother used to make for Sunday dinner, after Betsy spent the day in church praying, singing, and studying in Sunday school in Wilmington, North Carolina. Don fondly recalled his parents from Calabria, Italy, who "loved each other very much and were always together, were married at age 15 and 19. They were poor and used to work in the fields, and only cooked with fresh ingredients from their garden." Peppers and eggs, onions and potato sandwiches were a special childhood memory of a lunch his mother made for him and his five siblings to take to school. We did not make the stuffed derma recalled by Hilda, made by Tante Friede from Russia for the Jewish holidays. She spoke of her aunt's struggles with pogroms in the time of the czar, of her generosity and love, especially recalling Tante Friede visiting her when she spent many years in a state mental hospital—"She was to us our second mother."

CONCLUSION

Let me conclude with the words of Hilda, a schizophrenic client in a geriatric day treatment program, whom I asked to comment on art therapy. To quote Hilda: "Art therapy is a life saver. I put down on paper what I can't say in words, graphically, an instinctive impression of what I feel inside. I do very well and feel reborn in your presence, but when I go back [to my group home], digression sets in. In the structure of the group home, I feel like I'm drowning. Art therapy helps me. I know the solution."

REFERENCES

Arieti, S. (1976). *Creativity: The magic synthesis.* New York: Basic Books.

Blau, D., & Berezin, M. (1975). Neurosis and character disorders. In J. Howells (Ed.), *Modern perspectives in psychiatry of old age* (pp. 201–233). New York: Brunner/Mazel.

Buck, J. N. (1981). *The House–Tree–Person techniques: Revised manual.* Los Angeles: Western Psychological Services.

Butler, R. N., Lewis, M. I., & Sunderland, T. (1998). *Aging and mental health.* Boston: Allyn & Bacon.

Callanan, B. (1994). *Illuminating wisdom in older adults: An art therapy approach.* Paper presented at symposium New Directions in Art Therapy and Gerontology, Hofstra University, New York.

Crosson, C. (1976). Art therapy with geriatric patients: Problems of spontaneity. *American Journal of Art Therapy, 15*(1), 51–56.

Fenton, J. (2000). Unresolved issues of motherhood for elderly women with serious mental illness. *Art Therapy: Journal of the American Art Therapy Association, 17*(1), 24–30.

Gardner, H. (1976). *The shattered mind.* New York: Vintage Books.

Kerr, C. (1999). The psychosocial significance of creativity in the elder. *Art Therapy: Journal of the American Art Therapy Association, 16*(1), 37–41.

Landgarten, H. (1983). Art psychotherapy for depressed elders. *Clinical Gerontologist, 2*(1), 44–53.

Lang, E., & Heaney, C. (1993). *Proposal for enhancement of rehabilitation services: Geriatric treatment services, inpatient units.* White Plains, NY: New York Hospital–Cornell Medical Center, Westchester Division.

Silver, R. (2000). *Art as language*. Philadelphia: Brunner/Mazel.

Wald, J. (1983). Alzheimer's disease and the role of art therapy in its treatment. *American Journal of Art Therapy*, 22(2), 165–175.

Wald, J. (1984). The graphic representation of regression in an Alzheimer's disease patient. *The Arts in Psychotherapy*, 2, 165–175.

Wald, J. (1986a). Fusion of symbols, confusion of boundaries: Percept contamination in the art work of Alzheimer's disease patients. *Art Therapy: Journal of the American Art Therapy Association*, 3, 74–80.

Wald, J. (1986b). Art therapy for patients with dementing illnesses. *Clinical Gerontologist*, 4(3), 29–40.

Wald, J. (1989). Art therapy for patients with Alzheimer's disease and related disorders. In H. Wadeson, J. Durkin, & D. Perach (Eds.), *Advances in art therapy* (pp. 207–221). New York: Wiley.

Wald, J. (1993). Art therapy and brain dysfunction in a patient with a dementing illnesses. *Art Therapy: Journal of the American Art Therapy Association*, 10(2), 88–95.

Wald, J. (1999). The role of art therapy in post-stroke rehabilitation. In C. Malchiodi (Ed.), *Medical art therapy with adults* (pp. 25–42). Philadelphia: Jessica Kingsley.

Weiss, J. (1984). *Expressive therapies with elders and the disabled: Touching the heart of life*. New York: Haworth Press.

Zeiger, B. (1976). Life review in art therapy with the aged. *American Journal of Art Therapy*, 15(1), 47–50.

Zweig, R. (1994). *Overview on psychotherapy with older adults*. Lecture, White Plains, NY: New York Hospital–Cornell Medical Center, Westchester Division.

PART V

Clinical Applications with Groups, Families, and Couples

Art therapy, like other forms of therapy, often takes place in groups. There are groups in hospitals where people make art, outpatient groups where people may use art as a form of self-expression or for the benefits of social support within a group, and therapist-facilitated studios where people can come and make art and share it with others within a supportive environment. Clinics, community agencies, and shelters also offer art therapy groups as support and therapy for a variety of individuals, including survivors of trauma, people with alcoholism or drug dependencies, and individuals with serious or life-threatening illnesses such as cancer or HIV/AIDS. Family and couple art therapy is a specialized form of group art therapy in which family members are asked to express themselves through an art task in the same session to understand interpersonal dynamics or explore ways to interact more effectively.

Group situations, including group art therapy, naturally create the opportunity for communication, interaction, negotiation, and other types of personal exchange. The therapist may choose to reflect to the group some of the interactions that took place during the art activity, such as who took the leadership role, who directed the activity, and how well the group worked together. Participants may discuss what feelings arose in them in making decisions about creating art or discuss and reflect on the content of the finished work. Group art therapy also offers some special qualities that have "curative" potential to its participants. Irving Yalom, a psychiatrist respected for his work with groups, believes that there are "curative factors" found in groups and many of these are present in group art therapy. Some of these include:

- *Instilling hope.* Art therapy with groups involves being part of a supportive community of people. This experience of group support and sharing naturally

309

instills hope, particularly when group members relate positive experiences of overcoming problems, solving problems, and their own recovery from trauma, loss, illness, family conflicts, or addictions.

- *Interaction*. Groups provide the opportunity for social interaction between people. Most important, they provide social support, an aspect which has been connected to health and well-being. Art making within a group context can involve connecting group members with each other through group projects and/ or through the sharing of art products made during the session.

- *Universality*. Groups offer the opportunity for participants to learn that others have similar problems, worries, and fears and that people's experiences are more similar than different. While experiences may be universal, images people create also may carry universal meaning, but in a personal or unique way. Sharing common symbols and/or experiences is an important function of an art therapy group and helps to reduce isolation through communication and exchange of mutual concerns.

- *Altruism*. Group therapy emphasizes helping one another through difficult times. This sense of altruism can be a healing factor both for the person who gives help as well as for the person who receives the help. Art therapy groups reinforce positive support and exchange between group members by offering creative activities through which people can interact in positive and helpful ways (Malchiodi, 1998).

These "curative" characteristics apply to most group art therapy and a therapist may capitalize on any or all of these healing potentials found in group work through art experientials.

In some art therapy groups the therapist takes an active role in determining themes and directives for the group, designing group art activities with particular goals in mind and based on what the therapist has observed about the participants. The group may also be asked to identify problems or themes which they would like to explore through art. For example, in Chapter 27, I describe my work as an art therapist with a breast cancer support group; in that group, participants wanted to explore and communicate issues about medical treatments for cancer and its effects on their bodies through art. With this in mind we co-created an 8-week art therapy support group that met once a week to participate in an art activity developed by the women and myself. Each week a different theme was selected to use a focus for art making and discussion.

Many art therapy groups follow a similar format, including an opening discussion, an experiential process, and a postexperiential discussion. In the first part of the session, there may be an introduction by the therapist to the theme or activity of the group, such as those described by Liebmann in Chapter 25. In some groups, the participants use this time to develop a directive or theme with help from the therapist for experiential work. In nondirective groups, the participants may be working on ongoing projects such as painting, drawings, mixed media, or constructions. Chapter 24, on an interpersonal approach to group art therapy by Waller, gives an overview of both directive and nondirective groups. In Chapter 26, Klorer also provides guidance on the use of structured (directive) and nonstructured (nondirective) art therapy groups with children who have been sexually abused, along with setting treatment goals with developmental factors in mind.

The final three chapters of this section address art therapy with families and couples. Chapter 28 provides a practical foundation for readers on family art therapy and takes a strategic approach through case examples and common family therapy concepts such as metaphor, recursive patterns and second-order change, reframing, unbalancing, and therapeutic double bind. The techniques described provide therapists with a basis for understanding how art expression is integrated within the context of family treatment. Hoshino's discussion of multicultural art therapy with families (Chapter 29) adds the important component of cultural diversity to therapy and uses a case example to illustrate how family therapy can be enhanced through inclusion of art therapy. Finally, Riley explains couples art therapy (Chapter 30), demonstrating additional family therapy principles and how they can be integrated within the course of treatment of couples with a variety of presenting problems.

Riley (2001) observes that "when creative thoughts and opportunities emerge in the group process, it is essential to anchor them in an observable expression" (p. 4). She refers to this as making the "group process visible"; that is, art expression serves as a way to make tangible and viewable feelings, thoughts, perceptions, and world views, recording a moment in time, a pattern of interaction, or an issue that is not possible to communicate through words. The inclusion of image making in group therapy is a distinct advantage for the therapist and the members of the group because everyone can "see" what others are saying. In groups, families, and couples, the process of art making can enhance the course of therapy and is a testament to the progress of group or family members. As Riley (2001) notes, it speaks as a second language for the flow of the group's process and lets the therapist determine the best direction to take toward change.

REFERENCES

Malchiodi, C. A. (1998). *The art therapy sourcebook*. New York: McGraw Hill-NTC.
Riley, S. (2001). *Group process made visible: Group art therapy*. New York: Brunner/Routledge.

CHAPTER 24

Group Art Therapy: An Interactive Approach

Diane Waller

Group work is central to treatment in many different health and social services establishments. However, the word "group" can have many different meanings, and it is important to establish exactly what colleagues mean when they ask for an "art therapy group" to be set up. Many years of experience in supervising students in their clinical placement (practicum) has led me to believe that understanding the principles of group work is essential in developing and conducting art therapy groups.

The history of group psychotherapy parallels that of art therapy, beginning in both Britain and the United States during and after World War II. Art therapists in the United Kingdom and in the United States engaged in group work, but this usually took place in studio-type settings, called Open Groups, which made a creative haven in the bleak public psychiatric hospitals. Patients came and went freely; some spent all day and every day in the studio, others visited from time to time. The old-style studios of the 1940s and 1950s were rather like those found in art schools, where the students worked in silence, perhaps from a model, and the tutor wandered around making the odd comment to an individual. Usually the only sound was scratching of pencil, coughs, and sighs. All were engrossed in their own drawing and communication only happened in the breaks. During the 1970s, the "growth" movements coming from the United States, such as encounter, Esalen, and their British counterparts, influenced the course of group art psychotherapy. The work of Kurt Lewin, field theory, the Tavistock Clinic, and others shaped the course of group treatment.

The interactive (also known as interpersonal) model of group art therapy is flexible and effective in many different situations. It is based on concepts from group analysis (Foulkes, 1948), interpersonal therapy (Sullivan, 1953; Yalom, 1985), systems theory (Agazarian & Peters, 1989) and group art therapy (Waller, 1993; see also Skaife & Huet, 1998). The model is also influenced by process (or figurational) sociology (Elias, 1956) and social psychology (Lewin, 1948, 1951). This chapter presents concepts of interactive group psychotherapy; explains how to introduce group interactive art therapy; provides case examples of group interactive art therapy; and discusses overall considerations in running art therapy groups based on an interactive model.

INTERACTIVE GROUP PSYCHOTHERAPY

The interactive approach to psychotherapy which underpins group art therapy practice derives from the work of the neo-Freudians and in particular, Harry Stack Sullivan (1953). He believed that an individual's history influences every moment of life because it provides a dynamic structure and definition of one's experiences. Sullivan believed that early childhood personality developed through interaction with significant others but was always open to modification and change. Yalom (1985), Ratigan and Aveline (1988), Bloch and Crouch (1985), and Waller (1993) provide useful accounts of the theory of interactive groups; central features are highlighted here before discussing how these groups can be modified and enhanced by the introduction of art materials. The group framework retains substantially the same structure and curative factors as outlined by the authors previously, but another dimension and additional possibilities for expression and communication are available when images are produced.

Group interactive psychotherapy focuses on the actions, reactions, and characteristic patterns of interaction which constrain people in their everyday lives. Our personal world is continuously being reconstructed through interactions with others which determine our view of ourselves and others and affects expectations of others. In group therapy, the individual learns how his or her assumptions (conscious and unconscious) determine patterns of interactions and may have led to problems in relating. Concepts of responsibility, freedom, and choice are central to this model. Participants are encouraged to explore irrational belief systems (i.e., if I don't get married, pass an exam, get promotion by 30, then I am a complete failure) and discouraged from taking a passive victim stance. By incorporating systems theory, the model recognizes social, political, and economic realities including discrimination and racism and how internalization of these realities can lead to feelings of despair and powerlessness.

Taking responsibility for one's participation in the learning experience of the group, having a sense of one's influence on events, and learning to give feedback are prerequisites. Members reveal their difficulties through their here-and-now behavior, the "here and now" being where the therapy takes place. Disclosure may take place, possibly of "secrets" or significant events from the past and present outside the group, and this may be important in understanding the behavior of that individual in the group. The act of disclosing (and this may happen indirectly through image making) often releases tension and enables defenses to be lowered and relinquished. Feedback from members of the group and the therapist, illuminating aspects of the self which have become obvious to others, but which are not recognized by oneself, is essential. To be effective it must be well timed and delivered with sensitivity. In this respect the therapist is an important role model, demonstrating a positive critical approach as opposed to a negative and judgmental one, observing and commenting on behavior and images and their effects on the process of the group.

There are some fundamental processes of an interactive group that are often enhanced by the addition of image making. These include projection, mirroring, scapegoating, parataxic distortion, and projective identification. Projection involves group members having feelings and making assumptions about other members which are not based on their here-and-now experience. For example, one member might experience another as his critical mother and make assumptions about that person's feelings toward him. Mirroring entails a member having strong feelings and emotions about another's behavior, which is in fact an aspect of the member's behavior. Projection and mirroring are often accompanied by splitting—by experiencing a group member, the facilitator, or the whole group as all good or all bad. Scapegoating occurs when the group tries to put all its difficulties onto one member and to get rid of them. The members' tendency to distort their perceptions of others (parataxic distortions) provides valuable material for the group to consider. An important and often disturbing phenomenon is projective identification, which can result in one member projecting his or her own (but actually disowned) attributes onto another toward whom they feel "an uncanny attraction–repulsion" (Yalom, 1985, p. 354). These attributes may be projected so strongly that the other person's behavior begins to change. For example, murderous feelings may be projected so that the other begins to feel murderous, whereas the projector has no awareness of such a feeling. The group itself, as a social microcosm, also takes on patterns of behavior as if it were an individual and the facilitator must understand these processes and comment on them, with the aim being for members themselves to learn and to understand about these phenomena (see Rutan & Stone, 2001).

INTRODUCING ART THERAPY INTO AN INTERACTIVE GROUP FRAMEWORK

Given the curative factors of verbal groups outlined so clearly by Yalom (1985), why would we need to introduce art therapy and to attempt a synthesis of verbal and visual interactions? Why make an already complex model more so? Reference to the huge body of case material attesting to the effectiveness of art therapy with clients considered unable to benefit from verbal psychotherapy provides a rationale.

How Is Art Therapy Integrated within an Interactive Framework?

In practical terms, we take the framework of an interactive group, but instead of the usual 1½ hours that is often the norm in a verbal group, I suggest extending it to 2 hours, but it could be more or less, depending on the needs and capabilities of the clients. The group should be scheduled at the same time each week or several times a week in the case of inpatient work. The timetable depends on the institution, and finding facilities for art making is usually a challenge. Using art materials requires time, involvement in the process of making an image, letting the image speak to oneself and to the group, and then putting the images away and terminating the session. The group is bounded by time, place, and simple rules, such as coming on time, staying for the period of the group, engaging in the process, and not damaging self, others, or others' artwork. Art materials can be kept in one part of the room or laid out on tables, depending on the client group (e.g., if members have any physical or severe mental disabilities, materials should be easily accessible).

The facilitator may decide to conduct the group in the style of an interactive therapist, letting the group know that the materials are there to be used but not giving any direction as to how. Or, the therapist might spend a little time talking to the group, checking how people are feeling on that day, and identifying an open-ended theme for visual and verbal expression. The first moments in a group when the members are trying to decide how to proceed are often tense and the members want the therapist to tell them what to do. However, the interactive art therapist believes that the group has the resources to find its own solutions and will support any attempts to do this.

Once the initial phase of "being stuck" has passed, the group members usually finds various ways to engage together, either by dividing into smaller subgroups or by "giving permission" for members to work alone or by deciding to do a group artwork in the hope of bringing everyone together and avoiding dealing with "difference." Individuals will quickly fall into habitual patterns: being the one to suggest projects, withdrawing, moving away from the group to an isolated corner, disagreeing with whatever is suggested, quietly or not so quietly sabotaging the work, or being the peacemaker. All this is useful material for the therapist to note for comment and to later reflect to the group.

The Role of the Therapist

The role of the therapist is primarily to maintain the therapeutic task of the group: to encourage open communication and interaction, to note the process, and to intervene only when the group seems too stuck, when a member is in danger of being scapegoated, or to reinforce the boundaries. The group itself decides when to pause in the image making, talk, and process. If the members are reluctant to do this, the therapist must decide whether they are avoiding interaction or whether they are still deep in the image-making process and need more time. The therapist has to ensure that images and materials can be stored safely between groups (which is difficult if others are using the room). Where possible, it is important to draw attention to the limitations of the space, whether artwork has to be put away at the end of the session, and what will happen to it when the group is finished.

In Astrachan's (1970) model of groups based on general systems theory, the therapist appreciates the many diverse aspects of the role as "regulatory agent" in the group and is attuned to all parts of the therapy system, recognizing the likely repercussions on the system of the regulatory behavior he or she adopts. This would include defining and maintaining the boundaries of therapy. For example, when conducting an experiential art therapy training group at another university I noticed that at a certain point in the afternoon, without speaking, several members left the group. I was astonished as this would never happen in my own institution! After about 10 minutes they returned and got on with their art-making process in small groups. Nobody except myself seemed bothered.

In the feedback period I asked, "What was going on? How come people left the group?" They seemed surprised by my question, pointing out that it was everyone's right to go and have a smoke if they needed to. Having just spent several hours explaining the theory behind interactive group psychotherapy and the need to maintain clear boundaries, I was intrigued to find that the habits of several months (to go off midafternoon for a smoke) had prevailed and the boundaries so carefully explained had been broken. The students were equally amazed that they had done this without realizing.

The experience shed light on problems the group members had with their own patients' unexplained leaving of a therapy session. Some were annoyed with me, pleading "individual freedom," but others said how much such interruption in the group distracted them from their process and spoiled the work. They felt that it was safer when boundaries were maintained. From then on they did not leave the room, staying instead engrossed in the process of the group, and many reported not feeling a need to smoke. Had I not challenged this behavior, the system would have continued to exclude the new approach. The therapist attends to all the systems relevant to the patient and not only the therapeutic one (e.g., to the patient's work, marriage, relationship with parents, and relationship with a wider social circle and to social, cultural, and political events). The therapist must, in addition, bear all these factors in mind when viewing the visual products of the group members. All forms of interaction are potentially useful and none have priority over the rest (see Bloch & Crouch, 1985, pp. 80–81).

In summary, the role that the therapist has to play in a complex systems-based group is challenging in that there are so many layers of meaning to be observed and understood. Each member brings to the group a social system of which he is part and from which he is only temporarily disconnected while the session is in progress. Exploration of the patients' worlds and their relationship to the "here and now" of the group and to the social system of which the group is part can be very valuable and quite reassuring to individual members; they are not alone with their problems.

Case Example 1

Some examples from my own experience of training groups illustrate how a therapist might handle some of the interactions in a group. The first is of a 4-day intervention I made in an art therapy training program in an all-female group of Swiss students. I could not understand the aggressive, destructive attitude prevalent from the start of the art therapy group which caused the group members to disparage everything I or anyone else in the group said and to resist strongly any move anyone made toward the art materials. The students became increasingly frustrated because they could not allow themselves to move away from this position.

The group looked to me to tell them what to do, whereupon I suggested they try to think about what was happening from the point of view of their knowledge of the history of their group (I was a newcomer as they had been students together for 2 years). I suggested they bear in mind the all-female composition, and myself as facilitator, also female. At first they did not want to do this, again asking me to solve the problem, but I said they had the resources to do it themselves.

It turned out that the group had started off with three men, all of whom had left. The women were angry about this, feeling they had been abandoned and had driven the men out. They wanted men in the group so it would be a "serious" group. I wondered why this had to be. We then spent a long time thinking about the role of Swiss women, who only fairly recently had gotten the vote, and how they still felt men were more important. At the same time, they resented this feeling in themselves and felt angry when they encountered it in their workplace or home. So they disparaged each other and what I had to offer and projected their own feelings of inadequacy onto me. I was definitely beginning to take them in and had to struggle with a headache and feeling of wanting to escape. I resisted suggesting a theme, feeling it was important for them to arrive at a way to use the art materials themselves.

Eventually the group revealed feeling intensely competitive, which caused them to feel ashamed. They were worried about being judged by me and by each other. After a period of contemplation and reflection, they felt able to use the art materials to construct a network of visual communications, to which everyone contributed, and in which "difference" could be acknowledged and respected. It was created with great care and sensitivity, a truly cooperative effort which dispelled their fear that they could not work together. I felt that particular incident was a turning point for the group. The three-dimensional sculpture, consisting of words and images, was suspended from the ceiling, enabling its many facets to be explored by the group. It remained in the room overnight, and as this was a week-long group, provided a starting point for reflection the next day and for further work on the issue of female competition.

Case Example 2

Another example of the outside coming into the group occurred in Bulgaria several years ago, where I worked with a group of doctors and nurses in a seaside town during a freezing, cold April. The aim of the workshops was to give them a hands-on experience of art therapy using an interactive model, backed up by theoretical sessions. Every day we began the group at 9 A.M. and on the second day, only 2 out of 12 participants arrived. After 15 minutes had passed, another came rushing in to say that the others, who were staying at a local hotel, had to move to make way for some Western tourists. This was not an uncommon occurrence at this time because Western tourists would pay in convertible currency worth a lot to the Bulgarian economy. So they were literally on the streets, in the snow, trying to find somewhere to stay.

I felt immediately angry and guilty by association. The hospital in which we worked had felt unwelcoming and this was a setback and loss of precious time. We could not continue to work given such a disturbance. I visited the hospital director to report this incident, whereupon he shrugged his shoulders, regarded me with hostility, and said there was "nothing he could do." As an outsider from the West and a representative of the World Health Organization, I used my position to call the hotel and protest most strongly, insisting that these participants be given back their rooms (in fact, there were enough rooms and the hotel manager had thrown them out "just in case" more tourists arrived).

After some heated words, their rooms were restored. I did not think of the consequences but was shaken severely by the incident. We revised the timetable to deal with the crisis. When the group members arrived they were furious, legitimately outraged. However, they had, as their facilitator, a person from "the West." Paradoxically, I had taken on projections of both rescuer and persecutor. I felt bad. Without speaking, but with angry gestures, group members seized a large sheet of paper and all the available paints (the liquid variety in bottles). They poured, smeared, stabbed, and pounded the paper, spilling paint onto the floor. It was violent and symbolically bloody. They found clay and made figures which were destroyed, smashed into the paper. The battle raged on; I watched, I did not intervene. It was, however, well under control within the materials.

Energy spent, the participants sat down and surveyed their work with satisfaction. A catharsis had happened. They had "killed" off the Westerners, from a neighboring Balkan country, and in so doing had remembered ancient battles and settled some old scores. They had also "killed off" the hotel manager and representatives of the state. I was not sure if I was killed off too because of my status as a "Westerner" or whether I had become a "non-Westerner" by virtue of taking their side against the oppressors. The image was disturbing in its violence and at the same time majestic in all its references to battles past and present. It needed much processing before there could be any reparation.

The group feeling was exhausted, wound-licking satisfaction. The world was split into good and evil. Then came an acknowledgement that it was not the fault of the tourists but an aspect of "the system" of which we were all a part. Killing off the Western tourists was satisfying initially but led to guilt and despair afterward. So it was with war. Later, after much reflection, a life-size painting was made of a woman, nationality unclear. She was going to New York and would stay there a long time but would come back. She was given money (dollars), a passport, and a gun to protect herself against U.S. gangsters. Importantly, she was given a headband in the colors of the Bulgarian flag. The group was totally engrossed in this image, making a bag for the dollars and sticking it on the paper, making the gun, fantasizing about her life in New York. It was a true reflection of my position, coming and going freely, when others found it hard to get a passport let alone dollars. The differences, the "East and the West," privilege and powerlessness, were all combined in this image. These two images, made by the whole group, contained such rich references that they preoccupy me to this day. I only have the photos, but the images and the incidents are still alive in my mind.

My role was to act as a container for the group's projections, but this role was modified by the fact that the group members put so much into the images that I did not bear the whole weight of the projections. I experienced projective identification, continuing well after that group; it was hard for me to leave the country and I felt uneasy once I got home. Yet I was, at the same time, desperate to leave—I was between "East" and "West." It was possible to reflect on the meaning for each individual of the group experience and how it touched on their personal relationships within a system where individuals found it hard to take responsibility due to the projection of "The State" as the all-knowing authority.

These are but two examples from many in which the power of the images has enhanced an interactive group process and where it is doubtful whether such a range of meanings could have emerged in a verbal group alone.

MAJOR CONSIDERATIONS IN GROUP INTERACTIVE ART THERAPY

The following section presents some of the major considerations in running art therapy groups based on an interactive model:

1. An interactive art therapy group may give adult patients their first experience of using art materials for many years, or ever. Risking exposure through making an image is a big step and cannot be made until group members trust each other. In the framework of an interactive group, with its emphasis on exploration and learning and where no individual is isolated with his or her "problem," image making provides an excellent opportunity for another dimension of communication.

2. Members are encouraged to experiment with art materials and to find ways of working together or individually in the group. In the same way that references from the "outside" are brought verbally into the group, visual references are also present.

3. The images can help members to understand the "here and now" of the group and how this is experienced by each member. For example, a group of recovering drug addicts made a clay model of a prison, with considerable anger toward each other and the clay. Later, they destroyed it by mutual consent and transformed the clay into a colorful mask which they subsequently left as a present for the host institution. They expressed their current experiences and feelings through both cathartic and reparative processes that may have been not easily expressed through words alone.

4. Sometimes the objects stand as powerful symbols for an important experience. In the previous example, the group members expressed their feelings of imprisonment but could transform it and used a mask as a symbol. Moving beyond the mask and being able to offer the beautifully crafted finished object to others is an example of psychological growth both for each individual and for the group.

5. Artwork can become a focus for projection. Certain materials, such as finger paint and clay, can tap deep emotions and people may feel out of control like infants overwhelmed by sensation. They might project all their hateful feelings onto a single

figure or work, then transform it through modifying feedback from the group. The artwork then becomes a focus for both projection and interaction. It is helpful to encourage members to "free associate" to each others' work and not to try to "interpret" the work, to persecute with questions, or to judge it. This can be achieved by the therapist "modeling" inquiring and reflective behavior.

6. Art materials have the potential to induce the experience of play, but the therapist must remember that playing is often difficult for adults. An appropriate environment can help, especially one in which people can move around freely. The room itself becomes a "potential space," in Winnicott's (1990) terms, and may affect how people participate within the group.

7. Once images are created, they can remain in the group throughout its duration. But they may be transformed or even deconstructed according to the way the group is experiencing itself on any one day. A lot of the potential for group interactive therapy may be lost by having to put away or dispose of artwork at the end of each session. It is important to have a storage place from where the images can be retrieved, if so desired, at the beginning of each session. Keeping the images as part of the group prevents a splitting into "words and images." Rather, the "figure and ground" are merged, the images are part of the interactive system and not an afterthought.

8. The value of creative activity, through giving form to emotions and ideas alongside others and with others, is an important aspect of interactive group therapy. I witnessed a transformation of a hard-working and exploited woman who was convinced she was uncreative and undeserving of a better life. She created a life-sized figure of a dashing Russian soldier as part of a session in which dyads helped each other to realize and make a fantasy figure. She was able to project onto the figure the soldier part of herself, a fighter and, through feedback and reflection, to own these assertive feelings herself. As a result, she gave notice to her exploitive employer, gaining a senior position in another company and flourishing in her work. This sounds quite magical, but it is a powerful process in that images are made within a group and are thus public (see Waller, 1999).

SELECTION FOR THE GROUP

The examples I have given have mainly come from training groups with participants who could be said to be well functioning. However, it is possible for this model to be used with any client group but important for therapists to understand the nature of the group being offered and to explain it fully to clients and colleagues.

There is often a misunderstanding among colleagues who might think the group is an art class or for "relaxation." They may have already told the client that it is a place where he or she will "learn to paint." It is therefore essential that the therapist interview each prospective client and discuss the kind of processes likely to take place. This is possible even with disturbed or confused patients, as we have found in working with patients with dementia (although with severely impaired patients the caregiver or advocate may need to be involved).

The initial interview gives both therapist and client the chance to assess the situation. Often therapists, and particularly trainees, are pressured to accept clients already chosen by another staff member, or simply available (even ones for whom other treatments have failed). Thus it is important to take the time to talk about the group; otherwise the client may not realize what kind of group he or she is joining. The therapist has a chance to assess whether that person is likely to be able to tolerate the challenge of an interpersonal group. It may be that he or she is too fragile or too disturbed to cope with this challenge and might need some supportive sessions prior to the group's starting.

Criteria for Acceptance into a Group

Most of the literature on selection for groups deals rather with deselection for verbal psychotherapy (i.e., who is not suitable) (Bloch, 1979). When thinking about once-weekly outpatient groups, be they verbal or art therapy groups, then clearly clients have to be able to tolerate the time in between groups, and to tolerate the strong feelings which may be aroused in the groups. It is important for any client to have some readily available backup between groups, and preferably support from their family and friends for undertaking group therapy.

Therapists working in the public health services have traditionally accepted into groups clients who would have been unlikely to receive psychotherapy elsewhere. These include people in acute psychotic or borderline states, those with chronic alcohol or substance abuse problems, people with dementia, and people with mental handicaps. It is possible to use the interactive art therapy model with all these client groups, modifying one's stance as a therapist appropriately. For some clients, and here I am thinking of a recent group of elderly patients with dementia, making images is difficult, given their multiple handicaps. But interaction for this client group is so valuable, as they are facing constant losses, including loss of relationships. The safe boundaries of the group help these clients to express some painful feelings which they rarely have the chance to do in the average hospital ward or care facility (Sheppard, Rusted, & Waller, 1998; Waller, 2002). Outstanding work has also been carried out with people with severe mental handicaps, despite misgivings from hospital staff (Strand, 1990).

Clients who could be helped by group interactive art therapy are many and varied. However, it is important in any group that nobody be isolated, or at worst, scapegoated. Ideally, there should be a balance of male and female clients, black and white, gay and straight, but in reality, this balance is often difficult to achieve. The therapist must therefore be vigilant in ensuring that "difference" is acknowledged and addressed openly. My only serious reservation would be in admitting clients who had a tenuous hold on reality, who might become violent when under pressure, or who had a history of becoming disturbed by images. Group size depends on the functioning of the clients. A minimum of 5 and maximum of 12 is good for a "small group" and is a practical number when working in hospitals and clinics. I have found that five or six are manageable groups with clients who have severe difficulties.

CAN INTERACTION BE ANTITHERAPEUTIC?

This question has to be addressed as, clearly, any treatment can be effective and successful or, on the other hand, have no effect or, worse, be damaging. Bloch and Crouch (1985) point out that interaction may not always be helpful and there is potential for heightened discomfort in the interaction between members. For example, in a week-long art therapy group for staff working in drug addiction, where unfortunately I did not have the chance to interview people beforehand, a disturbed participant was unable to tolerate the boundaries of the group and entered the group room late at night and violated the artwork of her small subgroup. On discovering this violation, the whole group was distraught, especially the other three members of her subgroup. She was not able to understand the seriousness of her act and denied its importance. The group wanted to remove her and I had to decide whether it would be more damaging to the group to exclude the member or to keep her. I decided to work with the crisis and managed to retain her in the group until the end of the week. Much time had to be spent processing this violation of boundaries and of group rules.

After this experience I never again agreed to work with a group when I had not assessed the members beforehand. Generally, it is up to the therapist to manage the group dynamics appropriately so that potentially damaging behavior is challenged and understood by the group. It is a difficult balancing act, to be alert to aggressive or sabotaging actions and to point them out without scapegoating the perpetrator or preventing the group members from taking responsibility. Continuing failure on behalf of any member to observe the group's boundaries, especially in terms of violence to others, self, or others' artwork, would necessitate that person leaving the group for his or her own and the group's safety.

Another antitherapeutic element which could apply to any group but which is only too common for art therapy groups is premature termination of members caused by external pressures, lack of understanding about the nature of the group ("it is only a painting group"), and even referral elsewhere by another clinician. The therapist's role in understanding, possibly predicting, and reflecting to the group about these antitherapeutic processes is clearly vital. Any factors, such as those mentioned earlier, which interfere with the therapeutic potential of a group have to be identified in order for the group to do its curative work.

CONCLUSION

The group interactive art therapy model, complex in its range of interlocking networks of verbal and visual communications, with its emphasis on the sociocultural and political context as well as the personal, is a promising approach for understanding not only any one individual's patterns of being but those of our complex multicultural and multitechnological world. It poses challenges for the therapist, who, in addition to understanding group processes, must also be responsible for art materials, for overseeing the making of the artwork, for arranging for it to be stored and protected between sessions, and for its "disposal" after the group has finished. It is a powerful process, not to be undertaken lightly. Once the firm boundaries have been established, what happens inside the group depends on the skills of the therapist and the abilities of the participants to use the materials and each other. It is a flexible model, offering many patients who are often considered "unsuitable" for dynamic psychotherapy, a chance to relate to others in a safe environment, one in which a lack of verbal ability need not be a drawback.

REFERENCES

Agazarian, Y., & Peters, R. (1989). *The visible and invisible group: Two perspectives on group psychotherapy and group process.* London: Tavistock/Routledge.

Astrachan, B. (1970). Towards a social systems model of therapy group. *Social Psychiatry, 5,* 110–119.

Bloch, S. (1979). Assessment of patients for psychotherapy. *British Journal of Psychiatry, 135,* 193–208.

Bloch, S., & Crouch, E. (1985). *Therapeutic factors in group psychotherapy.* Oxford, UK: Oxford University Press.

Elias, N. (1956). Problems of involvement and detachment. *British Journal of Sociology, 7*(3), 226–252.

Foulkes, S. H. (1948). *Introduction to group analytic psychotherapy.* London: Maresfield.

Lewin, K. (1948). *Resolving social conflicts.* New York: Harper & Row.

Lewin, K. (1951). *Frontiers in group dynamics.* New York: Harper & Row.

Ratigan, B., & Aveline, M. (1988). Interpersonal group therapy. In M. Aveline & W. Dryden (Eds.), *Group psychotherapy in Britain* (pp. 43–64). London: Open University Press.

Rutan, J. S., & Stone, W. N. (2001). *Psychodynamic group psychotherapy* (3rd ed.). New York: Guilford Press.

Sheppard, L., Rusted, J., & Waller, D. (1998). *Art therapy with elderly clients suffering from dementia: A control group study.* Brighton, UK: Alzheimers Disease Society.

Skaife, S., & Huet, V. (Eds.). (1998). *Art psychotherapy groups: Between pictures and words.* London and New York: Routledge.

Strand, S. (1990). Counteracting isolation: Group art therapy for people with learning difficulties. *Group Analysis, 23*(3), 255–263.

Sullivan, H. S. (1953). *The interpersonal theory of psychiatry.* New York: Norton.

Waller, D. E. (1993). *Group interactive art therapy: Its use in training and treatment.* London: Routledge.

Waller, D. (1999). Introducing new psychosocial elements into already functioning systems: The case of art psychotherapy at the centro italiano di solidarieta, Rome. In D. Waller & J. Mahony (Eds.), *Treatment of addiction: Current issues for arts therapies* (pp. 59–78). New York: Routledge.

Waller, D. (2002). *Arts therapies and progressive illness: Nameless dread.* New York and London: Brunner-Routledge.

Winnicott, D. W. (1990). *The maturational process and the facilitating environment.* London: Karnac.

Yalom, I. (1985). *The theory and practice of group psychotherapy.* New York: Basic Books.

CHAPTER 25

Developing Games, Activities, and Themes for Art Therapy Groups

Marian Liebmann

There is much debate concerning the value of using themes in art therapy groups. I have participated in and facilitated both themed and unthemed art therapy groups and have seen benefits in both approaches. The choice of approach may depend on the client group, the purpose of the group, the time available, and the preferred style of the therapist.

This chapter describes how groups can be set up to address specific themes and issues which may be useful for certain client groups to explore. The first half of the chapter outlines the issues that need to be considered in setting up any group of this kind; the second half describes how this works in practice, with specific examples.

REASONS FOR GROUP WORK IN ART THERAPY

In some circumstances, there is a choice of using individual or group art therapy, so it is important to be clear about the reasons for choosing group art therapy. The reasons for using group work can be summarized as follows:

- Much of social learning is done in groups, so group work provides a good context to promote social skills.
- People with similar needs can provide mutual support for each other and help with mutual problem solving.
- Groups can provide a sense of belonging and identity.
- A themed group can help members look at particular issues from different perspectives.

- Group members can learn from the feedback of other members.
- Group members can gain insight about their family roles and try out new ones.
- Groups can be catalysts for developing latent resources and abilities.
- Groups are more suitable for certain individuals (e.g., those who find the intimacy of individual work too intense).
- Groups can be more democratic, sharing power and responsibility.
- Some therapists find group work more satisfying than individual work.
- Groups can be an economical way of using expertise to help several people at the same time (e.g., using valuable art therapy expertise, with a co-facilitator from another discipline).

There are, however, some disadvantages to group work:

- Confidentiality is more difficult to ensure, because more people are involved.
- Groups need resources and can be difficult to organize; they are not necessarily cheaper than individual work.
- Groups need a larger space than individual work.
- Less individual attention is available to members of a group.
- A group may be "labeled" or acquire a stigma by being more visible.
- Specialist supervision is needed to look at the group dynamics as well as the art therapy aspect of the work (Liebmann, 1986).

Art therapists working with groups need to be conversant with literature and practice in both art therapy and group work (Whitaker, 2001).

REASONS FOR USING THEMES IN ART THERAPY GROUPS

In certain settings, all art therapy is conducted in groups, and it is important to maximize the benefits of group work. As mentioned earlier, it can be useful to organize a group around a particular theme. Many people have great difficulty in starting artwork in a therapy setting. A theme can provide a focus with which to begin. Initial themes can help people learn what art therapy is actually about. This is especially true if group members are not familiar with art therapy, or if they see the group in terms of "art lessons."

Some groups are insecure and need some kind of structure if they are to operate at all. In addition, there is often pressure of time, and a suitable theme can help the group to focus more quickly. Sharing a theme can also help to weld a group together. Finally, staff in multidisciplinary settings such as schools or hospitals may find it easier to understand the purpose of the group if it has a particular theme and to refer clients accordingly.

The group can be involved in the choice of theme if this is appropriate. Themes can be worked on at many levels and used flexibly to meet different needs. Certain themes, for example, can be useful in helping group members to relate to each other. Sometimes they can help people out of well-worn "ruts" by enabling fresh work and discussion (Liebmann, 1986).

Using themes requires the same experience and sensitivity as any other mode of art therapy. If they are used inappropriately, they may evoke feelings which are too much for the group to handle at that time. At the other end of the spectrum, some can lead to a superficial experience which leaves people dissatisfied. Between these two extremes lies a wide variety of group experiences using themes which can be interesting, revealing, and enjoyable and can lead to personal growth.

SETTING UP A THEMED ART THERAPY GROUP

Aims and Goals

It is important to be clear about the goals of the group, because these goals will determine the way in which the group is carried out. Art therapy groups have been used for many purposes, including anger management, to support clients who have recently suffered bereavement or loss, to provide a means for two client groups from different institutions to come together by working on a common theme (for instance, the Life Journeys group described later in this chapter), to help elderly people come to terms with loss and alleviate isolation, and to enable mental health professionals to learn about the possible contribution of art therapy to verbal counseling. There are some groups that are seen as needing a directive group approach to challenge their ways of thinking, such as sex offenders (Hagood, 2000).

Facilities and Resources

Facilities and resources include availability of a therapist proficient in art therapy and a co-therapist, a suitable room, art materials, water, peace and quiet, and time. A contract may need to be set up detailing these.

Group Members

A system for referrals is needed, unless the group is being run for a "captive audience" (e.g., residents in a group home). This system may include information leaflets for other staff or agencies, liaison with referrers, application forms, interviews, and assessment for suitability. It may also involve talks to explain the benefits of art therapy, the purpose of the group, and the client group it is aimed at. Sometimes an art therapy workshop for staff is the best explanation of all, especially if a new art therapy group is being introduced into an institution. It may be necessary to recruit more members than the number aimed at—in my inner-city community mental health team, covering an area in which clients often miss appointments or change their mind, I have to recruit about 15 applicants to achieve a group membership of 6.

Open and Closed Groups

An important decision to be made is whether a group is to be closed or open. A closed group usually runs for a fixed number of sessions (usually 8 to 12, though some may run for longer) with the same members, so that they can get to know each other well and build up trust, leading to a greater willingness to share. An open group allows people to join and leave as they wish, and thus may remain on a fairly superficial level. They allow more disturbed clients to engage at a safe level with which they can cope. Open groups are often the only alternative in an institution in which client turnover is rapid, such as a psychiatric inpatient ward or a hostel for homeless people. Another variation is for members to join or leave an established group at intervals, thus maintaining the ethos of the group.

Ground Rules

Every group needs "ground rules" (sometimes called a "group contract" or "working agreement") to establish how it will operate, what is OK and what is not. Some ground rules may be settled beforehand by the therapist (e.g., attendance at every session is expected); some will need to be negotiated with the group. Typical ground rules encompass time limits, breaks, respect for others, confidentiality (and its precise definition for that group), speaking for oneself, tea breaks, smoking, and so on. Art therapy group ground rules, in addition to those mentioned, include respecting others' artwork, owning one's interpretations (e.g., "When I look at your picture, it reminds me of . . . " rather than "What you've drawn means . . . "), and valuing all contributions of group members.

Therapist Roles

Therapists need to decide if they are going to join in with the art activity. It is more usual in themed groups for the therapist to do so, to model participation, but this depends on the other demands of running the group. If therapists do join in, they need to do so in a way that does not inhibit clients' ability to participate. A co-therapist is advisable for most groups, to share roles, to act as a role model, and to "pick up the pieces" if there is a group member who is too upset to participate or who unexpectedly rushes out of the room.

Choosing and Developing Themes

Themes develop in response to the aims and goals outlined previously, and will depend on the client group and number of sessions. If there is a series of sessions, then the earlier sessions need to concentrate on introducing the clients to art therapy, helping them to feel safe and introducing the agreed theme in a fairly gentle way. The more challenging themes can be introduced in the middle of the series. The last two or three sessions need to concentrate on review of the learning, next steps, and closure of the group.

Similar considerations apply even to single-occasion sessions. There needs to be a way of "warming up," then using a theme which evokes some personal material, then finishing with a theme (perhaps a group picture) which leaves people in a good state to go on their way. Sometimes each session in a series has a warm-up activity followed by a main theme.

Sometimes the program for the group can have themes at the beginning (to get people going) and end (to help with ending), with space in the middle sessions for clients to use as they wish. Or, as the group begins to gel, clients can contribute ideas for themes themselves.

If the art therapy group is to take place on a continuous basis, with a theme for each session, there are a number of ways to develop themes in a sensitive way:

- Work out the best theme to pursue from the feelings and issues that arose in the previous session.
- When the art therapy group is part of a larger program (e.g., in a day center), use what has happened during the week to suggest a helpful theme. If there is a particular concern or problem in such a setting, an art therapy group on this theme can be helpful.
- Look at the paintings from the previous session to suggest the next suitable theme.
- Have a choice of themes so that the group can be involved, and to give flexibility.
- Begin each session with a "round of feelings" (often a good way to start any group), leading to client discussion of an appropriate theme reflecting current concerns.

However themes are chosen, whether by therapists or clients or both, it is important to choose a theme that has enough breadth to be worked with on many levels, allowing group members to disclose as much or as little of themselves as they wish, and allowing a wide variety of painting and drawing styles, including figurative, abstract, painted, drawn, three-dimensional, and so on. For anyone who may find a particular theme threatening or otherwise especially difficult, I usually make it clear that "doing your own thing" is always an acceptable alternative.

RUNNING A THEMED ART THERAPY GROUP

Pattern of Sessions

Most group art therapy sessions have a similar format:

- Introduction and warm-up
- Main art activity
- Discussion and ending of group

The precise time lengths of each section depend on the total time available (often $1\frac{1}{2}$ to 2 hours with client groups, perhaps $2\frac{1}{2}$ hours with groups of professionals), the client group, and the purpose. If there is a strong social aim, then a coffee/tea break may be included between the activity and the discussion, or refreshments may be available at the start of the group. For some groups, the actual painting/drawing/making is the main activity, with discussion having a minor role. For others, the discussion emerging from the artworks is just as important as the art activity, and time needs to be allowed for everyone who wants to share his or her work. In some settings there is a need for more discussion at the beginning, to share experiences during the previous week and choose a theme for the session.

The Art Process

This is the time when group members are usually totally absorbed in what they are doing. It is important that there are no interruptions which might "break the flow." This time is the essence of the art therapy process, when nonverbal processes take over and people are working things out using paint, crayons, or clay. Some people may find it difficult to start and may need a little help from the therapist.

Many groups have an understanding that people do not talk while engaged in the art process, and this silence can intensify the experience. However, in some groups talking is encouraged, for instance, clients with learning disabilities, or adolescents, who may "open up" with the help of art therapy.

Discussion

The physical arrangements are important here—everyone in the group needs to be able to see what is being discussed, and it is helpful if all members can also have eye contact with each other. Some groups stay in the same positions as for the art process, while others are lucky enough to be able to move to a designated talking area with comfortable chairs. The paintings can then be placed on the floor in the middle of the circle. If the artwork is a group painting or mural, the group can gather round it.

Leading a discussion about the artworks produced is another whole group session, and there are many models for sharing:

- Everyone takes turns, either by following on round the circle or by each individual choosing when it feels right. Sometimes groups adopt a formal "equal time-share" agreement; in others, not all members want the same time and the time is shared informally. Many people like the democratic aspect of this arrangement, and it creates the expectation that quieter members will have their turn, as well as those who are used to claiming their space and may dominate the discussion. However, it is important that there is a "right to pass" for anyone who does not want to share what he or she has done.
- Focus on one or two pictures. This overcomes a disadvantage of the aforementioned model, by allowing more time for one or two pieces of work, leading to a deeper discussion of these. Group members then take turns over time.
- Focus on group dynamics. In this model, discussion may range widely, loosely based on the work produced, and leading to expressions of feelings about relationships within the group.

One of the benefits of group art therapy is that the discussion can involve all members of the group rather than just the therapist. The images are visible to the whole group, and this helps to facilitate discussion about difficult issues (Liebmann, 1986).

Interpretation

There are many ways of interpreting pictures and each therapist may work from a particular perspective. However, many art therapists work in an eclectic way, drawing from many different philosophies, and the presence of other group members will expand this range even more. Most psychological theories are based on some cultural assumptions; thus, it is important (especially in a multicultural working environment) to avoid simplistic one-to-one meanings: There are many ways of interpreting the simplest mark. It is important for anyone making an interpretation to "own" it and say where it is coming from.

The basic essential is for art therapy clients themselves to make their own interpretations. In a group in which people feel safe, others can add their views, and the original client can decide whether these contributions add to his or her own understanding—often they do, but sensitivity is needed here. Asking people to reflect on their pictures and see if they "speak back" to them can be useful too. Toward the end of a series of sessions, an "artwork review" can help clients to notice themes running through their work over several weeks and then respond to these insights with a further picture.

Endings

Whether the art therapy group is a series of sessions or a single occasion, the ending is very important. Each session needs to bring members back to the "here and now," able to carry on with normal life. This can be done by closing the discussion and clearing up, by a verbal "round," or for a series of sessions, by a group ritual, such as a group painting or group "visual gifts" exercise.

Evaluation

It is good practice to evaluate art therapy groups as they progress. This can be done in several ways: keeping records of client contributions and therapists' thoughts and feelings, discussing each session with the co-therapist, having regular clinical supervision, having a comments book for group members, having "quick evaluation" forms for group members at certain intervals, group reviews at intervals, and feedback forms at the end of the series.

DEVELOPING THEMES: EXAMPLES IN PRACTICE

Anger Management

This group was set up in response to a request from mental health clients for help managing their anger. Several of these clients had difficulty in expressing themselves verbally, so an art therapy group was thought to be a way to move forward. Referrals came from mental health practitioners, and the group started with six men and four women, dwindling to a steady number of five male clients after 2 or 3 weeks (a normal attenuation in the inner city area in which I work). My co-therapist was a community psychiatric nurse, who took part in the group and also kept an eye on one or two particularly vulnerable members of the group.

I had had experience running verbal anger management groups and adapted some of the strategies and sessions for use in the art therapy group. The sessions covered the following topics, moving from "exploratory" themes to ones concerning deeper feelings and family issues, and finishing with some positive ways of dealing with these issues:

1. Introductions and ground rules
2. Relaxation and guided imagery
3. What is anger?
4. Anger—good or bad?
5. What's underneath the anger?
6. Early family patterns
7. Anger and conflict
8. Feelings and assertiveness: "I messages"
9. Picture review
10. Group painting, evaluation, and ending

Each session included an opportunity to share feelings at the beginning and a "round" connected with the week's topic (e.g., for week 2, "A place I feel relaxed in," for week 6, "The sort of things people in my family got angry about"). After reading about an art therapy group for homeless people in New York (Cameron, 1996), I decided to include a regular period of relaxation each time, at the end, both to ensure that group members would have a way of coping with any strong feelings brought up in the session and to teach another way of dealing with anger. I also prepared handouts, which some group members found useful.

There were several beneficial aspects about using art therapy for this group. The art process provided a real outlet for feelings, which could then be faced and worked through. Members were also able to express themselves individually, and the sharing time allowed them to appreciate the many different responses to the theme. Different sessions resonated for different members.

For one member, a chaotic young man with little control over his temper, the second session remained the most meaningful for him—he drew a peaceful scene of a lake with trees and rushes surrounding it. He said he was able to go back to this internal image whenever he felt anger welling up uncontrollably. Another man, in his 30s, having suffered from depression for 5 years (after the loss of his job and breakup of his marriage) painted very colorful and expressive pictures. In session four (Anger—good or bad?) his picture (see Figure 25.1) showed anger pouring down the middle of the paper, then splitting into two directions—one going inward (to the left) and turning into festering resentment inside him, the other going outward (to the right) into energy that could get things done. He realized for the first time after doing the picture that he had a choice about how he used his anger. He said, "I'm realizing my anger can be a tool or a weapon."

Looking at family connections with anger was a crucial session for several people, and three members of the group made connections about their stepfathers. The session on assertiveness and the importance of "being who you truly are" provided a way forward from that.

During the pregroup interview and assessment I had asked everyone to list his or her problems with anger and to rate the seriousness on a scale of 1 to 5. Typical problems were the following:

- Aggressive outbursts
- Bottling anger up
- Blaming selves
- Angry with life
- Physical tension
- Unable to identify feelings

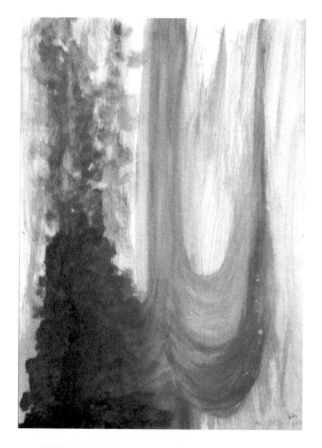

FIGURE 25.1. Anger: resentment or energy.

By the end of the group, clients felt they had made some progress with the problems they had, with most problems mentioned shifting 1 to 3 points toward the less severe end of the scale.

Conflict Resolution

This group followed from the anger management art therapy group and included one or two of the same clients, but also some new ones, and a more equal gender balance, with two men and three women clients, all with mental health problems, mostly depression and with an expressed inability to handle conflict. The structure of sessions was similar to that of the previous group but also included two sessions of interactive work so that we might be able to discuss conflict as it arose.

In the first of these sessions, clients worked in pairs on the same piece of paper, without talking. In one pair, Paul was energetically drawing all over the paper, when Maggie drew a brick wall. Paul withdrew, feeling hurt and rejected. After the drawing, Maggie explained that she just needed her own space to be quiet in, she was not rejecting Paul. This helped Paul realize that he had a pattern of feeling rejected and mostly did not wait to even ask why people acted as they did; he just assumed the worst and acted on that assumption.

In the second session (see Figure 25.2), all five clients worked on the same piece of paper. Two of the women (top middle and top right) worked in an individual way, oblivious of the others. The two men worked on the left, filling up the space between them, quite happy to merge at the boundary. The third woman, Jacki, started at the bottom on the right and worked her way toward the left, then stopped and worked her way back again. Afterward she said she had wanted to join in with the colorful scene on the left but had then thought, "Oh, that's the boys' corner, they won't want me," and so took herself away. I asked Jacki if she wanted to check out this view, and she did. The two men said they would have welcomed her contribution. The following week Jacki told us she had used this realization to sort out a conflict in her rock music band, a situation which had been going on for 6 months.

Life Journeys

Sometimes themes can develop over the period of the group's life. The idea of Life Journeys developed from three sources: several mental health clients who were assessed for art therapy and expressed a wish to "get a grip on their life," a trainee art therapist keen to run a group within her limited time on placement, and a course I had attended on narrative therapy.

I had also received a request to provide art therapy input to a day center near my workplace (an inner-city community mental health team) but had limited time available: I thought a themed group would enable clients from both facilities to benefit from an art therapy group. A 10-session group (plus pre- and postgroup interviews) would fit into the autumn timetable and the trainee art therapist's placement and be of use to the clients in mind.

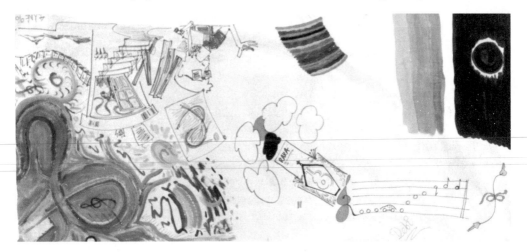

FIGURE 25.2. Group picture: conflict resolution.

We announced the group to staff of both agencies with a short description:

"An opportunity to look at where you have been, where you are and where you are going, using a variety of art materials. A group for people wanting to explore their journey through life. In this small supportive group, we will be using art materials to help you with personal self-expression and to look at the story or journey of your life. You do not have to be good at art—just willing to try. You can explore and develop your creativity and try out possible futures on paper."

We emphasized the need for a firm commitment, took applications, and arranged interviews. We accepted all the applicants but some with provisos regarding their behavior in the group, based on their interview or previous knowledge. We ended up with six regular members of the group.

In discussion about the group, we saw the group process as moving people on from the past through the present to the future. We decided to work from childhood (first five sessions) to adulthood (second five sessions). We would start each session with a "round" connected with the theme of the week. We finalized the first five sessions:

1. Introductions—hopes and fears, ground rules, what art therapy is and is not, art therapy exercise on names.
2. Lifeline—draw your life as a line/road/river with about five or six events.
3. Early childhood—a favorite place (in the widest sense).
4. Childhood—an event or continuing circumstance which, looking back, had a big or lasting effect on your adult life in some way.
5. A time you made a successful step toward independence.

We reserved the last two sessions for a "picture review" and closing session. We wanted to see how the sessions went before planning the precise details of the remaining three sessions. Then we worked on themes for these, so that the second half of the group went as follows:

6. The first time you felt "grown up."
7. Crossroads—a choice or decision which made a difference to your life—past or present.
8. The future: imagine where you would like to be in 5 years' time—including the very first step.
9. Review of pictures and paint/draw a response.
10. Closing: good-bye gifts—draw a basket/box/bag and then draw a gift in everyone else's container. Evaluation forms.

One participant, Mike, in session 7, did a picture of his elderly ailing dog (see Figure 25.3), his constant companion. The difficult decision he faced was whether to take the dog to the vet to be put out of its misery (with an injection in its leg) or to take it to his parents (the couple at the top left) who had a bungalow on one level, easier for the dog to manage than the stairs to Mike's flat. Either way, Mike was going to miss his dog a lot. In session 8 he drew his dream of traveling around the world, with money from a good job in computers, and the first step of going back to his university computer course. In session 9, as he reviewed his pictures, he realized that one element was missing: alcohol. He drew a picture of nine cans of alcohol and realized that the key to any real change was to stop drinking. At the end of the group he said the themes helped him a great deal—without them he would have felt totally stuck.

Another member of the group particularly appreciated a themed group, as she said it helped her to get going and to bridge the gap between the "mad" bit and the "sensible" bit of herself, in the company of others. She said she found individual work threatening because it reminded her of the secrecy of abusive situations from the past.

Women's Group: Using Themes to Start a Group

This women's group ran for 1½ years at a day center for women and their children on a deprived housing estate on the outskirts of the city. The group was started to provide an opportunity for those who found verbal expression difficult. At the women's request, I brought a theme each week, based on what they had done the previous week, or a theme developed out of the round of initial feelings (Liebmann, 1997).

An early theme to help the women begin to use paints was "Cover the paper with as many colors as possible as quickly as possible," which gave them permission to use the colors more boldly and spontaneously. Another theme I chose for one of the early sessions was "If I were an animal, what would I be?" with a background habitat. We worked round a table and the women worked on cats (always a favorite, combining independence with being fed and looked after), dogs, and birds. Suddenly one of the more vulnerable women disappeared under the table—was she all right? I could just see her, engrossed in the activity, so I did nothing. At the end of the painting time, she emerged

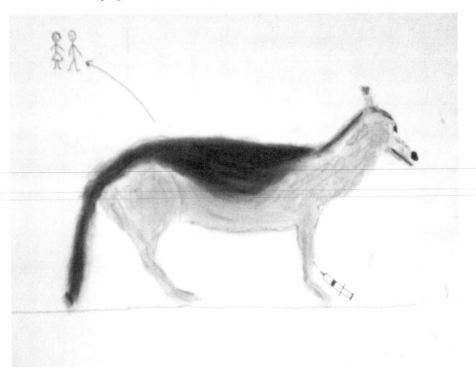

FIGURE 25.3. Decision about an ailing dog.

flushed and triumphant, with four sheets of paper stuck together. "There wasn't room on the table to do what I wanted." she explained. She had drawn a huge white wild horse, galloping over open fields, a complete contrast to her life hemmed in by several children, debts, illness, and a difficult and demanding husband. This picture became a turning point for her and something she could hold on to: At the end of the group she realized she was indeed strong and free inside herself.

On one occasion, the initial round of feelings demonstrated that all the women were feeling rather fragile that day. I suggested a theme of "a safe place" and later found out that the day center was in uproar that week because someone had broken the confidentiality rule and everyone felt unsafe. The theme met the women's needs to reclaim a feeling of safety.

With this group, the themes were useful in helping the women to get started. As they grew in confidence, they began to know how they wanted to use the art therapy sessions. Thus I gradually provided less support in the way of themes, or only provided a theme as a backstop if they were feeling totally blank. It seemed a natural progression from using some structure to being able to work independently.

SHORT SESSIONS

Art therapy can be useful in helping clients to look at any issue. This may take place in a single session or in two linked sessions which are part of another piece of work.

An example was a request, from a mental health day center running an ongoing women's group, for help in looking at anger and assertiveness. I worked together with the psychologist who had received the request.

We devised two linked sessions. The first one was centered around artwork on the theme "A situation when I feel/have felt angry," with some introductory and rounding-off exercises. The aim of this session was to help the women to be less afraid of their anger. The second session, a month later, included artwork on how the women would have liked the situation to turn out, followed by the psychologist introducing some simple assertiveness techniques. The role of art therapy here was to provide a vehicle for self-expression and material to work on in the second session. All the women were able to participate and felt they gained from the sessions. The artwork played a large role in helping the women feel less isolated with their anger.

CONCLUSION

This chapter has looked at the reasons for using group work involving themes in art therapy and at how to set up such groups. The examples show how themes can be developed for particular client groups and situations. Using themes appropriately takes experience and skill—both in art therapy and in knowledge of the needs of a particular group.

There are many ways of running groups. Some groups may use themes at certain times and not at others. What is important is that therapists think about what they are trying to achieve with their clients and choose the right mode at the right time. Well-chosen themes can provide clients with an avenue to explore issues in a particular way, with benefits to themselves and other group members.

ACKNOWLEDGMENTS

I would like to thank all the clients for their participation and their willingness to let me write about their work. Also, I wish to thank the following colleagues who read and commented on the first draft of this chapter: Karen Lee Drucker, Liz Lumley-Smith, Diana Van Loock, and Fiona Williams.

REFERENCES

Cameron, D. F. (1996). Conflict resolution through art with homeless people. In M. Liebmann (Ed.), *Arts approaches to conflict* (pp. 176–206). London and Bristol, PA: Jessica Kingsley.
Hagood, M. (2000). *The use of art in counselling child and adult survivors of sexual abuse.* London and Bristol, PA: Jessica Kingsley.
Liebmann, M. (1986). *Art therapy for groups.* London: Croom Helm.
Liebmann, M. (1997). Art therapy and empowerment in a women's self-help project. In S. Hogan (Ed.), *Feminist approaches to art therapy* (pp. 197–215). London and New York: Routledge.
Whitaker, D. S. (2001). *Using groups to help people.* (2nd ed.). London and New York: Brunner-Routledge.

CHAPTER 26

Sexually Abused Children: Group Approaches

P. Gussie Klorer

"Sex is when somebody get on top of you and do the nasty stuff. My brothers do that all the time. They put their thing between my legs and play all the time," 5-year-old Tasha announced authoritatively to her therapy group as she painted a picture. Tasha did not seem to be traumatized by the abuse; after all, her mother told her she could have sex any time she wanted.

By age 11, Tasha was "therapy wise" and could repeat safety rules, identify types of good and bad touch, and tell you who to tell if someone touched your private parts. Yet Tasha's behavior invited sexual advances from boys in her neighborhood, and she was at risk to be a repeated victim, even more so after 6 years of therapy, when the more mature preadolescent boys in her class began to notice her sexualized struts across the classroom.

Ideally, treatment for a child like Tasha includes group, individual, and family therapy. The goals of each of these treatment approaches will vary but together will help to address the needs of the child emotionally, cognitively, and behaviorally. The focus of this chapter is the group therapy component of treatment, which should be seen as one aspect of an overall treatment plan. Because sexual abuse is an issue children typically do not like to talk about, art and play therapy are often the methods of choice in group therapy. There are many advantages to using art, which this chapter highlights. There are also limitations, particularly in the area of assessment, which are mentioned here.

THE USE OF ART IN DETECTION OF CHILD ABUSE

Substantiating child sexual abuse is difficult for many reasons. Because of threats from the perpetrator, guilt feelings, a fear of not being believed, or a desire to protect the perpetrator, verbal disclosure is not always the child's typical mode of response. Determining the presence of sexual abuse is particularly difficult in the absence of medical evidence, and physical evidence is only present in 15% of all cases (Walker, 1988). According to Myers (1996), there are four things on which to base confirmation of abuse: (1) the child's sexual behavior and knowledge of sex, (2) the child's nonsexual behavior commonly associated with abuse, (3) medical evidence, and (4) disclosure. Behavioral indicators alone may be a clue, but they can be misread or can indicate knowledge rather than actual abuse experience.

Art therapists would like to think that the child's art can indicate abuse, but this, too, is inexact and cannot be used without corroboration of medical, physical, or other types of evidence. In the past few decades, efforts have been made to justify the use of art as a diagnostic tool in the area of child sexual abuse (Blain, Bergner, Lewis, & Goldstein, 1981; Cohen & Phelps, 1985; Culbertson & Revel, 1987; Goodwin, 1982; Kaufman & Wohl, 1992; Kelley, 1984; Manning, 1987; Peterson, Hardin, & Nitsch, 1995; Sidun & Rosenthal, 1987; Yates, Beutler, & Crago, 1985). Clinicians who regularly use art in therapy know that there are certain symbols that seem to be prevalent in abused children's art. The studies cited previously have found significance in certain graphic indicators, such as repressive defenses and lack of impulse control (Yates et al., 1985); omission of hands and fingers, head only, circles, and heavy line pressure (Sidun & Rosenthal, 1987); smoke coming from chimney, absence of windows from ground floor of the house, asymmetrical limbs on person, absence of feet, and disproportionate heads (Blain et al., 1981); heavy line pressure, absence of clothing, complex head, absence of feet and arms, vacant eyes, and large heads (Culbertson & Revel, 1987); inclement weather (Manning, 1987); presence of penis, compartmentalization, box-like figures, teeth, large noses, open mouths, bald heads, long hair, and transparencies in genital area (Kaufman & Wohl, 1992); inclusion of genitals, concealment of genitals, omission of genitalia, omission of central part of the figure, and encapsulation of figures (Peterson et al., 1995); emphasis on pelvic area, emphasis on upper portion of body, small figures, and omission of hands (Kelley, 1984).

Unfortunately, as this partial listing demonstrates, the attempts to find a unified pattern of signs indicating abuse have been inconsistent. None of the studies mentioned earlier identify the same grouping of graphic indicators as indicators of abuse. In some cases, the lists of significant items are vastly different, with virtually no item in common. A more recent study of the House–Tree–Person drawings of sexually abused children and a nonabused comparison sample revealed that it was not possible to discriminate between the two groups of children (Palmer et al., 2000). In addition, complications in this kind of research demonstrate that interrater reliability on the presence or absence of items can be problematic (Cohen & Phelps, 1985). Clearly, more studies need to be conducted and replicated. Children's drawings alone are not sufficient to diagnose child sexual abuse (McGlinchey, Keenan, & Dillenburger, 2000).

ASSESSMENT TOOLS

Although drawings are clinically useful and provide a tremendous amount of information, particularly when the child is not talking, there is not a particular sign that will always point toward an assessment of abuse. Despite the inability to identify characteristics that will always be abuse indicators, art is still an invaluable tool in understanding how a particular child views the world as the result of abuse, the child's defenses, strengths, coping mechanisms, and cognitive and emotional functioning. Art can also be used to help a child to talk about what happened and to communicate feelings about issues for which words may be woefully inadequate. Drawings may help the therapist to determine the child's reactions to abuse, such as degree of sexual-acting-out behavior, anxiety, fear, identification with the aggressor, or withdrawal tendencies, and what pattern of defenses have been used. Drawings will give additional information that will help the therapist to determine the appropriateness of a particular therapy group for a child.

Drawings that are particularly helpful are those that assess the child's perception of self (self-portraits or Draw-a-Person tests); drawings that assess the child's perception of the environment, such as House–Tree–Person and Favorite Kind of Day drawings (Manning, 1987); and drawings that assess the child's perception of him- or herself in the family or home environment (family drawings or kinetic family drawings). What is often proven to be most beneficial, however, are "free choice" drawings, through which children reveal much more simply by choice of materials and subject matter. Here, the therapist can begin to understand the child's own repertoire of symbols which will be important throughout the course of treatment.

Several assessment tools are particularly useful in work with abused children. The Child Sexual Behavior Inventory (CSBI; Friedrich, Grambsch, Broughton, Kuiper, & Beilke, 1991; Friedrich et al., 1992) is abuse specific and defines normative and clinical contrasts. The Child Sexual Behavior Checklist (CSBCL; Johnson, 1991b) helps the clinician categorize the child into one of four membership groups, ranging from normal, exploratory play to children who use force, bribery, or coercion to engage other children in sexual acting out. Putman (1997) and colleagues have developed several dissociation checklists: the Child Dissociative Checklist, the Dissociative Experiences Scale—II, and the Adolescent Dissociative Experiences Scale. These tests help to determine the child's reaction to trauma and the presence of dissociative symptoms.

THERAPY GOALS

Many treatment issues are prevalent among children traumatized by abuse. Surprisingly, the sexual abuse is often not what is traumatic, particularly when there was no force or pain involved. For some children, in fact, the abuse was the only time they felt love, and the abuse was experienced as pleasurable, albeit, the confusion that accompanied this pleasure may be overwhelming. It is the betrayal of the relationship, according to Finkelhor and Browne (1986), the betrayal of trust, that is most traumatic for the abused child. This may lead to attachment difficulties, emotional distress, and posttraumatic symptoms.

Other issues that arise in therapy are the cognitive distortions that are seen in how the abused child perceives the world. For some, the world is perceived as more dangerous than it is, and the self is perceived as helpless and without recourse or options (Briere & Elliot, 1994). This can be seen graphically in children's artwork, when they depict themselves with weak, ineffectual arms and as small figures amid chaotic and dangerous environments.

Depression, anxiety, and anger are also common in this population. Here, gender differences are noted. Boys are more often reported as acting aggressively, fighting with peers and siblings, and are more likely to recapitulate their experience by victimizing others. Girls, on the other hand, tend to show more depressive symptoms and seem to exhibit other kinds of "sexually reactive behavior"—sexualized or seductive behavior that puts them at greater risk for revictimization (Cosentino & Collins, 1996; Gil & Johnson, 1993; Johnson, 1989, 1991a, 1991b). In artwork, these differences are also noted. One often sees the male abuse victim drawing violent battles and monsters, clearly identifying with the aggressor, which Kramer (1971) states is a defense the child uses in order to feel less frightened and powerless.

The most worrisome art is that which indicates high identification with the aggressor, but when the child is not exhibiting any behavioral signs of aggression. The child who causes the most concern is the angelic child whose art is very disturbed. These children are like seething volcanoes ready to erupt, and their behavior when they do erupt is likely to be uncontained, violent, and unpredictable.

When recommending a child for group therapy, the severity of abuse reactions needs to be considered. One would not want to expose a child whose abuse experiences were not traumatic to children who have been deeply traumatized. The range of behaviors and reactions to abuse is proportional to the duration of the trauma, the age of the child at trauma onset, use of force, and severity of abuse (Briere & Elliot, 1994; van der Kolk, 1994). Studies show that not all abused children are harmed. A surprising number cope, survive, and even flourish (Beutler, Williams, & Zetzer, 1994; Levitt & Pinnell, 1995). A child who is not showing signs of trauma and stress—for example, a child who was fondled once by a babysitter but whose other life experiences have been appropriate, boundaried, and loving—may not need therapy at all, or may terminate therapy quickly, once safety rules and prevention skills are learned. For others, such as Tasha, the abuse issues are long term and are complicated by family dynamics and problems that are multigenerational and ingrained in her personality. The former child, if she is placed in a group, should be with group members whose experiences are similar to hers, and the group focus will likely be psychoeducational, to address basic rules of safety. Tasha's group should also be with group members of like experiences, and the group goals will encompass not only rules of safety but some of the deeper issues that come with long-term abuse.

Victims of ongoing abuse appear significantly more disturbed, with symptoms ranging from depression to psychosis, than children reacting to a single event of abuse (Kiser, Heston, Millsap, & Pruitt, 1991). In severe cases of sexual abuse over prolonged periods, dissociation may have been employed as a defense. Dissociation is characterized by the child's ability to store traumatic memory in an alternate state of consciousness. As the child is experiencing the event, the child learns to leave his or her body, splitting off the memory and the affect that accompanies it, and becoming numb to both the memory and the experience (van der Kolk & van der Hart, 1991). The most severe forms of dissociation occur when the abuse is frequent, unpredictable, and inconsistent and the child has been exposed to some form of love (Braun & Sachs, 1985). This suggests that in object relations terms, attachment coupled with abuse is a more severe stress trigger than abuse with no attachment.

When a child has dissociated the event, words may not be available. When the experience cannot be organized on a linguistic level, the failure to arrange the memory in words leaves it to be organized on a somatic level, expressed through somatic sensations, behavioral reenactments, and nightmares (van der Kolk, 1987, 1994). Art, then, is a natural tool to employ when working with children who do not have words for their experiences. Rarely do children draw or enact in art the actual facts of the abuse. Rather, the issues are enacted symbolically through repetition of themes that are idiosyncratic to each child. Each child develops his or her own symbols and stories. Through repetition of themes, the child begins to gain mastery over the overwhelming feelings. The therapist's role is to provide a psychologically safe environment in which this work can occur.

GROUP ART THERAPY FOR SEXUALLY ABUSED CHILDREN

When designing a treatment plan for a sexually abused child, group art therapy should be considered. Although some issues are best dealt with in individual therapy, group therapy helps the child feel less alone, guilty, and responsible for the abuse and empowers children to help one another, through telling their own stories and giving advice to one another. It allows for trying on new roles of behavior, enacting issues within a secure setting, and problem solving with others.

An important issue to consider when setting up a group is the developmental ages of the children. Because of vast variances in cognitive skills between children who are even close in age, and because the issues will be processed differently depending upon the child's developmental age, children should be grouped according to developmental rather than chronological ages.

There are different kinds of groups with differing goals. Ongoing groups, which accept new members at any time, time-limited groups, structured groups, and unstructured open-studio type groups are but a few.

Ongoing Groups versus Time-Limited Groups

Ongoing groups are groups that accept new members at any time. These groups can be structured or not structured. Ongoing groups have the benefit of older, seasoned members helping newer members to adjust. Some ongoing groups have been in existence for years, with a consistent core group and more peripheral members coming and going. This kind of group can offer long-term stability and friendship to a child who does not have a group of friends or family support and can be invaluable in terms of the child feeling less isolated and "different" from peers. For example, a 3-year ongoing group of adolescent females in a residential treatment program developed their own methods of introducing new group members. Typically, one of the older members would announce to the new person that this group was "special," and membership was limited to "girls who have something in common." The girls would giggle nervously, and then someone would volunteer that she had been sexually abused, bringing on nods and affirmation from others. The new girl was never asked directly about her abuse, but it was acknowledged that she was part of the exclusive "club." Because of the longevity of this group, the girls would define their own topics of discussion each week.

Time-limited groups usually have the same composition of group members throughout. Time-limited groups are often structured and are designed to have a period of trust building, to introduce the sexual abuse issue, and to bring the issue to some type of closure. The time limit allows the child some breathing room, knowing that there will be a limit to the stress. Despite its short duration, often children mourn the loss of this kind of group when it is over. Because of the intensity of the issues, the group can become tightly bonded in a few short weeks.

Structured versus Nonstructured Groups

Children will not necessarily want to talk about sexual abuse. If talking about what happened and learning about sexual abuse prevention are part of the group goals, structured activities and directed conversation are likely to be more successful than nonstructured, open-studio type groups. Structured groups allow for introduction of the issues in a direct but safe and contained way. Art and other activities can be designed to assist in the structuring of the issues to be discussed. For example, directing the children to draw the perpetrator, or draw what happened, or draw how they felt at the time of the abuse, gives the children the opportunity to express feelings that may be difficult to talk about. It allows them the ability to "hold" the feeling, while letting it out. It allows them the opportunity to "see" the feeling while allowing them distance from the feeling.

Structured groups allow the therapist the opportunity to plan a gradual introduction to sexual abuse issues. Research suggests that structure in a group setting is necessary to obtain a disclosure, as children do not volunteer this information easily. According to Mordock's (1996) study, it was rare for a child to disclose if the therapist never mentioned the abuse. Consequently, if disclosure is therapeutically indicated, structure will be important. The group may begin with getting-to-know-each-other activities and become increasingly more focused on sexual issues, with a different but related topic presented each week.

"Treatment manual" approaches to sexual abuse groups are often used, and these approaches often use art and play activities as part of the protocol. These highly structured approaches, with a set script for each week throughout the group's duration, are appealing, especially to the clinician with little experience in this area, but are also used by seasoned therapists who have discovered through trial and error what "works." Structure can be extremely helpful when children are exhibiting behavioral problems, and behaviors can be exacerbated when issues of a stressful nature are being discussed. Treatment manual approaches are also invaluable when the groups are part of a research study, such as the protocol presented by Berliner, Saunders, and Benjamin (1996). The structured, sexual abuse-specific protocol consisted of weekly topics and a series of activities in the form of games, short films, and role-play related to each week's topic. The study suggested that cognitive behavioral, abuse-specific treatment is associated with improved outcome for most sexually abused children.

Ideally, a therapist could use a combination of approaches, adhering to the treatment manual activities when necessary but being flexible enough to follow the needs of the group as it unfolds. Groups tend to take on a personality of their own, and if the therapist can provide a structure with attentive, flexible directives, the group can often surprise the therapist in its progression and processing through some extremely difficult issues surrounding abuse. For example, the therapist of an ongoing, structured group of adolescent females suggested that the girls make a mural, as a follow-up to a discussion the previous week about the hazards of unprotected sex. The group members immediately rebelled, saying they didn't "feel like it," they were "tired of talking about it," "this was stupid," all the while avoiding even picking up the materials to begin. Upon further exploration, it was revealed that a favorite houseparent was leaving, and the feelings of sadness were overwhelming. The therapist switched the focus, allowing the group to make a good-bye mural for the houseparent. As the mural was being created, deeper issues of abandonment, echoed in each of their early histories, became a much more relevant topic of discussion.

Nonstructured groups can have an advantage over structured groups in that the children will likely feel less threatened when the issue is not directly approached, but the issue may also never come up in a direct way. Mordock (1996) found that children in play/talk and play groups reveal their abuse in metaphors, stories, drawings, symbolic play, behavior, or behavioral cues. For some children, particularly at latency when avoidance of sexuality is developmentally the norm, the topic is so loaded that just the mention of a group for sexual abuse can trigger extreme acting-out behavior, even from children who do not usually respond as such. It might accomplish more to not make abuse the focus of the group. A graduate art therapy student, facilitating a group for potentially explosive sexually abused girls between the ages of 8 and 10, decided to call her group "The Girls' Group," and the children unanimously decided that it would be about "what girls should know." This allowed the group to form a group identity and safely approach some of the abuse issues but decreased the anxiety levels significantly.

The goals for a nonstructured group might be to form friendships, talk about feelings, learn to trust group members, and ultimately, use art to metaphorically express sexually laden issues. When the issues do come up in a story or metaphor, it allows the children the safety of staying within the metaphor if necessary. When a group "discovers" that all group members have been abused, it can lead to spontaneous disclosure.

For example, a group of three girls, ages 7, 8, and 9 were seen together in art therapy. All three had been sexually abused, but this was not presented by the therapist as a reason for the group. The group was semistructured, with flexibility to change the directive if the group seemed to have their own ideas from which a theme could be generated. One week the girls were asked to draw their families. The 9-year-old drew her mother, stepfather, two stepbrothers, and herself, but each figure was nude, with extremely graphic and exaggerated sexual characteristics. The two younger girls, horrified, looked toward the therapist to ascertain her reaction, and said in tattling tones of voice, "Look at what Allison did!" The therapist acknowledged the drawing, and told them that in art therapy such drawings were permissible, although we would probably not choose to hang them in the dining hall on the bulletin board display. The other two girls then proceeded to draw their own families in various displays of undress. Typically, children copy when the drawings have touched on their own issues in some way, and that was certainly the case in this instance.

After the drawings were completed, a discussion about families ensued, and the oldest girl, who had disclosed incest to the therapist in her individual therapy, admitted that her brothers and stepfather had "touched her." This brought relief and immediate disclosure from the other two girls. Once the issue was brought into the open, the group took on a new excitement. The girls began inventing games to play wherein they could process what had happened to them. For example, suddenly the anatomically correct dolls, which had largely been ignored, became a favorite focus of the group. The girls would play-act with the dolls, setting up abusive situations and enacting scenarios of rescue by the police, including putting the perpetrator in jail. This spontaneous play led into more structured sessions surrounding safety issues.

Structured tasks can be designed to address needs as identified by the group. A creative therapist will look at what issues the group is struggling with and design a directive that will help the group address that particular issue in a safe way. For example, when a group of high school-age girls were discussing their relationships, the standard opinion appeared to be that "boys are jerks." The art directive, tying into this issue, was to make two collages, one about their current relationships and one about the qualities of an "ideal" relationship. This helped to make visual the differences between what they hoped for and what they were settling for and brought new insight into the discussion. As one girl so aptly put it, "It's not that all boys are jerks, but why do we pick such jerks?"

SETTING REALISTIC TREATMENT GOALS

Organizing group members by developmental ages can help the therapist determine how issues will be processed. The issues that accompany child abuse will be ongoing and will be processed differently at each successive stage of development (Klorer, 2000). Using "Tasha" as an example, one can see how children progress through treatment stages, processing the abuse to the extent of their cognitive abilities and attending to the developmental issues at hand. (Tasha is a fictitious client, a compilation of three individuals with similar case histories.)

From the ages of about 5 to 7, Tasha is assertive and talkative about her own sexual abuse. In group therapy, she tells children about an uncle who abused her, whom she does not like because she was afraid of him. She does not see her brothers as abusive, and easily tells her therapy group what sexual things they do to her, not yet recognizing that it is wrong. She is a bright girl and quickly learns sexual abuse prevention rules.

From kindergarten to about second or third grade, art and play are wonderful, age-appropriate forms of therapy. Tasha's therapy group consists of free-choice play and art, allowing the children to express idiosyncratic and symbolic images. These sessions are interspersed with psychoeducation sessions aimed at teaching the children new responses. Through repeating or copying images, the children learn how to respond to abusive situations. Goals such as identifying kinds of good and bad touch, naming who to tell if someone touches your private parts, and talking about safe and not-safe situations, are all things that are taught in Tasha's group therapy. The children like it when the therapist reads books to them about safety issues, and they enjoy the repetition of the same books being read and reread. Much work is done in the area of identifying simple feelings, such as happy, mad, scared, and sad feelings, and the children play-act and draw these feelings in a group setting. Treatment issues that are particularly relevant involve children of this age internalizing guilt, shame, and sadness. Because at this age the boundary between fantasy and reality is blurred, children at this age sometimes feel that what happened was their fault. However, Tasha also has the ability to differentiate self from nonself. Separating out feelings about the perpetrator and the self is a key treatment issue.

As Tasha approaches latency, she starts denying all abuse. She "can't remember" things that she had previously disclosed about her brothers. She is extremely protective of them and insists that they don't do anything "bad" like that. However, Tasha continues to be the best in her therapy group at talking about abuse in general terms. Her favorite game is a board game about sexual abuse prevention. She also likes to play-act feelings, draw feeling faces, and have others guess the feelings.

During these middle years, from about 7 to 12, Tasha has more opportunity to resolve traumatic issues on a metaphoric level. Socially, she moves into more complex systems of relationships, rather than operating only in dyads. At this time, group therapy is seen as a vital part of the treatment plan in order to help children like Tasha feel less alone. Children no longer rely on repetitive memory, as in the previous stage, when it was appropriate to read and reread the same books, but rather will be capable of creating their own stories and solutions to hypothetical situations that are presented. Consequently, in terms of abuse prevention, psychoeducational process can become more advanced. Tasha is able to identify specific persons to whom she could go if in trouble, identify specific situations that are not safe, identify kinds of touch (good, bad, and confusing), and identify and take ownership of her own feelings. The beginnings of moral development, right versus wrong, are introduced in her group. The child no longer needs to use splitting as a coping mechanism. Rather, good and bad are integrated into one concept, which means that the child can tolerate more stress and ambiguity than he or she once could. Tasha can explore feeling two different ways at the same time, accepting the concept of loving or liking certain things about the perpetrator but hating the abuse.

At latency, children tend to repress frightening feelings. Expressive therapies continue to be used as a means of helping children express those feelings and issues that are avoided and denied. It is important that the therapist stay with Tasha's level of denial and support the process of allowing the issues to unfold as she experiences them. Providing both verbal and nonverbal opportunities for expression of complex feelings helps Tasha learn to discriminate between gradations of feelings.

Tasha's teacher reports that Tasha is sexually provocative in her walk but totally unaware of it. By the time Tasha is 12, she has been in several groups for sexually abused girls, along with individual therapy. She is a group leader, able to teach new girls in the group about prevention. She knows the "right" answers to hypothetical situations that are presented. She has not engaged in any sexual acting out for 1 year. She terminates therapy at age 12, feeling that she "doesn't need to talk about all this stuff anymore."

Tasha comes back to therapy at age 16, when she begins to explore what is "normal" in terms of sexual relationships with boys. She is overweight and wants the attention of boys. In her therapy group, she talks about wanting a boyfriend but is sexually promiscuous with several boys rather than just one. Her group points this out to her as being possibly detrimental to her goal. She counsels other girls about the importance of using condoms; however, she does not always use them herself. She wants to hear what the girls have to say about her behavior and tries out new roles periodically, to see how they fit.

In adolescence, the ability to deal with hypothetical situations is developed. Repression no longer works as well as it did in earlier stages, and issues of sexuality are rampant. Issues that were previously expressed through metaphor now demand to be expressed more directly. Children who had previously terminated therapy often come back at this time, because suddenly they find themselves needing to approach issues that can no longer be avoided. Group therapy is a key strategy in working with adolescents. Often, they can help each other more than the therapist can help them. Sharing feelings, processing relationships and sexual issues, making connections between past and present behavior, and identifying with the group helps Tasha to sort through her conflictual feelings. The group will allow the adolescent an opportunity to try on different roles and modes of interaction as part of identify formation.

It may not be until adulthood that Tasha will be capable of the insight necessary to see the long-term effects of her early, severe abuse in terms of her relationship choices. This does not suggest that previous therapy has been unsuccessful, nor does it suggest that continued therapy is always necessary. Therapy should be reinitiated whenever the child is showing signs of stress, usually evidenced through behavior. Many children are able to resolve the issues at hand according to their developmental capabilities and therapy can be terminated, with the understanding that it can be resumed if necessary as the child matures and develops new understandings about what happened.

CONCLUSION

When designing treatment goals for group art therapy with sexually abused children, the therapist needs to take into account a number of factors; the age and sex of the child, the severity of the abuse, the extent of trauma, and the child's cognitive stage of development. Decisions about the kind of group, be it structured, unstructured, time limited, or ongoing, should be made taking group goals into account. A recognition that the issues may be long term and will processed continually as the child matures and develops will help the therapist conceptualize realistic treatment goals according to the child's ability to process at a particular stage of development. This approach supports the health of the child, attempts to depathologize the child, and normalizes the child's reactions to abuse.

REFERENCES

Berliner, L., Saunders, L., & Benjamin, E. (1996). Treating fear and anxiety in sexually abused children: Results of a controlled 2-year follow-up study. *Child Maltreatment*, 1(4), 294–312.

Beutler, L., Williams, R., & Zetzer, H. (1994). Efficacy of treatment for victims of child sexual abuse. In R. Behrman (Ed.), *The future of children: Sexual abuse of children* (pp. 156–175). Los Altos, CA: Center for the Future of Children, the David and Lucille Packard Foundation.

Blain, G. H., Bergner, R. M., Lewis, M. L., & Goldstein, M. A. (1981). The use of objectively scorable house–tree–person indicators to establish child abuse. *Journal of Clinical Psychology*, 37(3), 667–673.

Braun, B., & Sachs, R. (1985). The development of multiple personality disorder. In R. Kluft (Ed.), *Childhood antecedents of multiple personality* (pp. 38–64). Washington, DC: American Psychiatric Press.

Briere, J., & Elliott, D. (1994). Immediate and long-term impacts of child sexual abuse. In R. Behrman (Ed.), *The future of children: Sexual abuse of children* (pp. 54–69). Los Altos, CA: Center for the Future of Children, the David and Lucille Packard Foundation.

Cohen, F. W., & Phelps, R. E. (1985). Incest markers in children's artwork. *The Arts in Psychotherapy*, 12, 265–283.

Cosentino, C., & Collins, M., (1996). Sexual abuse of children: Prevalence, effects, and treatment. In J. Sechzer, S. Pfafflin, F. Denmark, A. Griffin, & S. Blumenthal (Eds.), *Women and mental health* (Vol. 789, pp. 45–65). New York: New York Academy of Sciences.

Culbertson, F. M., & Revel, A. C. (1987). Graphic characteristics on the Draw-a-Person test for identification of physical abuse. *Art Therapy: Journal of the American Art Therapy Association*, 4(2), 78–83.

Finkelhor, D., & Browne, A. (1986). Impact of child sexual abuse: A review of the research. *Psychological Bulletin*, 99, 66–77.

Friedrich, W. N., Grambsch, P., Broughton, D., Kuiper, J., & Beilke, R. L. (1991). Normative sexual behavior in children. *Pediatrics*, 88(3), 456–464.

Friedrich, W. N., Grambsch, P., Damon, L., Koverola, C., Hewitt, S., Lang, R., & Wolfe, V. (1992). Child sexual behavior inventory: Normative and clinical comparisons. *Psychological Assessment*, 4, 303–311.

Gil, E., & Johnson, T. C. (1993). *Sexualized children: Assessment and treatment of sexualized children and children who molest*. New York: Launch.

Goodwin, J. (1982). Use of drawings in evaluating children who may be incest victims. *Children and Youth Services Review*, 4, 269–278.

Johnson, T. C. (1989). Female child perpetrators: Children who molest other children. *Child Abuse and Neglect, 13,* 571–585.

Johnson, T. C. (1991a, Fall). Children who molest children: Identification and treatment approaches for children who molest other children. *The American Professional Society on the Abuse of Children,* 9–11.

Johnson, T. C. (1991b, August/September). Understanding the sexual behaviors of young children. *SIECUS Report,* 8–15.

Kaufman, B., & Wohl, A. (1992). *Casualties of childhood: A developmental perspective on sexual abuse using projective drawings.* New York: Brunner/Mazel.

Kelley, S. (1984). The use of art therapy with sexually abused children. *Psychosocial Nursing, 22*(12), 12–18.

Kiser, L. J., Heston, J., Millsap, P. A., & Pruitt, D. B. (1991). Physical and sexual abuse in childhood: Relationship with post-traumatic stress disorder. *Journal of the American Academy of Child and Adolescent Psychiatry, 30*(5), 776–783.

Klorer, P. G. (2000). *Expressive therapy with troubled children.* Northvale, NJ: Jason Aronson.

Kramer, E. (1971). *Art as therapy with children.* New York: Schocken.

Levitt, E., & Pinnell, C. M. (1995). Some additional light on the childhood sexual abuse–psychopathology axis. *International Journal of Clinical and Experimental Hypnosis, 43*(2), 145–162.

Manning, T. M. (1987). Aggression depicted in abused children's drawings. *The Arts in Psychotherapy, 14,* 15–24.

McGlinchey, A., Keenan, M., & Dillenburger, K. (2000). Outline for the development of a screening procedure for children who have been sexually abused. *Research on Social Work Practice, 10*(6), 721–748.

Mordock, J. B. (1996). Treatment of sexually abused children: Interview technique, disclosure, and progress in therapy. *Journal of Child Sexual Abuse, 5*(4), 105–121.

Myers, J. E. (1996). Expert testimony. In J. Briere, L. Berliner, J. Bulkley, C. Jenny, & T. Reid (Eds.), *American professional society on the abuse of children handbook on child maltreatment* (pp. 319–340). Thousand Oaks, CA: Sage.

Palmer, L., Farrar, A., Valle, M., Ghahary, N., Panella, M., & DeGraw, D. (2000). An investigation of the clinical use of the House–Tree–Person projective drawings in the psychological evaluation of child sexual abuse. *Child Maltreatment, 5*(2), 169–175.

Peterson, L. W., Hardin, M., & Nitsch, M. J. (1995). The use of children's drawings in the evaluation and treatment of child sexual, emotional, and physical abuse. *Archives of Family Medicine, 4,* 445–452.

Putman, F. W. (1997). *Dissociation in children and adolescents: A developmental perspective.* New York: Guilford Press.

Sidun, N. M., & Rosenthal, R. H. (1987). Graphic indicators of sexual abuse in Draw-a Person tests of psychiatrically hospitalized adolescents. *The Arts in Psychotherapy, 14,* 25–33.

van der Kolk, B. (1987). *Psychological trauma.* Washington, DC: American Psychiatric Press.

van der Kolk, B. (1994). The body keeps the score: Memory and the evolving psychobiology of posttraumatic stress. *Harvard Review of Psychiatry, 1*(5), 253–265.

van der Kolk, B., & van der Hart, O. (1991). The intrusive past: The flexibility of memory and the engraving of trauma. *American Imago, 48*(4), 425–454.

Walker, L. E. A. (Ed.). (1988). *Handbook of sexual abuse of children: Assessment and treatment issues.* New York: Springer.

Yates, A., Beutler, L. E., & Crago, M. (1985). Drawings by child victims of incest. *Child Abuse and Neglect, 9*(2), 183–190.

CHAPTER 27

Using Art Therapy
with Medical Support Groups

Cathy A. Malchiodi

Art therapy has been used in medical settings with cancer patients in a variety of ways including psychotherapy (Barron, 1989; Dreifuss-Kattan, 1990; Hill, 1945; Hiltebrand, 1999; Long, Appleton, Abrams, Palmer, & Chapman, 1989; Luzzatto & Gabriel, 2000; Malchiodi, 1993; Rosner, 1982) and as a modality to enhance health and well-being (Lusebrink, 1990; Malchiodi, 1993, 1995, 1998, 1999). Art expression has also been explored in conjunction with guided visualization (Hiltebrand, 1999; Lusebrink, 1990) and as a method for stress reduction and relaxation (DeLue, 1999). Luzzatto and Gabriel (2000) conducted one of few studies of group art therapy within a medical setting, examining a series of specific directed activities with short-term, posttreatment cancer patients at a major teaching and research hospital. Camic (1999) notes that arts have the potential to contribute to the treatment tools of the health practitioner, along with medical intervention, pharmacology, and cognitive-behavioral therapy.

This chapter describes a medical art therapy group with women who have been diagnosed with breast cancer and provides a model for clinical work in a time-limited group format in an outpatient, wellness program. It presents an approach to treatment based on health psychology, the role of art expression in group work with people with cancer, and issues and concerns that can be addressed through experiential work. Examples of art therapy directives to stimulate and enhance self-expression and exploration among participants are offered within the context of a 10-week group format, demonstrating the importance of experiential work at various stages of group process.

THE ROLE OF MEDICAL ART THERAPY
FOR PEOPLE WITH CANCER

The use of the imagination as a form of healing is believed to be an ancient practice, and contemporary research has indicated that images play an important role in health and well-being (Achterburg, 1985). Health care professionals have included drawing as a way to provide a subjective measure of how an individual is dealing with cancer and to assist patients in participating in their own treatment (Simonton, Simonton, & Creighton, 1978). For example, the patient might be instructed to draw an image of cancer cells or tumors and then to either mentally visualize or draw an image of those cells being destroyed in some way. These directives have focused on interpreting images drawn by people with cancer for psychological and physical meaning as well as how to use these images to induce physiological change and stress and pain reduction.

Art expression is particularly helpful to individuals with cancer because people who are seriously ill often have two explanations for their condition, one verbal and one nonverbal (Malchiodi, 1998). The verbal explanation is often their medical description of the illness which involves a rational recounting of their condition based on medical knowledge. The other, the nonverbal one, is a more personal and often private perception of their illness. This personal explanation may or may not be conscious and may involve apprehension, confusion, misunderstanding, fear, or anxiety. It is also more likely to be revealed through a nonverbal modality such as art rather than directly communicated with words (Malchiodi, 1998).

Medical art therapy grew in part from the belief that art expression taps the unspoken and from the clinical work of art therapists with a variety of patient populations in medical settings. Medical art therapy has been defined as the clinical application of art expression and imagery with individuals who are physically ill, experiencing bodily trauma, or undergoing invasive or aggressive medical procedures such as surgery or chemotherapy (Long et al., 1989) and is considered a form of complementary or integrative medicine (Malchiodi, 1993, 1995, 1998, 1999). Although many practitioners view art therapy as a way to understand the psychosocial impact of illness on the individual, for those who participate in medical art therapy groups it has additional benefits: personal empowerment, stress reduction, social support, and the opportunity to reauthor one's life story.

Personal Empowerment

Art expression is a way to convey painful, confusing, and contradictory experiences of illness that are difficult to communicate with words alone. In addition, the very act of drawing, painting, or constructing can be a personally empowering experience in contrast to the loss of control that generally accompanies illness. For example, patients who are seriously ill often lose control of their time during their hospitalization because of the hospital's schedule and necessary medical treatments; they also may lose control of their bodies due to disease, medical intervention, surgery, or disability. In these circumstances art expression can help people regain some measure of control in their lives by providing an active process involving the freedom to choose materials, style, and subject matter; to play freely with color, lines, forms, and textures; and to create what one wants to create. This element of choice can contribute to feelings of autonomy and dignity when other aspects of life seem out of control.

Picirrillo (1999), in her work with people with HIV/AIDS, observes that a sense of mastery results from art making and a perception of one's ability to control events, at least to some extent. In this way, art making can provide an experience of normalcy and personal empowerment, even if only for the time one is engaged in creative activity. The benefits of achieving a sense of mastery can include increased self-esteem, enhanced self-confidence, and development of adaptive coping skills.

Stress Reduction

Benson (1975) pioneered medicine's understanding of the "relaxation response," a phenomenon that is now being embraced within psychosocial treatment of people with serious illness. In the late 1960s, Benson found that a physical state of deep rest that changes the physical and emotional responses to stress (e.g., decrease in heart rate, blood pressure, and muscle tension and increase in immune system functioning) and, if practiced regularly, can have lasting effects on mind and body.

Art making is believed to be a way to reduce stress and, for some people, to induce the "relaxation response." DeLue (1999) investigated the making of mandala drawings for their calming effects and as a technique for stress reduction. In work with individuals who have experienced trauma, it seems that drawing and other art activities stimulate the brain in a way that, in conjunction with verbal intervention, may be specifically helpful in resolution of stress reactions, intrusive memories, and other posttraumatic effects (Malchiodi, 2001). Because drawing is a sensory activity, one that involves tactile, visual, kinesthetic, and other senses, it is naturally self-soothing and involves repetitive activity that can induce relaxation and well-being similar to what Benson has reported in his studies (Malchiodi, 1997; 2002).

Social Support

The health psychology principle of social support is intrinsic to any group work with people with serious physical illness and is central to clinical application of medical art therapy to people with cancer. Group art therapy has the potential to enhance social support through both the sharing of art expressions with others and the natural interaction that is central to group participation. In contrast to individual art therapy, medical art therapy in a group format offers the additional benefits of interpersonal contact and an opportunity to share one's feelings with cohorts who have had similar experiences.

Reauthoring Life Stories

People who are confronting serious, life-threatening illnesses such as cancer often seek meaning for why they became ill. Art expression provides a medium for transforming feelings and perceptions into a new life story and, as a result, creating a new sense of self. This "re-authoring" of one's life story may be different for each person, and it often includes one or more of the following aspects: development of new out-looks; discovery of answers to the unanswered questions (e.g., Why did God do this to me?); revisions in the way one lives life; creation of solutions or a resolutions to personal struggles; creation of a new "postillness" identity; or discovery of an expla-nation for why one's life has been altered by illness, disability, or physical trauma.

Oliver Sacks (1990), the well-known British neurosurgeon, describes the impor-tant quality of "awakening" that the arts provide physically ill or disabled individu-als: "Awakening, basically, is a reversal . . . the patient ceases to feel the presence of illness and the absence of the world, and comes to feel the absence of his illness and the full presence of the world" (p. 53). I find that during art making people often shift away from the presence of illness in their lives, momentarily forgetting that they are sick or disabled. They essentially become "awakened" to experiences other than their illness and, through art expression and the guidance of the therapist, are able to develop and express new perspectives and reframe the story of the cancer in new ways.

GOALS OF GROUP WORK FOR PEOPLE WITH CANCER

People with cancer react to the impact of illness in a variety of ways. Some are deter-mined to fight their cancer and survive; others simply accept their condition and its outcome. Some are hopeful even while enduring invasive treatment or surgery; others surrender to the disease, quickly succumbing to both psychological and physical im-pact. Most have some or all of the following concerns as a result of their illness: un-derstanding the diagnosis, disease, and prognosis; understanding and coping with treatment such as surgery and medication, and their side effects; adapting to new life-style, postdiagnosis; facing loss of control, unknowns of the disease, and recurrence; coping with changing moods, energy levels, and functioning; and adjusting relation-ships to family, friends, and coworkers.

All these concerns are important in group work; however, for women with breast cancer, interest in making art as therapy is often motivated by additional factors:

- *Confronting mortality.* Cancer patients often respond to their illness with a profound search for wholeness, a desire to reexamine their life stories, and, as mentioned earlier, to reauthor them. Art may be offered as a way to summa-rize life experiences, to reclaim personal power, to create a lasting visual leg-acy, and to communicate through art, "I am" and "I exist."
- *Finding meaning.* Taking an existential approach to art therapy (as described in Chapter 3, this volume) can help cancer patients find new purpose and sus-pend the preillness image of the self, using art as a way to explore changes in lifestyle and relationships. Questions such as, "What is the meaning of illness to you?" and "How can you create meaning for your illness in the present time?" are important to this exploration. Art expression, by its very nature, can assist people in suspending current thinking by offering an alternative way to communicate feelings and the experiences of disability and distress.

- *Crisis resolution.* A diagnosis of cancer is a traumatic event for most people. Art expression is proving to be a powerful tool in crisis resolution (Malchiodi, 2001) and not only offers a respite from traumatic experiences and emotions but is useful in reducing symptoms of posttraumatic stress, such as fear, anger, and anxiety.
- *Authentic expression.* Communicating the complexities of life-threatening illness in words is difficult at best, and many cancer survivors prefer not to burden family and friends with their experiences. An overarching goal of art therapy with this population is to facilitate authentic expression, using illness as an opportunity for communication and self-awareness, and thus help people to come to terms with the circumstances of their lives and to live life more fully and deeply.

BREAST CANCER/MEDICAL ART THERAPY GROUP

Art therapy groups for people with cancer may have various orientations; some are intended as psychotherapy, some have psychoeducational goals, and others are offered as recreational groups. The group process described in this chapter is based on a wellness model (Myers, Sweeney, & Witmer, 2000), emphasizing a shift from a focus on disease to the individual's ability to experience health and well-being, even though medically ill. This model emphasizes the importance of social support, personal control and self-efficacy, self-actualization and creativity, emotional expression and awareness, and health psychology paradigms.

The title "Creativity and Wellness Group," is used to describe the group rather than a name including the words "therapy" or "treatment." The group is intended as a place to enhance healthy functioning and deemphasizes the "sick role" that therapy or treatment often implies. Rather than viewing the group as something "done to" a client, it is offered as a program in which the participants maintain an active role in taking responsibility for their well-being. The philosophy of the facilitator is holistic in that art expression taps the body's, mind's, and spirit's natural tendency toward health and well-being (Malchiodi, 1995, 1998, 1999).

Any woman of any age who has experienced breast cancer is eligible for the group. However, most woman who attend the group are generally in the active stages of treatment for an initial breast cancer; a few women have experienced recurrence of their cancer and metastasis (spread of the initial cancer to other parts of the body such as the bones or other organs). The group generally starts with 12 participants and, through attrition during the first 2 weeks, reduces to 7 or 8 women who complete all the sessions. The group typically runs for 10 weekly sessions, $1\frac{1}{2}$ hours in length.

Because each group is tailored to the needs of the individuals who attend, it is not possible to provide an exact template for a specific series of weekly activities. However, there are particular topics that most participants find helpful to explore through art and activities that facilitate exploration of issues related to the specific needs of cancer patients. Like most groups, goals for each session are based on the logical progression of the participants' experience from the initial or introductory session through the middle or intermediate sessions to closure or termination of the group.

Initial Session

While some therapists may elect to start a therapy group by asking participants to tell the story of their illness, I prefer to begin with more wellness-oriented approach and facilitate an exploration of their personal experiences with creativity. Many adults I see in groups and individually have not experienced art making since their childhood and invariably feel that they are not creative or "not an artist." To begin to create a sense of safety within the group and within each individual it is important to help the women identify their own capacity for creativity and art making.

Invariably, by asking questions such as "Did you have a favorite art or craft activity when you were young?" and "What kind of beliefs did your family have about art?," participants recognize that each has creative potential. Some have designed and constructed intricate quilts; others may use their creativity to design a special table setting for a family event or make an artistic memory book of photos commemorating a child's graduation or a reunion. I also ask group members about their earliest memories of art activity (such as a childhood memory) to help them identify any moments of successful as well as feelings of failure in art. These questions facilitate an exploration of personal creativity and bring to the surface any fears or anxieties participants have about making art within group setting.

In the first session I also introduce the idea of relaxation through simple guided imagery. As described in other chapters of this book, guided imagery is used in conjunction with art therapy to facilitate self-expression, to gain insight, and to reduce stress. Therapists have also used guided imagery to increase reflective distance, encourage relaxation, stimulate creativity, and enhance concentration (Camic, 1999). With this particular group I present a short exercise that involved relaxed breathing while mentally scanning the body (sequentially from feet to head) for any feelings or sensations that arise. If time permits and the group is willing, I ask each to make a simple image with colors, lines, and shapes on white paper describing any feelings or sensations recalled from the relaxation experience and the body scan (this activity is also discussed in the next section).

In the next two sessions participants may still feel a little anxious about making art, so it is helpful to proceed slowly and sensitively to the group's needs for safety. To facilitate a level of comfort I choose experiential work that helps group members to become acquainted with the materials they will be using and to offer activities that are simple and direct and ensure a measure of immediate success. I often suggest that participants start the second session by making simple scribbles, either with oil pastels or a piece of string dipped in black ink and dragged across paper. The scribble technique has been described throughout this book and is based on Winnicott's (1971) Squiggle and Cane's (1951) technique. After completing a series of scribble drawings, the women are asked to look at their scribbles, choose one, and then find images, either real, imaginary, or abstract, to color in with oil pastels. This experiential usually encourages a sense of playfulness and produces results that encourages a personal sense of creative skill.

When all members have completed their images, the therapist may offer the option to speak to the group about their pictures. Figure 27.1 is an example of this activity by one of the group members and is an image called "Trees of Life." The woman, 45 years old and recently completing a course of chemotherapy and radiation for a breast tumor, explained to the group that now that her treatment was ending she felt like "a young tree budding in the spring." She considered this particular image reflective of her renewed feelings of energy as she began to resume her work as a schoolteacher and begin some projects that she had to delay because of her illness.

Intermediate Sessions

Although there are many directions this type of group may take, there are some specific topics that tend to recur in medical art therapy groups with women who have had cancer: body image as a result of illness and/or treatment, coping with the experience of life-threatening illness, and questions about the meaning of life brought up by the experience of cancer.

Body Image

Because treatment for most women with breast cancer involves some sort of surgery, whether a less invasive lumpectomy or a complete mastectomy (breast removal), body image is a major concern for many patients. A simple body image, predrawn on 8½" × 11" paper is offered to participants and can be used in conjunction with the

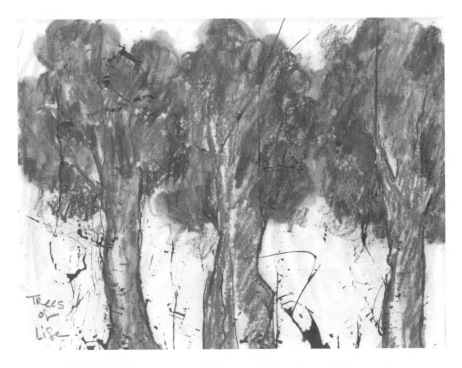

FIGURE 27.1. "Trees of Life" created from a scribble drawing.

guided imagery process mentioned earlier in this chapter. After completing a visual body scan and relaxation, group members are asked to recall any sensations or observations about their bodies and to record these using colors, shapes, or images on the body outline.

With some groups whose members want to explore body image in a deeper way I offer participants the opportunity to create a life-size image of themselves. This activity requires at least 1 hour and may not be suitable for group members who are debilitated from the effects of illness or treatment regimes. Group members are each provided with a large piece of white craft paper, approximately 3′ × 5′, and are asked to create a life-size image of themselves on the paper using drawing and collage materials. Some participants choose to have another group member trace around their body, providing an actual outline to fill in with images (see Figure 27.2).

Coping with Illness

A recurring concern of most women attending the group is how to cope with the ongoing physical, psychological, and interpersonal effects of illness. Although art therapy is certainly not a panacea for any disease, the creative process of art making can have beneficial impact on perceptions and responses to cancer and its impact on mind, body, interpersonal relationships, and spirit.

One activity that the participants find particularly helpful is creating imagery within a simple circular form, or mandala. While drawing a mandala has been used as a form of art-based assessment to evaluate psychological status (see Appendix I, this volume), as previously noted, mandala drawing is also a useful activity to reduce stress. I generally initiate this activity with a brief definition of the mandala and then present each participant with a set of oil pastels and two predrawn circles, one on white paper and one on black paper. Kellogg (1993) believed that it was important to introduce the opportunity to draw a mandala on both white and black of paper because each background encourages a different use of color and form. Participants are asked to first create a mandala image of their choice on white paper, followed by a second one on black paper. Although there is a predrawn image of a circle on each paper, they are encouraged to "go outside the lines" if they desire. To facilitate the experience of relaxation it is helpful to play some quiet music during the activity.

Participants are also encouraged to keep a visual journal—a simple drawing or sketch book in which they visually record thoughts and feelings about their experiences. The purpose of engaging in this activity is threefold: (1) it encourages participants to continue art therapy outside the sessions; (2) it can be used a form of relaxation during times of stress; and (3) it serves as a record of experiences that can be brought back to group for discussion. Overall, the visual journal is a way to cope with illness between group meetings and provides an additional tool for illness management during times of distress.

Meaning of Life

For many of the women in the group the question of why they became ill becomes important, as well as additional questions such as "What am I going to do with

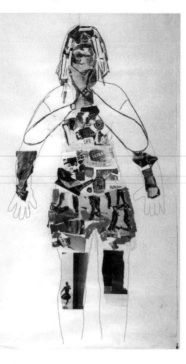

FIGURE 27.2.   Life-size body collage created by support group participant.

the rest of my life? What would I like to change about my life? What are the personal beliefs that guide my life?" To facilitate an exploration of these questions participants are asked to create a "personal shield." To begin the process the women select from various shields precut from cardboard or use paper or cardboard to make a shape representing a shield. Drawing and collage materials (scrap paper, yarn, magazine images) are provided to create images for the shield. I ask participants to draw or cut out images to glue to their shields in response to any or all of the following questions:

1. What is your greatest source of strength?
2. What are your greatest sources of comfort?
3. In one sentence or image, how would you describe the purpose of your life?
4. What goal is most important to you right now?
5. What belief guides your life?

These can be difficult questions to answer because each evokes powerful emotions and unfinished business. These topics stimulate self-examination and self-awareness and initiate group discussion of deeper issues through both images and verbal exchange. Some members interpret questions as related to spirituality, although a belief in religion or a higher power is not necessary to explore these particular issues. However, the experiential provides those participants who need to explore spiritual dimensions the opportunity to express their concerns and identify ways they draw strength from religion or personal beliefs.

Closure

Because this group is time-limited rather than ongoing, there is a final session and termination is a normal and expected part of the process. In the final session it is important to address the needs of the group in order to have a sense of closure and to express good-byes to other participants. For this reason the therapist must consider how to facilitate the group's experience of termination through a structured process.

One of the more popular processes I use during the final session is what I have come to call an "intention box." This is simply a large cardboard box which I prepare before the session by painting it (the colors are up to the therapist, although I like to paint it blue on the outside and yellow or gold on the inside) so it is ready to be decorated by the group during their meeting. In recent years I also take the box to a group of Tibetan Buddhists who live near the facility where the group meets and ask them give their blessing to the box and the women in the group. The women appreciate this gesture because it gives the box as special meaning and adds the important quality of ritual to our work as a group.

At the group's final meeting I ask each group member to create two small symbols from paper and art materials: (1) an image representing what that person feels about her experiences in the group and (2) an image of an intention that she wishes to make for herself. When complete, each person comes up and glues the image about feelings about the group to the outside of the box, so that eventually the box is covered with symbols. After this is completed, each group member comes forward, one by one, and places her image of a personal intention in the box and makes a statement to the group either about her intention or about the group in general. This is often a powerful experience for the participants, helping each person to summarize her thoughts and feelings about the group and establish goals for the future now that the group is ending.

CONCLUSION

Medical art therapy groups provide a means of expression not found in other forms of psychosocial treatment and offer the opportunity to explore concerns intrinsic to the experience of cancer in a creative, personal way. For women with breast cancer, art expression within a group therapy context not only addresses the common concerns of this patient population but also encourages communication of the "unspoken aspects" of illness, enhancement of stress reduction, and facilitation of a search for meaning. It is a powerful partner with verbal therapy and group treatment that helps those threatened by disease or disability relate their experiences in an atmosphere of social support, personal empowerment, and authentic expression.

REFERENCES

Achterburg, J. (1985). *Imagery in healing.* Boston: New Sciences Library.
Barron, P. (1989). Fighting cancer with images. In H. Wadeson (Ed.), *Advances in art therapy* (pp. 148–168). New York: Wiley.

Camic, P. (1999). Expanding treatment possibilities for chronic pain through the expressive arts. In C. Malchiodi (Ed.), *Medical art therapy with adults* (pp. 43–62). London: Jessica Kingsley.

Cane, F. (1951). *The artist in each of us.* Craftsbury Common, VT: Art Therapy.

DeLue, C. (1999). Physiological effects of creating mandalas. In C. Malchiodi (Ed.), *Medical art therapy with children* (pp. 33–49). London: Jessica Kingsley.

Dreifuss-Kattan, E. (1990). *Cancer stories: Creativity and self-repair.* Hillsdale, NY: Analytic Press.

Hill, A. (1945). *Art versus illness.* London: Allen & Unwin.

Hiltebrand, E. (1999). Coping with cancer through image manipulation. In C. Malchiodi (Ed.), *Medical art therapy with adults* (pp. 113–136). London: Jessica Kingsley.

Kellogg, J. (1993). *Mandala: Path of beauty.* Bellair, FL: Association for Teachers of Mandala Assessment.

Long, J., Appleton, V., Abrams, E., Palmer, S., & Chapman, L. (1989). Innovations in medical art therapy: Defining the field. *Proceedings of the American Art Therapy Association 20th Annual Conference* (p. 84). Mundelein, IL: American Art Therapy Association.

Lusebrink, V. (1990). *Imagery and visual expression in therapy.* New York: Plenum Press.

Luzzatto, P., & Gabriel, B. (2000). The creative journey: A model for short-term group art therapy with posttreatment cancer patients. *Art Therapy: Journal of the American Art Therapy Association, 17*(3), 265–269.

Malchiodi, C. A. (1993). Medical art therapy: Contributions to the field of arts medicine. *International Journal of Arts Medicine, 2*(2), 28–31.

Malchiodi, C. A (1995). *Art making as complementary medicine.* Unpublished syllabus, 26th annual conference of the American Art Therapy Association, San Diego, CA.

Malchiodi, C. A. (1997). Invasive art: Art as empowerment for women with breast cancer. In S. Hogan (Ed.), *Feminist approaches to art therapy* (pp. 49–64). London: Routledge.

Malchiodi, C. A. (1998). *The art therapy sourcebook.* Los Angeles: Lowell House.

Malchiodi, C. A. (Ed.). (1999). *Medical art therapy with adults.* London: Jessica Kingsley.

Malchiodi, C. A. (2001). Using drawing as intervention with children who have experienced trauma or loss. *Trauma and Loss: Research and Interventions, 1*(1), 21–28.

Malchiodi, C. A. (2002). Using drawing in short-term assessment and intervention of child maltreatment and trauma. In A. Giardino (Ed.), *Child maltreatment* (3rd ed., pp. 125–146). St. Louis, MO: G.W. Medical.

Myers, J., Sweeney, T., & Witmer, J. (2000). The wheel of counseling for wellness: A holistic model for treatment planning. *Journal of Counseling and Development, 78*(3), 251–265.

Picirrillo, E. (1999). Hide and seek: The art of living with HIV/AIDS. In C. Malchiodi (Ed.), *Medical art therapy with children* (pp. 113–131). London: Jessica Kingsley.

Rosner, I. (1982, October). *Art therapy in a medical setting.* Unpublished presentation at the 12th annual conference of the American Art Therapy Association, Philadelphia, PA.

Sacks, O. (1990) *Awakenings.* New York: HarperPerennial.

Simonton, O. C., Simonton, S., & Creighton, J. (1978). *Getting well again.* Los Angeles: Tarcher.

Winnicott, D. (1971). *Playing and reality.* New York: Basic Books.

CHAPTER 28

Family Art Therapy

Shirley Riley
Cathy A. Malchiodi

Art therapy with families emerged during the past several decades as the natural consequence of the development of family therapy theories. The integration of theory, has been a central concern to practitioners using art expression with families (Riley & Malchiodi, 1994) and many theories have been used as a framework for family art therapy, including psychodynamic, systems theory, humanistic, strategic, structural, solution-focused, and narrative approaches. Major influences on the growth of family art therapy from the field of art therapy include family art evaluation and art-based assessment of family systems (Bing, 1970; Kwiatkowska, 1967a, 1978; Landgarten, 1987; Levick & Herring, 1973; Mosher & Kwiatkowska, 1971; Rubin, 1978; Rubin & Magnussen, 1974; Zierer, Sternberg, Finn, & Farmer, 1975); art as an intervention with families (Kwiatkowska, 1962, 1967b, 1975, 1978; Landgarten, 1987; Mueller, 1968; Sobol, 1982) and child/parent dyads (Landgarten, 1975; Malchiodi, 1998; Rubin, 1978); couples art therapy (Riley, 1991; Wadeson, 1973, 1976, 1980); and integrative approaches to family art therapy (Riley & Malchiodi, 1994). Each has drawn on the major theories of family therapy, using these theories as the basis for art expression to effect change, identify system dynamics, and understand the communication patterns of family members.

The overall benefits of art therapy, such as nonverbal communication, visual problem solving, and active participation in treatment, have been discussed throughout this text. These advantages are also evident in family art therapy; however, there are several unique advantages to using art therapy in family work, including the following:

- Family art therapy allows every generation to have an equal voice through art expression; even the youngest child who may often be resistant to verbal therapy can participate actively in treatment. The experience of using art as the means of expression places all family members on even ground within the therapeutic context.

- Infusion of the art process in family therapy allows participants to simultaneously express their thoughts and feelings through individual and group art activities. Individual and family beliefs can be communicated within a single art expression.
- For the client in individual therapy, visual expression can be an important vehicle for communicating family issues to the therapist. A simple drawing or collage can be the means by which the client "brings the family in" and it offers an opportunity to discuss roles within the family and issues in the client's family of origin (Riley, 1985).
- Family art therapy enhances communication among family members and uncovers, through the process as well as the content of the art task, family patterns of interaction and behavior.
- Through art therapy the family is offered a means to communicate with each in a new way. Habitual patterns of response may be reflected in the therapeutic process, but the family has the opportunity to use its creative potential to solve problems, open themselves to a broader perspective, and to support changes in behavior.

This chapter provides a brief overview of family art therapy and its clinical application. Because family art therapy is predicated on a variety of family therapy theories, for the purpose of this chapter a strategic approach is illustrated through case examples and the following concepts: the use of metaphors, recursive patterns and second-order change, reframing, the use of ritual, unbalancing, and therapeutic double bind. The techniques described provide therapists with a basic foundation in how art expression is integrated within the context of family treatment.

THE USE OF METAPHORS

Haley (1963, 1973) believed that metaphors are analogies through which the therapist and client can communicate in a powerful, direct, but nonthreatening way. They can be visual, verbal, or both. Metaphors can be helpful in giving directives because when an intervention is presented in the form of a metaphor, the client may not even realize that one has been made (Haley, 1976). By using the client's metaphor, the therapist shapes an intervention that is unique and fits the situation presented by the client.

A young woman named Ann, age 26, entered art therapy with concerns about her 4-year-old marriage and unacknowledged anger toward her widowed mother. She and her husband Neil had recently moved out of her mother's apartment and into their own home, some 30 miles away. Ann's hobby was gardening, and she especially enjoyed spending her weekends working on the grounds of her new home.

Conflict had recently appeared in the couple's relationship and Ann was growing anxious over Neil's increasing demands on her time and attention. Ann's mother had also become more demanding, insisting that the couple visit her on the weekends, which interfered with Ann's gardening.

Early in treatment, Ann began to make sketches of her lawn and garden. Her yard was an elaborately developed image she explored in drawing after drawing and became the basis for metaphor and a discussion of her emotional state. Her lawn had recently become "brown and dry" and the flowers on its perimeter were "dying off." During one session, Ann told the therapist that the lawn was being taken over by crabgrass (Figure 28.1). At first she mused, "Wouldn't it be wonderful if one could just say 'to heck with it' and grow an untraditional weedy lawn?" She carefully considered this solution but finally rejected it and started to plan how to eradicate the crabgrass from her yard.

The therapist expanded Ann's metaphor beyond the boundaries of her drawings and designed an intervention to fit. She instructed Ann to go to the library with Neil to research the best method of eliminating the crabgrass. After they had done the reading, Ann reported that they had decided not to pull up the crabgrass after all because its roots would remain, only to grow and spread. Their choices were limited: They could till the soil and destroy the healthy grass, or apply chemicals that would kill the crabgrass, roots and all, but not the rest of the lawn. They decided to do the latter.

Their library research and yard work left Ann and Neil little time for anything else. The therapist coached Ann in explaining to her mother that she and her husband would have to limit their visits to Sunday-morning breakfasts because the lawn project had to be finished before the winter rains began. In addition to helping with the research, Neil hired a man to do the heavy yard work. Ann enjoyed having her

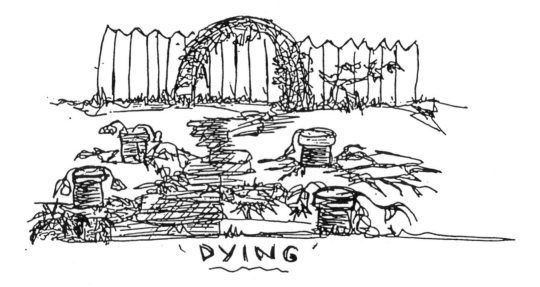

FIGURE 28.1. Crabgrass.

husband's support, and together she and Neil were able to curtail her mother's demands.

Neil was pleased because Ann no longer withdrew from him. In fact, she genuinely welcomed his involvement with her project. Now that Ann's mother held less sway over their daily lives, he could draw closer to his wife and express more support for her interests. Ann reciprocated by showing renewed affection.

Ann experienced a change in her relationships with her husband and her mother. In therapy, through the visual metaphor of a lawn full of crabgrass, she managed the difficult separation from her mother and reestablished intimacy with her husband. It would have been arduous indeed to teach her insight into her "unresolved separation from her family of origin," clarifying the problem of generational boundaries and helping her understand her "displacement of anxiety." It is doubtful that insight alone would have achieved the desired change in behavior.

RECURSIVE PATTERNS AND SECOND-ORDER CHANGE

Symptoms and the client's previous attempts to ameliorate them are important pieces of the diagnostic puzzle for the therapist. The presenting problem should not be seen as a pathological weakness within the client but, rather, as recursive patterns that serves some function in maintaining the interactional sequence (Bross & Benjamin, 1982). This dynamic was clearly evident in the case of Elaine, a 42-year-old woman who was distressed because she constantly took on the responsibilities of friends and family. As a result, she felt abused and angry because the burdens imposed upon her were beyond her strength. She was aware that she resented the commitment she had made, but she nonetheless continued to assist others with their unresolvable difficulties.

The therapist asked her to draw an image of how she appeared to herself as she continued to accept these unmanageable loads. Therapist and client were both surprised by what emerged: the figure of a heavy woman festooned with smaller persons clinging to her whole body (Figure 28.2). This figure bore no physical resemblance to Elaine, and after contemplating the figure for some time, Elaine told the therapist, with much emotion, that it represented her grandmother. This grandmother had raised her from infancy, when her mother died, until she was about 12 years old.

The grandmother's credo was "sacrifice yourself for others and never say no to a request." Elaine was tearful and then angry as she remembered how her grandmother had taught her to always accommodate others. She then recalled being molested by her grandfather, a memory that had been repressed until the drawing called it forth. Suddenly, she understood why "doing for others" held such a distressing and malevolent meaning for her. As the session was concluding, Elaine decided to bury her grandmother once and for all and drew her lying in a horizontal position (see bottom of illustration). She declared that in so doing, she was "burying" the behavior that had kept her grandmother's beliefs alive. This intense, symbolic action was accomplished with great tension and an aura of finality.

In Elaine's revelation and decision to bury her grandmother, we see an example

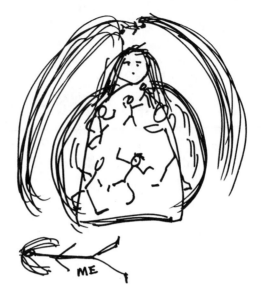

FIGURE 28.2. Figure of heavy woman.

of what Watzlawick, Weakland, and Fisch (1974) call "second-order change," the leap to an entirely new context in which to view a problem or relationship. This can be a mechanism for instigating systems change. Within a relatively stable system governed by a self-regulating feedback mechanism, minor fluctuations ordinarily occur and are accommodated within the previously set limits of the system (Hoffman, 1981; Watzlawick et al., 1974): Slight alterations are made in the system without changing the system itself. Elaine's recovered incest memory dramatically altered her view of her grandmother's prescriptions and made her see self-sacrifice and accommodation in a new light. The fundamental shift in Elaine's attitude toward the family values instilled in her at an early age propelled her into a new context and range of behaviors.

REFRAMING

Second-order change is sometimes initiated by a change in the client's world view, which can be achieved through the tactic of *reframing*. "To reframe . . . means to change the conceptual and/or emotional setting or viewpoint in relation to which a situation is experienced and to place it in another frame which fits the 'facts' of the same concrete situation equally well or even better, and thereby changes its entire meaning" (Watzlawick et al., 1974, p. 95).

In reframing behavior, therapists frequently acknowledge that the behavior of an individual, even when it is dysfunctional, is an attempt to preserve the status quo of a system to which the individual belongs. For example, in exploring the family myths and roles that shaped their behavior, a client will sometimes recognize that he was the child "designated" by the family to engage in destructive behavior in order to save the family system. This "bad" child's actions might have distracted the parents from other issues, such as substance abuse or an unsatisfactory marriage, and forced them to join together in dealing with the child, thus strengthening their parental relationship. The child's "bad" acts can be reframed as "self-sacrifice for the good of others," which redefines the client's position in the family and may alter the client's perception of the situation.

If the client still clings to a role as "the family problem," the therapist can encourage him or her to experiment with separation in a graphic way. After having the client make a family drawing, the therapist presents the client with a pair of scissors and tells him or her "Cut yourself out" of the family. Once the client has made a "hole," he or she can speculate on how the remaining family members will relate to each other once the client is out of the picture. The client can also think about what he or she can now do as the cut-out member, liberated from the family frame. This simple metaphorical intervention can assist a client in addressing the neglected developmental task of individuation.

Giving an event or behavior a meaning that suggests value or worthiness is a form of reframing called *positive connotation* (Papp, 1983) and can drastically alter a client's perception of what he or she is doing. For example, clients frequently see themselves as sick, damaged, or dysfunctional and incapable of solving their problems. The therapist, however, usually sees the client's request as a healthy move, an indication that the client has forsaken the helpless stance and can give it this positive connotation. When the client expresses a willingness to try art therapy, an unfamiliar treatment modality, there is an additional opportunity to endow client action with connotations of strength, courage, and determination to solve one's problems. (One caveat about positive connotation: It is not appropriate to use with clients who present issues of violence to self or others or who have a history of impulsive behavior.)

An effective use of positive connotation occurred in the case of a 40-year-old businesswoman who aspired to be a novelist. Her second husband did not use his talents and had been only partially employed during the 5 years of their marriage. There was affection between them and they did not want to divorce, but the wife had become progressively depressed as her children grew up and moved out. Her executive job seemed "cold" and "not creative enough." She complained that she "worked like a horse" because if she did not, her family would starve, and there was never time to write.

In the second session, the therapist redefined the wife's depression as "an omen for change" and told her that unconscious desire to be creative and publish a novel was demanding that she take a sabbatical. Because this wish had been denied for so long, depression had set in. Moreover, by continuing to sacrifice her career as a writer, the wife was keeping her husband from assuming his proper role in the family. In fact, by neglecting her talents, she was giving off the misleading impression that she was too businesslike and assertive. The therapist congratulated the wife because, in spite of all these conflicting circumstances, she continued to deprive herself and carried on as the primary financial provider.

These interventions paved the way for another strategic technique, restraining

(Madanes, 1981; Papp, 1980). After "diagnosing" depression, the therapist cautioned the wife that due to the complexities of family and work issues, any attempt at change would be premature. A rapid move to alter herself or the marital relationship could lead to unknown problems.

In the third session, the wife appeared less depressed and made a drawing of "last week's feelings and this week's feelings." Whereas "last week's feelings" were compressed and drawn mainly in black, "this week's" were expansive looking and contained bright reds and oranges. The client was puzzled because even though her routine at home and work had not changed, her perception of it had inexplicably altered. She had decided to continue working until her husband got a job. However, she would go "on sabbatical" for a few hours every evening by withdrawing to her study to work on her novel. She was glad that the depression had given her a helpful message.

When this client recognized that by overachieving she dominated her husband, she decided to work at making the marriage a more equal partnership. As that change occurred, the husband surprised her by taking on part of the financial burden. The client continued to work and write, and decided to remain in art therapy so that she could explore other issues.

RESTRAINING THROUGH A RITUAL

The paradoxical technique of restraining is often used to counter the common belief that either change must be complete and all-encompassing or else everything must stay exactly the same. After defining the symptom as benign and essential for family survival and advising a client to follow the interactional sequence which leads to the presentation of the symptom, the therapist cautions the client *not* to change.

Prescribing the symptom was the approach taken in the case of Steve, a 20-year-old who sought treatment for compulsive handwashing. Steve washed his hands countless times during the day and even woke several times each night with an irresistible compulsion to wash them again. When he entered therapy, Steve was still living at home with his parents and blamed his compulsion for his inability to look for work. His parents continued to let him live with them and had only recently asked that he help out with the household expenses.

The therapist hypothesized that the parents were covertly supporting the youth's handwashing compulsion because it diverted attention from their alcoholism: The symptom served both the parents' and child's need to postpone Steve's developmental task of leaving home. In art therapy, Steve drew many pictures in which he recalled ways he had previously expressed anger, such as shattering the bathroom mirror with his fist. He continued to complain about his handwashing, which now was causing his skin to crack and bleed, but the reason for the compulsion remained a mystery.

To interrupt this sequence of compulsive behavior, the therapist designed a *ritual* (Haley, 1976). The young man was told that his handwashing was symbolic of his need to "wash his hands of his family"; that is, to separate from them as a young adult. Therefore, the symptom could be addressed only with his family's help. The therapist told Steve that every time he experienced a compulsion to wash his hands, he should ask the family to join him. All family members were to accompany him to the bathroom and wash their hands, too. By experiencing the handwashing themselves, Steve was told, family members would be inspired to find a cure for the problem. This ritual required that Steve wake everyone in the family several times during the night.

A week later, Steve reported that his family had initially been helpful and cooperative, joining him in the bathroom throughout one full day and night. Then they grew extremely annoyed at being awakened from their sleep. In anger, the parents refused to continue to cooperate in the task and thereby made the first move to detriangulate their son. Steve slept through the next night "by accident," and other family members did not have to get up with him. For the rest of the week, he managed to sleep all night without waking to wash his hands.

In a subsequent session, the therapist suggested that Steve trace and cut out an outline of his hands. Steve then pinned the hands on the wall of the therapy room, where he asked to leave them for a week. He was job hunting, he explained, and constant handwashing would be inconvenient and embarrassing. He wanted the therapist to be in charge of his hands while he was looking for work.

Shortly after this intervention, Steve found a job. Within several months, his handwashing was at a near normal level, and he had moved from his parents' home into an apartment with a friend. Treatment stopped because the symptom was now resolved.

UNBALANCING

A paradoxical intervention was also made in the treatment of Mary, a young woman who was seen individually for short-term therapy. Mary was unhappy with her husband, who had become progressively more controlling. The couple had been married 3 years and enjoyed a loving relationship, but their roles were rigidly complementary with a potential for oppression. Eduardo, the husband, came from a Hispanic family in which males were supposed to be dominant. Mary had adopted the role of a submissive and protected woman.

Mary and Eduardo had one child, a toddler. The couple agreed that Mary was inadequate as a mother to this little girl, but Mary was eager to improve. The child had stimulated her desire to be competent and respected in her new role as mother. The goals of therapy were to help Mary individuate from her family of origin, in which she served the role of submissive and dutiful child, to help her to become a "mother" rather than a "daughter," and to redistribute the power in the marriage so that it would be shared more equally.

Early in the therapy, the focus was on Mary's anger at her husband. To illustrate how he provoked her, she related an incident that had occurred when she was chopping onions. Eduardo grabbed her paring knife, insisting that she use a French chopping knife instead because it was "safe" and "the correct tool for chopping onions." This had infuriated Mary because the paring knife was one of her favorite utensils;

moreover, Eduardo had intruded on her territory, her preparation of the family meal. After describing this scene, Mary drew a picture of a stick figure who was berating her (Figure 28.3). She identified the scolding figure as either her husband or her mother, who "act and say the same." In discussing her husband's overprotectiveness, Mary made a connection between her current problem and the distress and resentment she felt as a child, cared for but smothered by an overinvolved mother.

To redefine the interactional sequence between husband and wife, the therapist gave the following directive:

> "Each time your husband comes into the kitchen and asks you to change the way you prepare dinner, stop what you are doing and go over and give him a kiss or a hug. You may then return to preparing the meal in the same way you were doing. Do not change."

Mary responded with a startled and confused look, but smiled as she left the room.

The therapist structured this intervention so that it would address the motives behind the husband's controlling behavior while interrupting the couple's interactional pattern. Because Eduardo was behaving in a caring and protective manner toward Mary, the kiss rewarded him for his positive intentions. But when Mary replied to Eduardo's interference with an unexpected display of sexual affection, his characteristic exercise of paternal control became unbalanced. Mary felt supported by the therapist's directive, which kept her in charge of her own method of cooking. But it

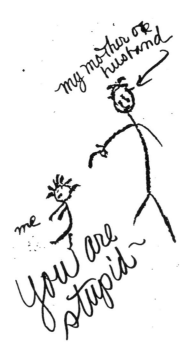

FIGURE 28.3. Stick figure.

also served to interrupt a redundant and toxic pattern of repetitive behavior while giving each spouse a positive reward.

THERAPEUTIC DOUBLE BIND

The use of a paradoxical intervention is based on the concept of the *double bind* (Weeks & L'Abate, 1982), a means of understanding communication and behavior in families with a schizophrenic member (Bateson, 1972). The double bind describes a relationship in which there are two or more members, a repeated interactional sequence, a primary negative injunction enforced through punishments or other threats to survival, and a secondary injunction in conflict with the first. Another essential condition is that the subject of the double bind be prohibited from leaving the arena of the relationship. In a family in which this sequence produces dysfunctional behavior, the double bind is said to be pathogenic. But sometimes, a bind can be created to work therapeutically, as when a paradox is introduced that forces the client and/or family system to make the leap to a new level of functioning. Even though the subject of a therapeutic double bind receives confusing messages, he or she is in a win-win situation and is rewarded regardless of the choice made.

In the following case, a paradoxical intervention was built around imagery that appeared in client artwork. A couple entered therapy with complaints about each other's parenting, and argument about who contributed more to the household, and mutual accusations of poor communication skills. The symptoms seemed vague and out of focus until the couple revealed that they had physically abused the husband's son by a previous marriage during a visit 6 months before entering therapy. The wife had committed the actual abuse, but the husband had stood by watching and did not intervene. In therapy, the wife uncovered memories of abuse in her family of origin, and this helped her understand her own abusive behavior. But the husband continued to puzzle over why he had passively held back from protecting his son.

In an individual session, the therapist asked the husband to draw a picture of his relationship with his mother (Figure 28.4). He portrayed himself on his knees, bowing and protesting ineffectually as his mother loomed over him, pointing an accusing finger and saying, "You're weak, selfish, stupid, but I need you even though you wrecked my life, you bastard!" It was clear that even as an adult, he continued to believe that his mother was correct and that there was some basic flaw in his nature for which he "deserved" abuse. In early childhood, he had continually experienced devaluation and rejection and had a poor self-concept and low self-esteem, and his mother's belittling words still rang in his ears. Now, however, he could evaluate his mother's parenting abilities more realistically, and in so doing felt much anger but also intense guilt.

In a subsequent session, the husband was asked to "draw his guilt." He explained the picture (Figure 28.5): "The guilt flows from my mother's pot, fills up the container, drips off the spigot. I catch the runoff and pour it back on myself." When asked what purpose this served, he replied. "If I take off the container, the volcano in my head will explode." Even after this dramatic disclosure of how he perpetuated his

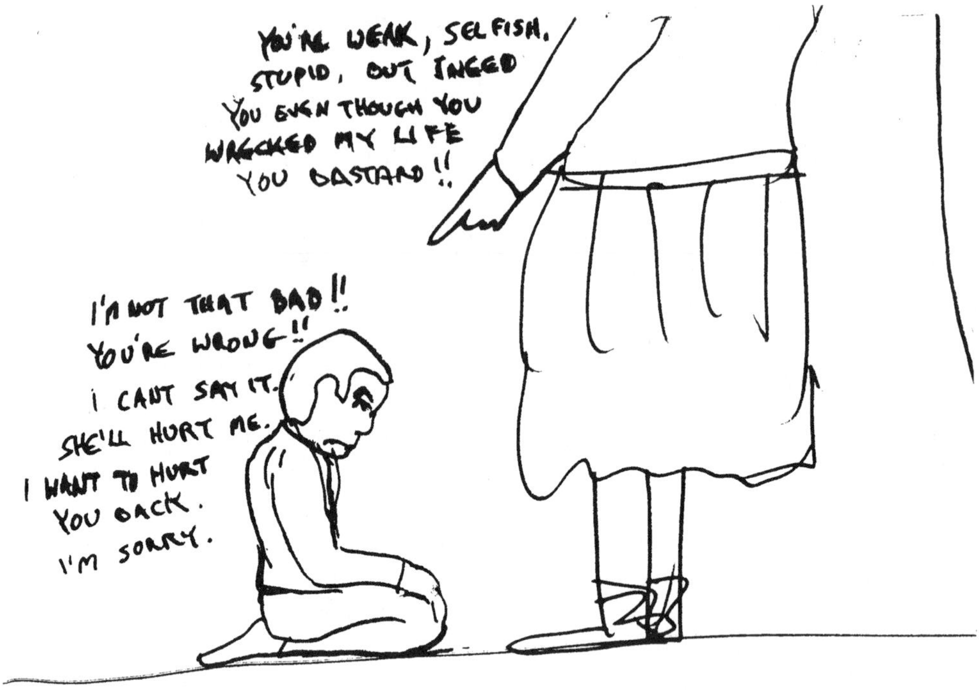

FIGURE 28.4. Relationship with mother.

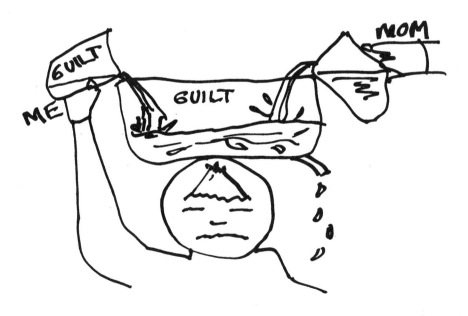

FIGURE 28.5. Guilt.

feelings of guilt, the husband continued to believe he had to behave in this "guilty manner" and was unwilling to attempt any change.

The therapist decided to make a strategic intervention in the form of a homework assignment. At the end of the session, she congratulated the husband for being astute enough to understand how important it was to keep the container of guilt balanced on his head. In order that he might fully experience his guilt and evaluate its role in his life, the therapist instructed him to go family members, friends, and acquaintances individually and ask them how he had failed them and what he could do to make reparations for his sins. The client was told to pay close attention to the heightened feelings of guilt this exercise would evoke. Reluctantly, the client agreed to perform the assigned task.

At the next session, the client brusquely informed the therapist that the homework was a "foolish plan." He had tried it several times but trying to please everyone was "nonsense." He was now convinced that he could "give and take equally in this world" and refused to complete the assignment. The therapist apologized for mishandling the homework and wondered aloud how it could have failed so miserably. The client counseled the therapist not to feel guilty because "guilt is a waste of time."

This tactic was successful in redefining the "guilt" symptom and provoking a recoil by the client, who discarded a feeling state based on years of conditioning. An alteration in perception enabled him to modify his world view and quickly achieved second-order change without requiring insight.

CONCLUSION

The integration of art expression within the context of family treatment not only enhances client–therapist communication but also offers the opportunity to explore family-related issues through visual means. Therapists can capitalize on this quality through the use of metaphor, both visual and verbal, to help clients and families achieve change, and can infuse art experientials with strategic techniques such as reframing, unbalancing, restraining, and other approaches. Most important, family art therapy allows the individual or family to "see" the presenting problem and take advantage of visual symbols for problem solving, personal change, insight, and understanding the family dynamics which brought them to treatment.

REFERENCES

Bateson, G. (1972). *Steps to an ecology of mind*. New York: Ballantine.

Bing, E. (1970). The conjoint family drawing. *Family Process, 9*, 173-194.

Bross, A., & Benjamin, M. (1982). Family therapy: A recursive model of strategic practice. In A. Bross (Ed.), *Family therapy: A recursive model of strategic practice* (pp. 2–33). New York: Guilford Press.

Haley, J. (1963). *Strategies of psychotherapy*. New York: Grune & Stratton.

Haley, J. (1973). *Uncommon therapy. The psychiatric techniques of Milton H. Erikson, MD*. New York: Norton.

Haley, J. (1976). *Problem-solving therapy.* New York: Harper & Row.

Hoffman, L (1981). *Foundations of family therapy.* New York: Basic Books.

Kwiatkowska, H. Y. (1962). Family art therapy: Experiments with a new technique. *Bulletin of Art Therapy, 1*(3), 3–15.

Kwiatkowska, H. Y. (1967a). The use of families' art productions for psychiatric evaluation. *Bulletin of Art Therapy, 6,* 52–69.

Kwiatkowska, H. Y. (1967b). Family art therapy. *Family Process, 6*(1), 37–55.

Kwiatkowska, H. Y. (1975). Family art therapy: Experiments with a new technique. In E. Ulman (Ed.), *Art therapy in theory and practice.* New York: Schocken.

Kwiatkowska, H. Y. (1978). *Family therapy and evaluation through art.* Springfield, IL: Charles C Thomas.

Landgarten, H. (1975). Group art therapy for mothers and daughters. *American Journal of Art Therapy, 14*(2).

Landgarten, H. (1987). *Family art psychotherapy: A clinical guide and casebook.* New York: Brunner/Mazel.

Levick, M., & Herring, J. (1973). Family dynamics—as seen through art therapy. *Art Psychotherapy, 1*(1), 45–54.

Madanes, C. (1981). *Strategic family therapy.* San Francisco: Jossey-Bass.

Malchiodi, C. A. (1998). *The art therapy sourcebook.* Los Angeles: Lowell House.

Minuchin, S. (1974). *Families and family therapy.* Cambridge, MA: Harvard University.

Mosher, L., & Kwiatkowska, H. Y. (1971). Family art evaluation: Use in families with schizophrenic twins. *Journal of Nervous and Mental Disease, 153*(3), 165–179.

Mueller, E. (1968). Family group art therapy: Treatment of choice for a specific case. In I. Jakab (Ed.), *Psychiatry and art: Proceedings of the IV International Colloquium of Psychopathology of Expression* (pp. 132–143.) Basel: Karger.

Papp, P. (1980). The Greek chorus and other techniques of family therapy. *Family Process, 19,* 45–57.

Papp, P. (1983). *The process of change.* New York: Guilford Press.

Riley, S. (1991). Couples therapy/Art therapy: Strategic interventions and family of origin work. *Art Therapy: Journal of the American Art Therapy Association, 8*(2).

Riley, S., & Malchiodi, C. A. (1994). *Integrative approaches to family art therapy.* Chicago: Magnolia Street.

Rubin, J. (1978). *Child art therapy.* New York: Van Nostrand Reinhold.

Rubin, J., & Magnussen, M. (1974). A family art evaluation. *Family Process, 13*(2), 185–220.

Sobol, B. (1982). Art therapy and strategic family therapy. *American Journal of Art Therapy, 21*(2), 43–52.

Wadeson, H. (1973). Art techniques used in conjoint marital therapy. *American Journal of Art Therapy, 12*(3), 147–164.

Wadeson, H. (1976). The fluid family in multi-family art therapy. *American Journal of Art Therapy, 13*(4), 115–118.

Wadeson, H. (1980). *Art psychotherapy.* New York: Wiley.

Watzlawick, P., Weakland, J., & Fisch, R. (1974). *Change: Principles of problem formation and problem resolution.* New York: Norton.

Weeks, G., & L'Abate, L. (1982). *Paradoxical psychotherapy.* New York: Brunner/Mazel.

Zierer, E., Sternberg, D., Finn, R., & Farmer, M. (1975). Family creative analysis: Its role in treatment. Part 1. *Bulletin of Art Therapy, 5*(2), 47–63.

CHAPTER 29

Multicultural Art Therapy with Families

Janice Hoshino

This chapter addresses the importance of incorporating a multicultural framework in art therapy practice in work with families and presents the ADDRESSING model (Hays, 1996a) as a framework for multicultural family art therapy. A case example demonstrating the use of art therapy with a family is provided to illustrate theory and practice within a multicultural context.

There is a growing literature on multicultural and diversity issues in art therapy, including supervision and training (Calisch, 1998; Cattaneo, 1994; Feen-Calligan, 1996; Rubin, 1999; Ward, 1999), gender and identity issues (Campbell, Dienemann, Kub, Wurmser, & Loy, 1999; Hogan, 1998), and specific cultural issues (Gilroy, 1998; Gilroy & Hanna, 1998; Hiscox & Calish, 1998; Lachman-Chapin et al., 1998; Westrich, 1994). Although these topics vary, all acknowledge that multicultural competence in art therapy practice is imperative.

A multicultural awareness in art therapy entails understanding how race, ethnicity, socioeconomic status, and religion may affect both attitudes toward drawing and the content of what is drawn. For example, Malchiodi (1998) notes that in her work with Chinese children in Beijing she found that they preferred to copy drawings rather than to draw spontaneously, despite the fact that their artwork was developmentally comparable to children's drawings in the United States. Sociological influences that affect the drawing process are frequently picked up at home. For example, a child who is taught to respect authority or not to make a mess may approach an art project with a certain amount of reserve or choose materials accordingly. Likewise, certain symbols or motifs may be more dominant in particular religions or cultures, and this may be reflected in a person's artwork. All these factors need to be taken into account before coming to any conclusions about an individual's artwork or the meaning thereof.

Therapists also need to refer to the considerable literature on cultural differences and their impact on the therapeutic process. The complexity of those individuals and families that come to therapists for treatment can be both intimidating and inspiring. How can a therapist truly understand the psychological ramifications of exclusionary behavior if he or she has lived in the mainstream, white culture of privilege? How can we change patterns of behavior and thinking of the mainstream culture which often polarize, generalize, and minimize the difficult journeys, migration factors, and acculturation issues of those who are culturally diverse? While respect has to be given to the uniqueness of experiences and issues that lead the family into treatment, therapists who are not culturally sensitive may fail to address multicultural issues. Certainly, some positive strides have been made in clinical training programs and subsequent publications around cultural development and competence in clinical training (Bean, Perry, & Bedell, 2002; Carter & McGoldrick, 1989; Dana, 1993; McDowell, Fang, Brownlee, Young, & Khanna, 2002; Sue & Sue, 1990) and in training techniques such as constructing culturally sensitive genograms (Keiley et al., 2002; Lustbader, 1993).

The search for a multicultural framework that is comprehensive, pragmatic to clinical practice and applicable to a myriad of populations and treatment settings is difficult. Although most cultural frameworks focus exclusively on ethnicity, McGoldrick, Giordano, and Pearce (1996) believe "that class, more than ethnicity, determines people's values and behavior" (p. 16). One model that addresses both ethnicity, class and ability is Hays's (1996a) ADDRESSING framework, which presents a "transcultural-specific perspective" (p. 334). The ADDRESSING acronym uses each letter to represent one of ten cultural factors and minority groups. They are: Age and generational influences, Developmental and acquired Disabilities, Religion, Ethnicity, Socioeconomic status, Sexual orientation, Indigenous heritage, National origin, and Gender. It "highlights the complex, overlapping nature of cultural influences and identities" (Hays, 1996b, p. 337), helps "to raise awareness of and challenge one's own biases and areas of experience, " and "to consider the salience of multiple cultural influences on clients of minority cultures" (Hays, 1996a, p. 74).

Many of the areas of the ADDRESSING model can be applied in practice. For example, when working with a family, the therapist considers age, examining generational and intergenerational influences on the family. While some embrace their ethnicity and heritage, therapists need to be attentive to those who reject their cultural background as some may do so as a result of discrimination or oppression; moving away from cultural roots is seen as a means of survival and necessity by these individuals. A visual genogram is a helpful activity to assist both therapists and family members in understanding generational and intergenerational influences and heritage. Hardy and Laszolffy (1995) outline a meaningful cultural genogram, including defining one's culture of origin, organizing principles and pride/shame issues, and identifying issues such as intercultural marriages. I have adopted their recommended use of symbols and colors in my work with art therapy students for many years. Genograms may also help in exploring the role and impact of gender, another characteristic of the ADDRESSING model, because gender may relate to issues such as power distribution, sex roles, division of labor and childrearing, acculturation issues in potential shifting roles in gender and identity, and inequity.

As mentioned previously, religion can be a source of strength, cultural identity, and growth in both individuals and families. Artwork may reflect religious symbols and have spiritual significance. Horovitz-Darby (1994) emphasizes the importance of addressing spirituality and the need for holistic, integrative forms of art therapy treatment.

As a biracial family art therapist, I always grapple with the following questions: What will ensure my sensitivity to the unique cultural issues that lie in front of me? How can I relay my respect and pay homage to the survival of the incredible experiences and issues of oppression that many of us can only barely imagine? What can I do, as a family art therapist, to help influence and guide their journey that will break destructive, generational patterns; increase understanding of alliances, triangles, and other family dynamics; and encourage preservation of meaningful traditions and rituals? The following case, laden with tragedy and cultural oppression with all the subsequent consequences, is, unfortunately, not too uncommon.

CASE EXAMPLE: MULTICULTURAL FAMILY ART THERAPY

The Indian Child Welfare worker referred this family of four Native American/Latino children to a small, rural community mental health clinic, located near the reservation on which the children reside with their foster parents. Two older children had been placed with their biological grandmother (see genogram, Figure 29.1). All six children had been removed for the second time from their biological mother, Donna, after it was discovered she was drinking heavily and neglecting her children. The four youngest children were placed with a biracial foster family that was closely aligned with their own ethnicity. Prior to the 1978 Indian Child Welfare Act (Public Law 95-608), "out of home placements of Indian Children in Foster Care or adoptive homes was far greater than was true of non-Indian children. The prior massive removal of Indian children from their families and Tribes was devastating not only to the integrity of Indian families and to the psychological and cultural identity of these children, but to the vitality of entire Indian Tribes" (Swinomish Tribal Community, 1991, p. 28).

The foster mother, Dotty, reported she had been caring for the children for 2 months. The children arrived frightened with dirty clothing, were underweight, and had severe head lice infestation that required shaving their heads. The oldest child, Trevor, age 6, was in first grade, and struggling academically and socially. His general demeanor in session was quiet and reserved with sad affect, yet he was very curious. In contrast, Dotty reported that he was "loud and rambunctious," refusing to listen, had no boundaries, and occasionally had tantrums when he did not get his way. Trevor "plays rough," hits to solve conflicts, and has been caught stealing and lying since he moved into the foster home.

Rosa, age 4, was all smiles, very enthusiastic about participating in all therapeu-

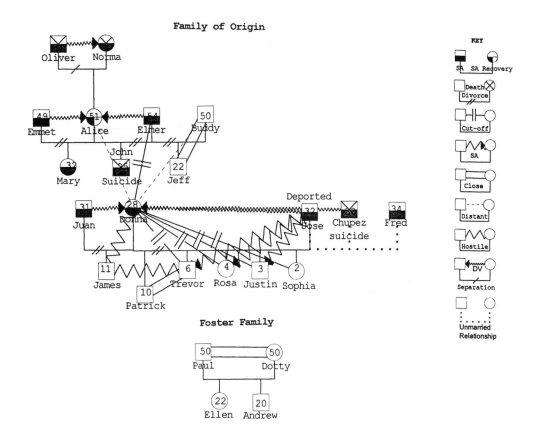

FIGURE 29.1. Genogram.

tic directives, and very spontaneous and talkative. Dotty reported that Rosa acted out less overtly but said that Rosa cried easily, was afraid to ask for help, and would pick her nose until it would bleed and pinch her skin and face when she was upset. She discovered Rosa kissing and touching both brothers' genitals behind a living room chair. Rosa typically assumed a caretaker role, particularly with her younger siblings.

Justin, age 3, was bright-eyed and curious, highly energetic, and tactile, wanting to touch and play with everything in the therapy office. Dotty noted that Justin had problems falling and staying asleep and had night terrors. Justin threw frequent tantrums and pretended he was shooting or cutting someone with a knife during play. Justin also picked his nose and face when upset, and when having a tantrum, he would cry out "Justin bad boy." She described Justin as the "most problematic" of all four children.

Sophia, age 2, had attached herself to Dotty almost instantly. Initially Sophia did not exhibit behavioral difficulties but later threw tantrums and hit her siblings. Over a period of several months Trevor, Justin, and Rosa disclosed that they had been sexually abused by two family members. Further, they witnessed their father beating up their mother.

The Biological Family

Most of the information on the biological family came from the Indian Child Welfare caseworker and maternal grandmother, Alice. The children's mother, Donna, age 28, had been born on and registered to a Indian reservation. Donna's mother, Alice, also born on a Reservation, had been married three times. Alice had a daughter from her first marriage and two children, John and Donna, from her second marriage. Both husbands were alcoholic and physically abusive toward Alice. Alice described herself and her mother before her as both "drunks." Alice divorced again, married a third time to another tribal member, and had her fourth child, a son. She reported that her third husband was sober, nonabusive, and a good father: "When I was out to the taverns, he was home with the kids making sure they were fed and got their schoolwork done." It is questionable if Donna was sexually or physically abused because Alice was usually out drinking and seldom home. Alice quit drinking at 48 years of age due to heart problems but admitted that both she and Donna drank throughout all of their pregnancies.

Donna married at 18 years of age to a nearby Latino man. She was pregnant with her first son, James. Donna's husband was both violent and alcoholic from the relationship's inception. They divorced 2 years later when Donna met Jose, who was also alcoholic and physically abusive. Donna became pregnant with her second son, Patrick. Their marriage of 8 years produced four more children: Trevor, Rosa, Justin, and Sophia. The eldest son, James, became the parentified child, who fed the children and changed their diapers. James is now happily living with grandmother Alice.

Donna's children were first removed after Jose assaulted Donna and her aunt. He was arrested and subsequently deported to his country of origin, although Donna refused to press charges. Donna then allowed her late brother's friend, a suspected sexual predator, to move in with her. He left a few months later and was incarcerated.

Donna attempted to take some classes but could not find child care and quit. She then lost her housing and the children were placed in foster care while she completed drug and alcohol treatment. Donna and her children subsequently moved in with a new boyfriend, but she began to use alcohol and neglect her children once again and they were placed in long-term foster care and made dependents of the Tribe. The two eldest boys now live with their grandmother, Alice, who maintains a sober lifestyle.

The Foster Home

The foster mother, Dotty, is originally from the Midwest and of Latino heritage. Determined not to repeat the patterns of her parents' failed, alcoholic marriage, Dotty received child development training and worked at a preschool. She met her husband, Tom, while he was in the Army. They have two children, Alicia and Donald. Tom was born on an Indian reservation and always wanted to move back home to his roots, which they did 12 years ago. They became licensed for foster care at the suggestion of the social workers at the Tribe, becoming known for providing a stable, loving home for long-term troubled or needy children.

Dotty's two children, 20 and 22, live at home and are invested in and spend time with the foster children. Both Tom and Dotty maintain their Latino and Tribal cultures through church, traditional ethnic cooking, dancing, and various other cultural activities. They also volunteer regularly for Tribal youth activities and other local area Pow Wow Ceremonies and cultural events.

Art Therapy Sessions

General Overview

The children regularly attended art therapy with their foster mother, Dotty. Initial assessment goals for treatment included identification of boundaries, communication patterns, roles, and structural patterns in the family. Whitaker (1989) contended that "all expressions of yourself are symbolic" (p. 51). Klorer (2000) further notes that "group tasks, such as a family mural or family sculpture, help the therapist understand the family's interactive pattern, and interventions can be made through the art process to facilitate attachment" (p. 171).

Artwork has been central to the therapeutic process and has been used in multiple ways. Riley (1999) notes that "language can be a barrier to understanding" (p. 56), as exemplified in this case study. Sessions often begin with free choice in materials; given the limited opportunities they have had with media, activities such as finger painting have opened up a new world for the children. Demonstration of media by the art therapist is given as needed. Dotty sometimes engages in free art with the children and other times opts to observe as the process unfolded.

A wide range of art material is offered as well as sandtray, puppets, clay, and found objects. Directives are also given, as deemed helpful by the therapist. Often, the children and Dotty are asked to engage in collaborative projects such as murals and joint projects. Assimilation issues, boundaries, alliances, cooperative efforts, and family processes are observed through these activities. Everyone in the family was receptive to both unstructured and structured activities, and sessions have typically included a mixture of both.

Initial Sessions

The children's artwork initially had several recurring themes and symbols. First was the recurring theme of roads: Drawings labeled "the road back to me" and "the road to (biological) Mom" (see Figure 29.2) seem to be indicative of their confusion and conflict over abandonment, unstable living arrangements, and life events. These roads have been a realistic theme that accurately portrays the long, windy roads that lead to where Donna resides. The opportunity to engage in art making provided the children with an opportunity to talk for the first time about their mother.

The children drew and talked frequently about missing their biological mother and expressed fear over her well-being and safety, as well as feeling divided loyalties and much ambivalence toward her. They continued to need reassurance from Dotty regarding stability and continuity, given the events around visitation with Donna.

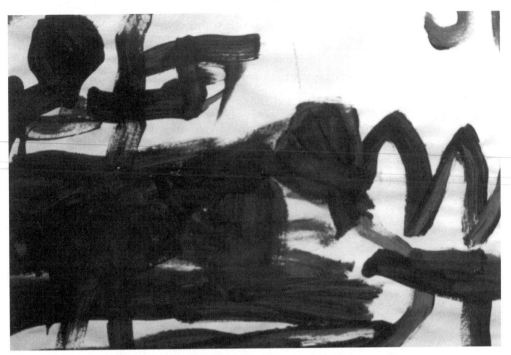

FIGURE 29.2. Drawing of roads.

Gray (2002) purports that, "attachment is key to regulating extreme frustration and anxiety" (p. 16).

During this time, the last scheduled visit to see their biological mother occurred and had been rather devastating for the children. Dotty drove the children more than 2 hours to see Donna, who let the children and Dotty wait in the car for 2 hours while she disappeared in a casino. Donna was finally successfully paged, but she decided to not see the children. The dominant issues of abandonment (by biological father, then biological mother), coupled with separations from the remaining family (the oldest two siblings and maternal grandmother) were generalized to the foster family along with many fears expressed by the children. This continued to be a primary topic in art therapy during the initial phases.

Forming a New Family

Art therapy also focused on the formation of a new family system. Although the children may never be formally adopted, as Tribal rites seldom allow for this, Donna has relinquished all parental rights and Dotty will remain the foster mother until they graduate high school. The first family mural, a collage medley, was great fun to all involved, although each member remained within his or her own separate space (see Figure 29.3). Likewise, their joint family drawing reveals each choosing to individually depict the family on the same page, creating a single image, in essence, of four different families (see Figure 29.4). This may also speak to the process of forming a new family, defining what "family" is, and transitioning to similar, but different cultural factors and traditions. Further, it should be noted that factors such as religion and ritual, learning of one's ethnic heritage, traditions, and language were cherished and taught more in the foster family than would have been taught in the family of origin.

Dotty recognizes the importance of tradition and ritual and plans to give Trevor and Justin the option of going before the Tribal Elders to dance so they can earn their feathers for a special dance costume, thereby learning the value of heritage and tradition. In addition to Native American dancing, Dotty, fluent in Spanish and English, is also teaching the children Spanish, by speaking Spanish, then translating into English. In short, Dottie is encouraging the children to shift from an assimilated identity to a bicultural identity (Lustbader, 1993) by learning rituals and tradition in art, dance, religion, language, and other factors relating to their ethnicity and heritage.

Subsequent Sessions

Art therapy sessions also provided the vehicle through which to report previously unknown incidences. For example, both Rosa and Trevor spontaneously drew blatant sexual abuse episodes on separate occasions. Art provided a means through which to begin communication and to address abuse, safety, and trust issues.

Despite these disclosures, it was exciting to witness how the children worked with new media or expanded their interests in materials already introduced. The chil-

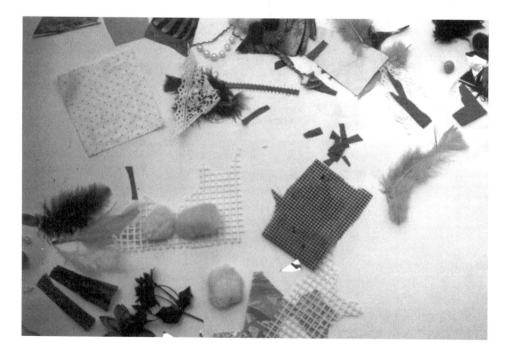

FIGURE 29.3. Collage.

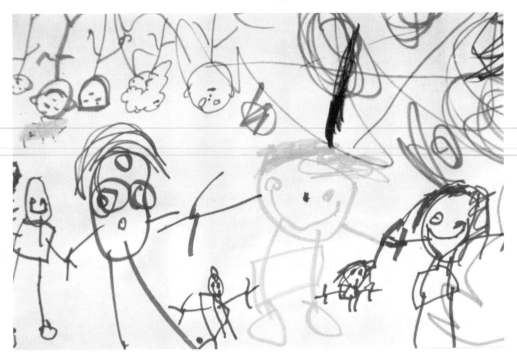

FIGURE 29.4. Group family drawing.

dren were generally provided with a free choice of materials. Because they have little say in where and how and with whom they live, free choice of art media and collage materials provided choices, something to which they were not accustomed. Landgarten (1993) notes: "The opportunity to exercise some *control* over the selection process can lessen inhibitions and resistant factors for so many clients" (p. 2). She further notes that collage is not culturally specific.

The children approached collage wanting a multitude of media, and used materials generously and confidently. They often talked freely about their artwork, school, home, Dotty, and their concerns as they worked. However, they were also adaptable and seem to enjoy all kinds of media such as clay, drawing, painting, and sculpting. Regardless of the media (either self chosen or provided), they seem to have the same effect on the children—they find the media simultaneously stimulating and soothing, and they visibly relax while working on their pieces. Last, the children also engaged in dramatic play around some of the images.

Another shift that occurred as sessions progressed was a change of themes: The recurring road symbols, so prominent in the early sessions, largely subsided. These have given way to drawings centered around the foster family system. Kinetic family drawings (draw your family doing something) illustrate a family together, in contrast to earlier drawings where members were separate and in their own space. The children seemed delighted to depict themselves helping Dotty with chores: Rosa readily drew herself helping Dotty clean and entitled the picture, "Cleaning with Mommy." Likewise, Trevor drew himself folding clothes with Dotty. The drawings also seemed to have a similar theme that shows all the foster children with Dotty and/or Tom together at home, while Dotty's 20-and 22-year-old children are present in the drawing, but separate from the family, a realistic portrayal.

Art therapy also provided an opportunity to examine and negotiate the newly formed family system. For instance, the children, through their drawings, depicted feelings of anxiety and concern around "getting dirty." This emergent theme was explored and gave Dotty the opportunity to work on defining and carrying out realistic expectations for children of this age. Overall, artwork became much brighter in color and happier in content than in the initial drawings.

During this time, Donna was seldom mentioned and the children did not report being fearful. Tragically, it has been reported that Donna has not changed her lifestyle. The children have drawn and continue to miss their two eldest siblings, who are doing well with their maternal grandmother.

Future Sessions

Regarding future sessions, art therapy will focus on the newly formed family system as it develops and solidifies and on maintaining and supporting cultural heritage and identity. Focus on symbolic importance and utilization of art in the preservation of rituals and heritage could also be explored. Including the older siblings and maternal grandmother in art therapy sessions is another possibility; reunification of the siblings may also ease the children's transition process. Last, it should be noted that the therapists involved have been circumspect in what thematic material has been introduced, given the numerous agencies, foster homes, interviews, and overall trauma and abuse to which these children have been exposed.

CONCLUSION

Art therapy generally transcends cultures, many of which do not value language as Western culture does. With the changing and expanding profile in diverse populations in the United States, art therapy seems a logical choice in serving these individual and families. Creativity and nonverbal imagery is inherent in all people, although some non-Western cultures embrace silence and symbols more fluidly than does Euro-American culture. This chapter speaks to the need of multicultural competence in therapists who use art therapy in treatment. The ADDRESSING model was introduced as a comprehensive framework to use while considering the many complexities of cultural influences. Finally, genograms can be imperative to sifting through these complexities as well. McGoldrick, Gerson, & Shellenberger (1999) contend they "appeal to clinicians because they are tangible and graphic representations of complex family patterns" (p. 1).

Multicultural competence does not mean a comprehensive understanding of every cultural variable, as this is an impossible task (although ongoing, continuing education is always highly recommended). It does speak to the need for continued self-evaluation around one's owns prejudices and areas of inexperience. In summary, therapists should be cautioned not to label or generalize behaviors prior to understanding the source of the behavior. In this way, the therapist is more likely to engage more genuinely with clients, thus being more sensitive and aware.

ACKNOWLEDGMENT

I thank Kim Henderson, MA, for collaborating with me on the case example discussed in this chapter.

REFERENCES

Bean, R. A., Perry, B. J., & Bedell, T. M. (2002). Developing culturally competent marriage and family therapists: Treatment guidelines for non-African therapists working with African-American families. *Journal of Marriage and Family Therapy, 28*(2), 153–164.

Calisch, A. (1998). Multicultural perspectives in art therapy supervision. In A. Hiscox & A. Calisch (Eds.), *Tapestry of cultural issues in art therapy* (pp. 201–220). London: Jessica Kingsley.

Campbell, J .C., Dienemann, J., Kub, J., Wurmser, T., & Loy, E. (1999). Collaboration as a partnership. *Violence Against Women: An International and Interdisciplinary Journal, 5*(10), 1140–1157.

Carter, E., & McGoldrick, M. (Eds.). (1989). *The changing family life cycle* (2nd ed.). Boston: Allyn & Bacon.

Cattaneo, M. (1994). Addressing culture and values in the training of art therapists. *Art Therapy: Journal of the American Art Therapy Association, 11*(3), 184–186.

Dana, R. H. (1993). *Multicultural assessment perspectives for professional practice.* Boston: Allyn & Bacon.

Feen-Calligan, H. (1996). Art therapy as a profession: Implications for the education and training of art therapists. *Art Therapy: Journal of the American Art Therapy Association, 13*(3), 166–173.

Gilroy, A. (1998). On being a temporary migrant to Australia: Reflections on art therapy education and practice. In D. Dokter (Ed.), *Arts therapists, refugees and migrants: Reaching across borders* (pp. 262–277). London: Jessica Kingsley.

Gilroy, A., & Hanna, M. (1998). Conflict and culture in art therapy: An Australian perspective. In A. Hiscox & A. Calisch (Eds.), *Tapestry of cultural issues in art therapy* (pp. 249–275). London: Jessica Kingsley.

Gray, D. (2002). *Attaching in adoption.* Indianapolis: Perspectives Press.

Hardy, K. V., & Laszloffy, T. A. (1995). The cultural genogram: Key to training culturally competent family therapists. *Journal of Marital and Family Therapy, 21*(3), 227–237.

Hays, P. A. (1996a). Addressing the complexities of culture and gender in counseling. *Journal of Counseling and Development, 74,* 332–338.

Hays, P. A. (1996b). Cultural considerations in couples therapy. *Women and Therapy, 19,* 13–23.

Hiscox, A. R., & Calisch, A. (1998). *Tapestry of cultural issues in art therapy.* London: Jessica Kingsley.

Hogan, S. (1998). Problems of identity: Deconstructing gender in art therapy. In S. Hogan (Ed.), *Feminist approaches to art therapy* (pp. 21–48). London: Routledge.

Horovitz-Darby, E. (1994). *Spiritual art therapy: An alternative path.* Springfield, IL: Charles C Thomas.

Keiley, M. K., Dolbin, M., Hill, J., Karuppaswamy, T. L., Natranjan, R., Poulsen, S., Robbins, N., & Robinson, P. (2002). The cultural genogram: Experiences from within an MFT training program. *Journal of Marriage and Family Therapy, 28*(2), 165–178.

Klorer, P. G. (2000). *Expressive therapy with troubled children*. Northvale, NJ: Jason Aronson.

Lachman-Chapin, M., Jones, D., Sweg, T., Cohen, B., Semekoski, S., & Fleming, M. (1998). Connecting with the art world: Expanding beyond the mental health world. *Art Therapy: Journal of the American Art Therapy Association, 15*(4), 233–244.

Landgarten, H. B. (1993). *Magazine photo collage: A multicultural assessment and treatment technique*. New York: Brunner/Mazel.

Lustbader, W. (1993). *Taking care of aging family members*. New York: Free Press.

Malchiodi, C. (1998). *Understanding children's drawings*. New York: Guilford Press.

McDowell, T., Fang, S.-R., Brownlee, K., Young, C. G., & Khanna, A. (2002). Transforming an MFT program: A model for enhancing diversity. *Journal of Marriage and Family Therapy, 28*(2), 179–192.

McGoldrick, M., Gerson, R., & Shellenberger, S. (1999). *Genograms: Assessment and intervention.* (2nd ed.). New York: Norton.

McGoldrick, M., Giordano, J., & Pearce, J. K. (1996). *Ethnicity and family therapy* (2nd ed.). New York: Guilford Press.

Riley, S. (1999). *Contemporary art therapy with adolescents*. London: Jessica Kingsley.

Rubin, J. A. (1999). *Art therapy: An introduction*. New York: Brunner/Mazel.

Sue, W. S., & Sue, S. (1990). *Counseling the culturally different* (2nd. ed.). New York: Wiley.

Swinomish Tribal Community. (1991). *A gathering of wisdoms. Tribal mental health: A cultural perspective*. LaConner, WA: Veda Vangarde.

Ward, C. (1999). Art therapy training and race and culture. In J. Campbell, M. Liebman, F. Brooks, J. Jones, & C. Ward (Eds.), *Art therapy, race and culture* (pp. 287–305). London: Jessica Kingsley.

Westrich, C. (1994). Art therapy with culturally different clients. *Art Therapy: Journal of the American Art Therapy Association, 11*(3), 187–190.

Whitaker, C. (1989). *Midnight musings of a family therapist*. New York: Norton.

CHAPTER 30

Art Therapy with Couples

Shirley Riley

This chapter proposes a variety of concepts concerning the treatment of couples and the introduction of the language of art as a facilitator of change. Art therapy is a preferred method of working with couples for a variety of reasons. Visual images of relational problems provide a fresh view of rigid patterns of behaviors and introduce a new mode of communication. Art expressions can make marital issues visible and provides the opportunity for both client(s) and therapist to establish goals and create a treatment plan.

In this chapter, the term "couple" is defined as two persons committed to a long-term relationship and who have, or had, the intention of remaining a couple for the foreseeable future. The term "marriage" is a convenience, to avoid describing the many varieties of committed relationships that exist in our present-day society. The developmental stage of both the partners and the relationship is considered as well as the messages and family dynamics that each person invariably brings into the marriage.

ART THERAPY LITERATURE ON COUPLE THERAPY

Couple therapy is practiced by many art therapists, but little of this work has been recorded in print. Wadeson (1980) discussed research with individuals with a manic–depressive disorder and their spouses. Her facility sponsored a 2-hour art therapy protocol using the results to reinforce the evaluation of the marital team; four art tasks were given to all the couples. The interesting, and not fully understood, results from these interdependent relationships were apparent in the drawings. The drawings of the spouse had an equal amount of depressive indicators as the diagnosed patient. This was not expected and added to the assessments' value. Riley discusses couple therapy (Riley & Malchiodi, 1994) by taking into account the more contemporary approaches to problem solving in marital discord.

Landgarten (1981) shows how art became a voice for a couple in conjoint treatment. She deconstructs therapy with a couple wherein the husband suffered from a severe stroke and the marital relationship suffered as a result of the illness. The husband had lost his ability to verbalize and had limited paralysis of his right arm. He consistently created artwork that pictured himself as a nonperson, no longer useful or valuable. Conjoint art therapy, through use of clear and well-defined art interventions, helped the couple to reexamine the roles in their relationship and establish an adjusted relationship which included the impact of the stroke on their interactions. The art provided the husband with a voice which had been damaged due to his illness.

THERAPEUTIC WORK WITH COUPLES

Angry, sad, depressed, lonely, the couple comes through the door of my office seeking relief from the discord in the marriage. Through the years of working with couples I am convinced that there is one dominant need for both the man and the woman that supersedes all the others that will surface during out time together. Each partner passionately wants the other to see the world through his or her lens. From this basic dynamic all the subsequent behavior emerges.

I have found that each member of the dyad is convinced that all would be well if the other could only see their perspective of the problem. To *see* is the key. To "see" is not possible with words alone; therefore, it becomes logical to introduce the visual form of therapy because it responds to the declared need of the client. Art therapy makes "seeing" a reality as it adds illustration to verbal descriptions of problems.

I also wear a lens when I work with couples that reflects a bias: I find the search for pathology unpleasant and not respectful. It does not help a couple if I am searching for a character flaw, but it does help to find small moments of cooperation or caring that provide a base from which we can build. My goal is to co-construct with the couple a vision of what they hope to find in a more satisfying relationship. To reach that end, my position is to listen carefully to their stories and make every effort to enter into their perceptions of what would lead to happiness. I do not impose my notions of successful living on their belief system. In addition, I must find the metaphorical language that they can hear, language that reflects their world view. To do this I rely on the information that becomes apparent in the art product and the metaphors that rise from the conversation about the art expression (Halford, 2001).

USING ART DYNAMICALLY WITH COUPLES

When the couple first comes into therapy I spend some time in introductions and a brief background exploration of their decision to come into conjoint therapy. I explain that we will be using two languages, one verbal and the other concrete, and that the art product will not be aesthetic but will have creative value for them. I also say that this dual form of knowing will help them achieve their goals more efficiently than the conventional mode of therapy. Introducing action (in this case, art making) stimulates many areas of cognition and emotional awareness that previously have not been evoked (Damasio, 1994; Goleman, 1995).

Getting Started

After the brief introduction I hand each person a piece of paper and ask each to explain, "Why have you chosen this time to come into therapy? Please help me understand your view by making some marks or symbols on the paper that reflect your goals." The language I use is deliberately vague and avoids artistic language. I usually offer oil pastels because they are receptive to light or firm pressure, they are colorful, and they are not difficult to control. It is surprising how many persons have never used this media and find it interesting in itself. Thus, we have started with an experience that is shared by the couple.

After the drawings are completed I ask the couple to exchange drawings. They are asked to consider for a short time the image their partner created and then explain the other's art as each understands it. My rationale is this: From the first moment I strive to find a safe activity that begins to destabilize the cycle of misinformation that has interrupted their ability to understand one another. When the recipient of the art explains the other's drawing, he or she does so without interruption. The partner then does the same. This forces the couple to listen to how the partner interprets and projects meaning on his or her art. After this period of exploration of the meaning of the spouse's image, the conversation revolves around how accurately each had explained the other's artwork. At times the partner understands the message in the art, but more often he or she does not.

This exercise is a way of starting a dialogue around the misconception that couples often hold, that they know what the other is thinking or feeling. Magical thinking and significance projected on behaviors are major deterrents to clear communication.

Middle Phase of Treatment

In subsequent sessions I often start with this same routine, asking, "Let's start by showing (drawing) what we shall focus on today" The same ritual of exchange of drawings and dialogue follows. There is a level of comfort that is experienced by repetition of an activity, and it also countermands the theory that some new art directive has to be offered in each session. Drawings change every time the identical question is asked; therefore, it is not necessary to have a laundry list of ideas to engage the client.

A difficult dynamic that is often encountered in these early sessions in couple therapy is that of blaming: finding the problem in the other and not acknowledging any personal responsibility. This issue can be made visible if the couple is asked to draw together the dominant problem that they both agree on, using the same paper.

The dual drawing is the beginning of a process that will lead to (1) selecting the difficulty as a team, and (2) creating a symbol for the problem. After the drawing is complete each partner is asked to identify the part of the drawing he or she created. The therapist then has the opportunity to explore the notion that because each person had a hand in creating this drawing, perhaps each had a hand in creating their difficulty in the relationship. Blame is placing the problem on the other person, drawing the problem is a mutual act; therefore, the results cannot be blamed on the other because it is a shared creation.

After the conversation about this continues I offer scissors and ask the couple to cut away the piece that they feel would be the first move to change the shape of the image. After the incision has been made (the clipped portion of the original drawing), we place it on another sheet of paper and focus on this reduced image of the problem. What is happening in this transaction is that action takes the place of words. Change is literally made through the cutting and shaping of the dual drawing and the message can be absorbed without interpretation.

The value of the language of art is that is allows the person to speak of painful issues through the safe protection of a drawing or lump of clay. Keeping the couple focused on the art piece and the activity instead of reviewing old patterns of blaming is the responsibility of the therapist.

During the earlier phase of therapy the story of the couple's troubles are told and retold many times. Each partner corrects and confronts the other with his or her version of the events. For every story there is a need for an illustration; the art accompanies and illuminates the story each time it is told. Adding a pictorial dimension to the story enriches the dialogue; by exploring the illustration other aspects of the story emerge. As alternative variations in the narrative arise it becomes evident that each of us lives the same event through different meanings and sees through different eyes. This conclusion helps the couple enter into the therapeutic phase of looking at family myths, rituals, and roles that have had an impact their relationship (Christensen & Jacobson, 2000).

The Four-Poster Bed

When two people marry, they join together their own multigeneration systems of beliefs and truths. Although this concept is generally is held by many therapists doing conjoint work, it is a ponderous and difficult message to convey. As a result of this dilemma I conceived an image and a task, which I call the "four-poster bed."

A copy of a drawing of the bed (Figure 30.1) is given to the man and the woman. They are asked to "show how many people are in bed with you when you sleep together." There are usually startled looks and some laughter, but the idea filters in rather quickly. I suggest they start by drawing figures reclining together in their favorite sleeping position, using stick figures if necessary. Then the question is, "Who is looking over the headboard? Who is under the bed? Who shares the bed?" and many more variations on this theme. I also encourage the individuals to draw separately from each other, even assigning this task as homework if the time is pressing.

The drawings are amazingly revealing. For example, I have seen mother sleeping

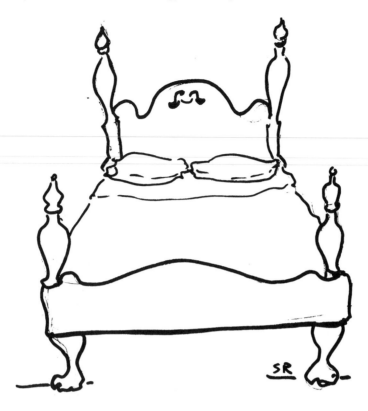

FIGURE 30.1. Four-poster-bed image.

between the couple, father peering over the headboard, grandparents offering a trundle board, children standing all around, telephones and computers in the bed, lamps on and off. In other words, countless clues to the family systemic messages are portrayed, ideas from the past that have to be either embraced or cast out in the process of making a new primary relationship.

The author of the drawing is then asked to explain where and how the family and objects got into the bed and to give each object a voice. Through this gestalt-type, reflective play I have heard mother cautioning her daughter about men and father warning son that women are insatiable. Not all messages are negative; sometimes the bedfellows send loving messages. Making these traditions and prejudices visible is a dramatic event in couple therapy.

By introducing family attitudes and belief systems in this manner through the bed image the couple can each see and recognize the behaviors they are carrying out from their past history. Many reactions and behaviors arise from a semiautomatic response level. Family messages that were implanted even before conscious memory have great power in the here and now. How certain traits or physical appearances or color, race, or religion is favored are messages that are often embedded in the client from the family's nonverbal conversation or attitude. The material that surfaces through the four-poster bed can fuel many sessions that are attentive to the interplay between generations, the dependency or withdrawal from the parental system, and old feelings of rejection or loss that have intruded on the here-and-now experiences in the marriage (Bobes & Rothman, 1998).

THE ART THERAPY GENOGRAM

It is often useful in conjoint treatment to propose an art therapy genogram. The therapist explains the notion of the family map and suggests that the relationships and generational patterns can be individually portrayed and augmented by using color and images to expand the content of the symbols. There is no attempt made to follow the traditional genogram schema as proposed by McGoldrick and Gerson (1985). For example, those family members who took a protective role could be colored green and those who were violent could be black. Color-coding behaviors gives the genogram life and helps the couple to trace inherited traits and behaviors (see Figure 30.2). Often the man and woman have not dwelt on their family background and it is interesting to them to get to know the other's lineage, the behavioral patterns, and relationships over the generations.

In addition, I ask the couple to represent the emotional climate of their family.

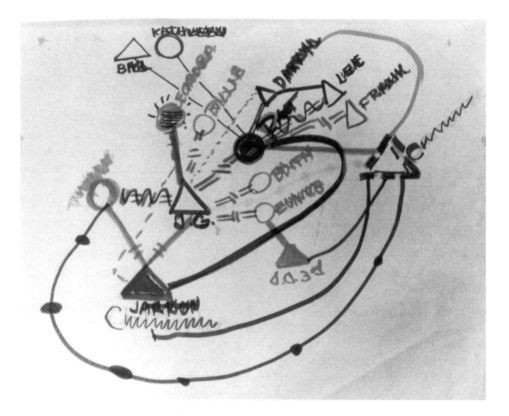

FIGURE 30.2. Example of an art therapy genogram.

This can be represented by filling in background color on the genogram drawing, for example, a color that depicts a hot, violent, or highly emotional family or a cool, distant one. In this manner the personalities, the relational patterns, and the socioeconomic cultural backgrounds can all be addressed in one representation. In addition, the number of instances of divorce or separation gives some witness to the commitments that are dominant in the family. I do not try to go beyond the grandparent generation, because in conjoint therapy we are attempting to focus more on the here and now. If grandparents are influential in their grandchildren's lives, they are important to include. The genogram also allows for memories to emerge of those who have died and those who have moved away; these people can be a part of the family map.

Genograms are used for many reasons in therapy. In couple therapy they are used to bring to the relationship an awareness that the two persons have a choice of how they wish to perpetuate the patterns they observe or choose new resolutions. In addition, the two can see how their families' interactions were similar and how they differed. From that information they can decide if any of these ways of relating are in existence in their present marriage.

CASE EXAMPLE

A couple, Alicia and Hishi, came into a crisis center in serious trouble. They were convinced that their marriage was over and that their previous attempts at couple therapy were a waste of time. Hishi complained that Alicia was loud, unreasonable, and demanding. Alicia replied that Hishi was distant and noncommunicative. They reported that they were fighting all the time. They contradicted themselves and asked the therapist to "save the marriage."

The history revealed that Alicia had immigrated to the United States with her family when she was 11 years old. Hishi was born in the United States; his father was African American and his mother Japanese. His parents had met when his father had military duty in Japan. The couple had been married for 7 years, most of the years in conflict.

The usual joining exercises and conversations (as noted previously) were offered to the couple. They cooperated with the therapist, but all the interventions seemed to no avail. They appeared not to hear one another even in the session and certainly did not when they were elsewhere. I was struck by the way they presented themselves. Alicia was talkative, rather loud, very animated, and ready to engage. Hishi, in contrast, sat quietly, rarely adding to the conversation, and when he did it was tentative and self-effacing. I was impressed by the contrasting behaviors and I wondered if it could have a great deal to do with their cultures. When the issue of contrasting cultural backgrounds was suggested, both Alicia and Hishi denied vigorously that that was of any importance. To explore these issues further, Alicia and Hishi were asked to show what I would see if I went to their family's home and opened the door when everyone was home. (Figures 30.3, 30.4)

Alicia said her family would be dancing to gay Argentine music, arguing, eating, and showing affection with abandon. Hishi was reluctant to show his family home.

He said he usually sat there alone, reading a book and listening to soft music. His mother was very reclusive and never adapted to this country. His father was seldom home and avoided the depressive environment.

The couple sat looking at these drawings for some time. For the first time I experienced them really being attentive to the other's story. It was as though they had never really understood each other before. The impact of Alicia's reds and oranges compared to the frailty of Hishi's pale greens and blues underscored the differences in their childhood experiences. To dramatize the contrast even more I asked Alicia to speak of her family in Spanish and for Hishi to reply in Japanese. These drawings and this interchange in foreign languages seemed to open the couple to "hearing" the difficulties in a different manner. They were open to discussing the impact of cultural roles and traditions, and they were less inclined to argue and more inclined to listen.

I present this case as an example of how the visual message can impact clients in unexpected ways. The art representations became problem solvers in a unique way, ones that broke through the communication barrier that this couple had erected between themselves.

COLLAGE

More sex, less sex, no sex, better sex, all the variations on one of the most rewarding and often the most contentious area of the marriage are bound to surface in most therapy with couples. How the individual was raised in regard to physicality and sex-

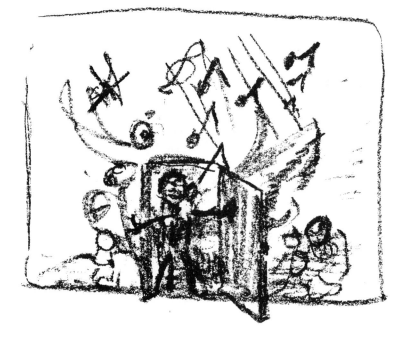

FIGURE 30.3. Alicia's drawing of family.

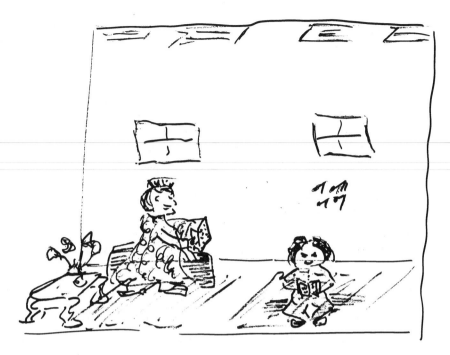

FIGURE 30.4. Hishi's drawing of family.

uality is an issue that often is a focus in the marital relationship. Telling the story of how family members felt about showing affection and making art that reflects this issue is a path to understanding. I suggest that collage be available for this exploration; as it is such a multileveled subject, it is a great challenge to represent. The images may tap into preverbal memories that are only recalled in an instinctive, symbolic manner. The magazine pictures can be translated into complicated imagery that would be a challenge for nonartists to draw.

Clients cannot actually remember the first year of their life, but creative expressions can often offer clues that rise from visual (preverbal) memory. Intrinsic memories reveal themselves in behaviors and reactions to sensual stimuli. How these desires and reactions are played out now is the concern of the couple therapist (Bowlby, 1969).

THREE-DIMENSIONAL MEDIA

A couple in art therapy were having a difficult time with the issues of closeness and distance. As he came closer to his wife, with overtures of remorse for past deeds, she move farther away and rejected his attempts at reconciliation. When he reacted with hurt and turned away from her, she pursued him and asked for affection. This push–pull interaction is not uncommon and usually stems from fear of intimacy on both sides. This dynamic is hard to address because it does not always happen in the therapy room, and, therefore, is difficult to observe.

Mary and John were each asked to make a "self-shape" in plasticine (a type of clay) in any manner they chose. Mary created an oblong sphere with some holes placed in the upper and lower parts of the shape. She chose to blend the neutral beige clay with a light green. John chose a fairly large piece of dark blue and made it into a brick with red bumps pressed on all sides. Mary explained that her blended colors represented her lack of definite views and the rounded shape her trying to fit in—the holes were the gaps in her relationship with John. John immediately took a tool and reduced the size of his clay piece, saying, "I do not want to overpower Mary." He then explained that he was "walled in by frustration, and the red bumps were the magnets he had tried to use to get his wife to come closer."

I provided a paper tray and suggested that it represent their marriage. I asked them to place their clay figures in relation to each other at a distance that was comfortable. They chose a moderate distance apart and said that worked as a comfort zone where each was occupied with their separate activities and did not need the other, except as support in the background. When the clay figures were moved closer together the couple were less comfortable. I asked the clay pieces to talk to each other why they needed the former amount of distance. Mary said she did not want to be drawn in by his magnets because if she were he would want to have sex and not talk about their problems. John said he felt he had to fill up her emptiness (the holes) and he thought that making love was a positive thing and words only led to more disagreement.

The clay figures continued to have a dialogue and move around the tray. Mary offered to take some of John's blue clay and make her clay hole smaller if he would remove some of the magnets and let her have them when she wanted them. The clay gave this couple a dynamic vehicle to demonstrate concretely inner anxieties that were unspoken up to now. The session concluded with an agreement that the "figures would stand still until next week," which to them meant that they would not do the chase, reject, or pursue until we had time to readdress this area of tension. The three-dimensional media allowed for movement, metaphorically redefining the shape of the problem by exchanging colors and giving the couple a chance to see how their transactions had become a pattern that was not useful. The clay figures could "converse" because they were once removed from reality.

PARADOX AND REFRAMING

Many times the couple therapist will be confronted with situations that either puts clients in a double bind or demonstrates a paradoxical bind that has entrapped the couple. Paradox cannot be confronted on the same cognitive level as other conflictual situations because it will not respond until the thinking has moved to another level (Haley, 1963).

A couple came into therapy with the complaint that she was "too old" and he persistently stayed "too young." There was an age discrepancy of about 6 years. Indeed, the wife was older and the husband was younger. They confronted me saying,

"You must solve this problem because it is ruining our marriage." I realized I could do nothing about age, nor could they. Without addressing this problem, I asked them to bring in their birth certificates to the session and then I asked them to re-create a single birth certificate. They cut them up and reformed them into a single collage. The couple was aware of the underlying implications of this task, and we did not have to dialogue about it or explore other issues that were embedded in their original request. The couple let go of this complaint as it had been solved on another plane of awareness and discourse.

Reframing is also helpful in situations in which there is great deal of energy being expended by the couple on keeping a point of contention alive and flourishing. By not trying to eliminate the problem but giving it a changed meaning, a positive meaning, a shift in the system can be created. For example, Jean was unhappy in her marriage because her husband was unresponsive to sex unless she was the aggressor and instigated intercourse. Jean was a rather mild-mannered woman who dressed and acted conservatively. She, however, did enjoy lovemaking and was also conflicted over the societal message that says that women should never ask for sex. She was drawing her depression and gradually allowing some of the anger to spill onto the page when I had a sudden flash, which I shared with her. I said, "Jean, I just was overtaken by an image of you that has me shaken! I see you as a Jungle Queen, who takes her man when she wants him!" She looked startled, then suddenly straightened up, threw her head back, rose, and said, "I believe you." I can truthfully say she stalked out of the room.

From that session on we had very little discussion about her husband's performance in bed. The husband was delighted, Jean was free of the restriction that told her that initiating sex was "unwomanly," and the couple's lovemaking greatly improved.

CONCLUSION

Couple therapy is one of the greatest challenges of treatment; however, the addition of art expressions greatly improves the chances for a positive outcome. The multiplicity of issues that arise in a relationship reflecting old beliefs from the past, roles that society has imposed, and the differing modes of thinking that a man and a woman bring to problem solving are exciting. These issues can be made visible through the use of art and, when made visible, transform abstract words into material that can be altered. The case examples offered earlier demonstrate the effect the art product has on understanding the difficulties and miscommunications that often have a negative impact on the individuals in a relationship.

The notion that the partner would be acceptable, even happier, if he or she "saw the world as I do" is the ongoing lament in many marriages. Without providing the lens with which to "see" the other's viewpoint, the therapy is stagnant. Art is the language that complements and illuminates verbal narrative and is the essential added ingredient. The use of art expression opens doors to material either too sensitive or forgotten and is the key to helping couples find alternative solutions to their conflicts and to create a preferred outcome.

REFERENCES

Bobes, T., & Rothman, B. (1998). *The crowded bed*. New York: Norton.

Bowlby, J. (1969). *Attachment*. New York: Basic Books.

Christensen, A., & Jacobson, N. S. (2000). *Reconcilable differences*. New York: Guilford Press.

Damasio, A. R. (1994). *Descartes' error*. New York: Avon Books.

Goleman, D. (1995). *Emotional intelligence*. New York: Bantam Books.

Haley, J. (1963). *Strategies of psychotherapy*. New York: Grune & Stratten.

Halford, W. K. (2001). *Brief therapy for couples: Helping partners help themselves*. New York: Guilford Press.

Landgarten, H. B. (1981). *Clinical art therapy*. New York: Brunner/Mazel.

McGoldrick, M., & Gerson, R. (1985). *Genograms in family assessments*. New York: Norton.

Riley, S., & Malchiodi, C. (1994). *Integrative approaches to family art therapy*. Chicago: Magnolia Street.

Wadeson, H. (1980). *Art psychotherapy*. New York: Wiley.

Art-Based Assessments

This brief section serves as an introduction to four art-based assessments: Diagnostic Drawing Series, Silver Drawing Test, Formal Elements Art Therapy Scale, and the MARI Card Test. Many therapists have used projective drawing tests such as the House–Tree–Person and Draw-A-Person in evaluation, but researchers in the field of art therapy have developed and are currently standardizing several art-based assessments. These assessments look at drawings through the structural quality, use of materials, client-generated narratives, and other aspects rather than specific items, elements, or omissions inherent to evaluating projective drawings tests.

Readers are cautioned that they may need additional training to use the assessments described in this section. A basic description of each assessment is provided with examples and references to additional literature for further study.

The Diagnostic Drawing Series

Anne Mills

THE DEVELOPMENT OF THE DIAGNOSTIC DRAWING SERIES

The creation of the Diagnostic Drawing Series (DDS) in the early 1980s was a response to three important questions facing the field of art therapy: (1) can we accurately differentiate diagnoses through art, particularly by generalizing from the art of a group of people? (Gantt & Howie, 1979; Levy & Ulman, 1974; Wadeson, 1971), (2) how shall we assess people through art? (Kwiatkowska, 1967; Rubin, 1978; Ulman, 1965), and (3) can the form of art tell us as much or more about the artist as its content? (Arnheim, 1954/1974; Rhyne, 1979; Ulman & Levy, 1968).

The DDS offers a way to contribute to accurate differential diagnosis and provides a structure for participating in sound diagnostic research because reliable diagnostic information was collected when the art was made (Cohen, 1983). The DDS art interview has a protocol that clearly specifies which art materials are to be used and how it is to be administered (Cohen, 1983). It is the first art therapy assessment with an accompanying rating system that focuses primarily on the structure or formal qualities of the picture (Cohen, 1986a).

In 1983 the DDS project won the annual Research Award of the American Art Therapy Association for its collaborative design, which helps art therapists work together despite geographical separation. It was then that instructions for administering the DDS became widely available, enabling art therapists from different parts of the world to administer the DDS in the same way. The resultant drawings could be compared to each other productively. In the mid-1980s the first DDS research was presented, the first publication on the tool appeared (Cohen, 1986b), and a DDS newsletter was launched to meet the growing demand for information on the tool by psychologists (Cohen, 1985; Turkington, 1985). In 1988 the first DDS research paper, which normed three psychiatric diagnoses and controls, was published (Cohen, Hammer, & Singer, 1988).

HOW TO ADMINISTER THE DIAGNOSTIC DRAWING SERIES

The DDS is designed to be administered on a tabletop and must be drawn with a package of 12 colors of soft chalk pastels with flat sides and no paper wrappers around the sticks. One box of chalk can be used to draw many DDSs. A white 18″ × 24″/45 × 60 cm drawing paper, preferably 70 pounds with a slightly rough surface, must be used. No substitutions are acceptable. The advantages of the DDS include the use of good quality supplies that art therapists use for their own art—large, attractive paper and chalk pastels that can be used in both a fluid and resistive way (Lusebrink, 1990, p. 85). This is respectful to the artist/client, and introduces the potential for truly expressive art making during what may be the first art therapy contact.

The artist/client is informed that (1) he or she may turn the paper in any direction; (2) he or she has up to 15 minutes to work on each drawing, if needed; (3) he or she will be asked to make three pictures, that there is a separate piece of paper for each drawing, and that the directions for each picture will be given one at a time; and (4) the pictures will be discussed when the artist is finished.

For the first picture the artist is asked to "make a picture using these materials" (paper and pastels). When presenting the second sheet of paper, the instruction is "draw a picture of a tree," even if a tree was drawn in the first picture. The third task is to "make a picture of how you're feeling, using lines, shapes, and colors." These three pictures are different types of tasks which allow the art therapist to see disparate strengths and difficulties (Figures 1, 2, and 3). If the artist/client is unable to start or complete any of the three pictures, the blank or incomplete drawing is saved as a part of the Series. To end the session and to gain important information, his or her thoughts and associations about the drawings should be discussed.

The DDS is designed to be administered in one 50-minute session; however, most people complete it in about 20 minutes. It can be used with individuals age 13 and older. A number of researchers have worked with younger children using a variety of versions of a modified DDS. Please note that the Handbook (Cohen, 1983) must be consulted prior to giving a DDS so that the art interview is administered properly. More detailed information on how the Series was developed, the function of the pictures as elements of the Series, and many other matters about the DDS are published elsewhere (Cohen, Mills, & Kijak, 1994).

DIFFERENTIAL DIAGNOSIS AND THE DIAGNOSTIC DRAWING SERIES

The word "diagnostic" is part of this assessment's name because, from the beginning of its clinical use, research has been done grouping DDS drawings by the diagnoses given to the artist/clients by psychiatrists. Because the possibility of error in psychiatric diagnosis was much under discussion around the time of the creation of the DDS, the decision was made that two agreeing diagnoses must accompany any Series accepted into the research. The attending physician's admission diagnosis on an inpatient psychiatry unit is used, as well as the diagnosis of a second psychiatrist. The second or "cross-reference psychiatrist is expected to have an interview of at least twenty minutes duration with each patient" and "*may not* read the chart prior to interviewing the patient or formulating the diagnosis" (Cohen, 1983, p. 3). If the two diagnoses are not in accord with each other, the art is not used for research purposes.

The DDS is "diagnostic" in that an art therapist trained in it and familiar with its research basis has the ability to contribute sound, clear-cut, practical information to the diagnostic process. The name of the assessment does not mean that simply administering the

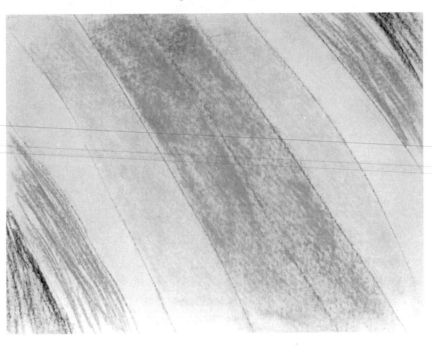

FIGURE 1. Diagnostic Drawing Series, Picture One, drawn in response to the request "Make a picture using these materials." The Series is by a nonpatient control (i.e., someone not psychiatrically hospitalized), a 25-year-old female.

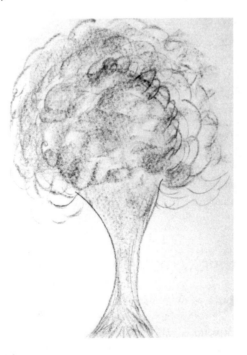

FIGURE 2. Diagnostic Drawing Series, Picture Two, drawn in response to the request "Draw a picture of a tree."

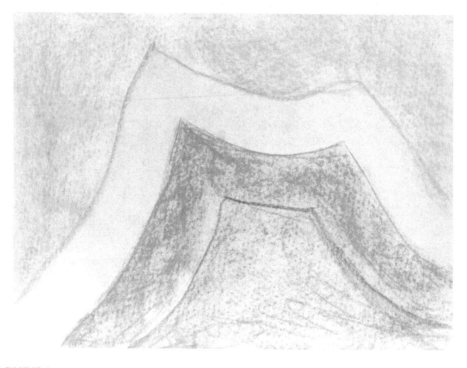

FIGURE 3. Diagnostic Drawing Series, Picture Three, drawn in response to the request "Make a picture of how you're feeling, using lines, shapes, and colors."

assessment will lead to a diagnosis. That is dependent on the DDS-specific knowledge of the assessors and whether they are allowed to give or contribute to a diagnosis.

The DDS is also "diagnostic" in that its objective is to "detect . . . and classify the client's pathology, focusing primarily on its causes, symptoms, severity, and prognosis" (Bruscia, 1988, p. 5). The point is to see what configurations have been drawn on the three pages and to inform clinicians how to identify them accurately (Dawes, Faust, & Meehl, 1989), not to interpret them in terms of a particular theory. However, clinicians can and do bring the skills and constructs that aid them in their work into assessment sessions. Information from the art interview as a whole may contribute to treatment planning. For example, one can and should see clients' strengths by means of their DDSs (Cohen & Mills, 1994). Strengths may be defined in part as the presence of formal elements associated with the DDSs of nonpatient controls, or the absence of criteria found in the DDSs of any diagnostic group.

UNDERSTANDING THE FORM OR STRUCTURE OF ART

It is important to understand that many of the marks in a picture are not symbolic (Kreitler & Kreitler, 1972). Moreover, in a drawing assessment, some of the most important information about the art and the artist is not symbolic, or metaphorical, or about the process of making the picture; rather, it derives from the form or structural level of the drawing. Relying on the content of the picture as the main way to grasp the art's meaning, though shown to have some use in developmental and intelligence measures, can produce misleading interpretations (Groth-Marnat, 1997).

Cohen, the primary creator of the DDS, studied under art therapist Janie Rhyne. He attributes the structural approach of the DDS to her research on form as content. Rhyne was the first art therapist to systematically study structural or formal elements—abstract lines and shapes—to determine meaning in art without relying on narrative content (Rhyne, 1979). DDS research revealed that a number of components of structure, such as placement of the image on the page, the quality of lines that are straight or undulate, or how much of the page is used, cluster in characteristic combinations to create a graphic profile of the artist/client and, by extension, diagnostic categories.

When viewing an image, whether in a gallery or in a clinical situation, we characteristically absorb an enormous amount of information about color, shape, pressure, and placement instantaneously but without being consciously aware of doing so. We slow down to note the faces, the story depicted, and the style (Zeki, 1999). It is now known that viewing art is an "active process in which the brain . . . discards, selects, and by comparing the selected information to its stored record, generates the visual image" (Zeki, 1999, p. 21). Different compartments process different aspects of visual data (e.g., form, color, and motion); each emphasizes a particular part of the field of view; all are essential. The association cortex compares these impressions with prior visual experience and quickly understands constancies and patterns. "The brain is interested in particularities, but only with the broader aim of categorizing a particularity into a more general scheme" (Zeki, 1999, p. 39).

Approaching the DDS through the structural level encourages viewers to slow down and teaches them to retrace the incredibly rapid process of the brain back from seeing the pattern, through the content and the story of the picture, to the formal elements that make up the picture. Figures 1, 2, and 3 illustrate how useful this is. Rather than trying to guess the artist's diagnosis (if any) by comparing one's impressions to visual memory, or trying to focus on possible symbolism in the Series, one considers the structural elements. In this Series there are structural elements that overlap with the ten criteria found to be statistically significant in a study of the nonpatient control sample (Cohen et al., 1988). Many of these same graphic indicators were found again and confirmed in other studies of adults (Couch, 1994; Morris, 1995) and children without psychiatric illnesses (Gulbro-Leavitt & Schimmel, 1991; Neale, 1994). It was easy to see that despite the age gap and developmental difference in the art in these various studies, the pictures were structurally similar. Investigators are able to compare the ratings of different groups because the pictures were collected in the same standardized way—comparing apples to apples, if you will.

Just as certain structural categories typified the DDSs of nonpatient controls and established a graphic profile for this group, each other group examined using the DDS has its own distinctive graphic profile. This process of looking at people who share something in common, such as the diagnosis of schizophrenia, is called norming and has been applied to 21 different groups using the DDS (Mills, 2002).

In addition to the presence of statistically significant criteria which suggest that Figures 1, 2, and 3 are drawn by a nonpatient, one also looks for the absence of the statistically significant elements associated with the art of people who do have psychiatric diagnoses. In other words, we can rule out the possibility that the DDS is made by a person with a psychiatric diagnosis because it contains no statistically significant characteristic of such groups (e.g., there is no unusual placement) and at the same time it does contain some of the statistically significant elements found in the work of nonpatient controls (e.g., full space use in Figure 3).

STRENGTHS AND LIMITATIONS
OF THE DIAGNOSTIC DRAWING SERIES

How can art be rated fairly, avoiding viewer projection and other pitfalls? If words could be defined and used to describe precisely the marks on the page (without having to rule that the marks mean "house"), one can report what is present and avoid guessing the artist's intentions or judging the artist's success. Art therapists have done this in creating the DDS Rating Guide. One of the most important contributions of the DDS may be the language it has marshaled to express in a precise and objective way what is seen on the page.

Numerous tests to see if people with and without training were able to perceive and rate formal elements accurately show that the rating system is highly reliable (Mills, Cohen, & Meneses, 1993). The same review noted that the DDS is also highly valid when used with a variety of types of people; that is, the drawing test and its Rating Guide do measure aspects of how people draw that help in understanding them and their art. It has been demonstrated that this objective art therapy vocabulary of formal elements is simple and accurate to use. Metaphorically, the language of the Rating Guide is the net used to catch the fish that interest the researchers: clusters of statistically significant graphic indicators across a large number of drawings in a sample (Cohen et al., 1994).

Again, this is not an X = Y reduction such as was once taught by some—that this kind of tree drawing means the artist probably has schizophrenia. Instead, it is the development of a graphic profile based on research on the art of many people in many categories, so that we know not only how the DDSs of those diagnosed with schizophrenia tend to look but also how they differ from those of people diagnosed with borderline personality disorder, for instance.

Of course, the structural level is not the only level that those trained in the use of the DDS look at in a picture or observe during an art therapy session. In clinical work with the DDS there is no intention, or indeed possibility, of reducing each artist's individual richness and variability. On the contrary, a construct has been formulated to describe a systematic way to incorporate all the information in a DDS session into a well-rounded clinical response. The author calls this approach "Cohen's Tri-level Model" and teaches it in DDS trainings. A related approach, the Integrative Method, has been published (Cohen & Cox, 1995).

Researchers have published studies which provide graphic profiles (the cluster of formal characteristics which are emblematic for a given group) of adjustment disorder and conduct disorder (Neale, 1994), schizophrenia (Cohen et al., 1988; Morris, 1995), eating disorder (Kessler, 1994), major depression (Cohen et al., 1988; Morris, 1995), dissociative identity disorder (Fowler & Ardon, in press; Mills & Cohen, 1993; Morris, 1995), dysthymia (Cohen et al., 1988), women with disturbed body image (Cohen & Mills, 1999), and children who have witnessed domestic violence (Woodward, 1998; Yahnke, 2000). Additionally, there are unpublished DDS studies of almost all of the above mentioned groups. More information on these studies, plus unpublished studies on nine other diagnostic categories, is available from the DDS Project clearinghouse (P.O. Box 9853, Alexandria, VA 22304) and will be available from the future DDS website.

Even though there are generalities in art and human creative behavior, and group commonalities are useful to know, individual peculiarities are still dominant. Therefore, no single Series is a perfect example of a given group and a single Series is unlikely to include all statistically significant indicators.

CROSS-CULTURAL CONSIDERATIONS

Instructions on how to administer the DDS are currently available in six languages. Researchers have increased their cultural competence by becoming aware of graphic responses by a wide variety of artist/clients making DDSs: that people who live in deserts have no difficulty drawing cacti in response to the instruction to draw a tree; or that Japanese people draw red suns, as that is how they conceptualize the sun (Yamashita, 1989).

A drawing system that judges the meaning of content (e.g., does the picture's story make sense?) could be problematic in that what is considered normal differs from culture to culture. The DDS rating system primarily looks at form. When content is rated, no value judgment is given (e.g., Is an animal present or not present? Not, does this look normal?). However, it is potentially useful to note, for example, when a DDS is drawn entirely in white on white paper or when blue is used to denote skin in drawing a person. Idiosyncratic color, as these examples would be rated, can help distinguish those with psychopathology from those with none, and so it would be unwise to ignore such important information.

CONCLUSION

A tool is only as effective as its user. Administered by a clinician sensitive to the full range of information it can elicit, the DDS can be a natural part of treatment that explores deeply personal individual themes, or sociopolitical issues, without imposing reductive interpretation. However, it can also be used toward more unidimensional clinical and research ends, according to professional needs. Proper training in the administration and analysis of the DDS is always recommended. Applying DDS research data to other drawing assessment tools is not recommended because there is no firm evidence that DDS research findings can be transferred accurately or meaningfully to other art.

The construction of the DDS art interview, its strengths as a diagnostic aid and descriptive system, the volume of studies spanning 1983 to the present, and a published literature base make it one of the best-known and more commonly taught assessments in art therapy (Hall & Knapp, 1993; Mills, 1995; Mills & Goodwin, 1991; Mills, 1995; Smitheman-Brown, 1998).

The DDS project continues to address the complex relationship between art production, personality, and psychiatric diagnosis. In so doing, it provides a solid structure for clinical use and invites continuing inquiry.

ACKNOWLEDGMENT

Special thanks to art therapist Pam Manner who collected the DDSs that appear in Figures 1, 2, and 3 and donated them to the DDS Archives. Photo: Mills.

REFERENCES

Arnheim, R. (1974). *Art and visual perception*. Berkeley: University of California Press. (Original work published 1954)

Bruscia, K. E. (1988). Standards for clinical assessment in the arts therapies. *The Arts in Psychotherapy, 15*, 5–10.

Cohen, B. M. (Ed.). (1983). *The Diagnostic Drawing Series Handbook.**

Cohen, B. M. (Ed.). (1985). *DDS Newsletter.**

Cohen, B. M. (Ed.). (1986a). *The Diagnostic Drawing Series Rating Guide.**

Cohen, B. M. (1986b). Een nieuwe tekentest (A new diagnostic test). *Psychologie, 4*, 26–29.

Cohen, B. M., & Cox, C. T. (1995). *Telling without talking: Art as a window into the world of multiple personality.* New York: Norton.

Cohen, B. M., Hammer, J. S., & Singer, S. (1988). The Diagnostic Drawing Series: A systematic approach to art therapy evaluation and research. *The Arts in Psychotherapy, 15*(1), 11–21.

Cohen, B. M., & Mills, A. (1994). *How to write an evaluation, using the Diagnostic Drawing Series.**

Cohen, B. M., & Mills, A. (1999). Skin/paper/bark: Body image, trauma, and the Diagnostic Drawing Series. In J. Goodwin & R. Attias (Eds.), *Splintered reflections: Images of the body in trauma* (pp. 203–221). New York: Basic Books.

Cohen, B. M., Mills, A., & Kijak, A. K. (1994). An introduction to the Diagnostic Drawing Series: A standardized tool for diagnostic and clinical use. *Art Therapy, 11*(2), 105–110.

Couch, J. B. (1994). Diagnostic Drawing Series: Research with older people diagnosed with organic mental syndrome and disorders. *Art Therapy, 11*(3), 111–115.

Dawes, R. M., Faust, D., & Meehl, P. E. (1989). Clinical versus actuarial judgment. *Science, New Series, 243*(4899), 1668–1674.

Fowler, J., & Ardon, A. (in press). Using the Diagnostic Drawing Series for the screening of dissociative disorders. *The Arts in Psychotherapy.*

Gantt, L., & Howie, P. (1979). Diagnostic categories and art work. *Proceedings of the Tenth Annual Conference of the American Art Therapy Association* (pp. 120–121). Alexandria, VA: American Art Therapy Association.

Groth-Marnat, G. (1997). Projective drawings. In G. Groth-Marnat (Ed.), *Handbook of psychological assessment* (3rd ed., pp. 499–533). New York: Wiley.

Gulbro-Leavitt, C., & Schimmel, B. (1991). Brief report: Assessing depression in children and adolescents using the Diagnostic Drawing Series modified for children (DDS-C). *The Arts in Psychotherapy, 18*(4), 353–356.

Hall, N., & Knapp, J. (Speakers). (1993). *National practice study of art therapists* (Cassette Recording No. 66). Denver, CO: National Audio Video.

Kessler, K. (1994). A study of the Diagnostic Drawing Series with eating disordered patients. *Art Therapy, 11*(2), 116–118.

Kreitler, H., & Kreitler, S. (1972). *Psychology of the arts.* Durham, NC: Duke University Press.

Kwiatkowska, H. Y. (1967, January). The use of families' art productions for psychiatric evaluation. *Bulletin of Art Therapy,* pp. 52–69.

Levy, B. I., & Ulman, E. (1974). The effect of training on judging psychopathology from paintings. *American Journal of Art Therapy, 14*(1), 24–27.

Lusebrink, V. B. (1990). *Imagery and visual expression in therapy.* New York: Plenum Press.

Mills, A. (1995). Outpatient art therapy with multiple personality disorder: A survey of current practice. *Art Therapy, 12*(4), 253–256.

Mills, A. (2002). *Diagnostic Drawing Series Resource List.**

Mills, A., & Cohen, B. M. (1993). Facilitating the identification of multiple personality disorder through art: The Diagnostic Drawing Series. In E. Kluft (Ed.), *Expressive and functional therapies in the treatment of multiple personality disorder* (pp. 39–66). Springfield, IL: Charles C Thomas.

Mills, A., Cohen, B. M., & Meneses, J. Z. (1993). Reliability and validity tests of the Diagnostic Drawing Series. *The Arts in Psychotherapy, 20*(1), 83–88.

Mills, A., & Goodwin, R. (1991). A survey of assessment use in child art therapy. *Art Therapy, 8*(2), 10–14.

Morris, M. B. (1995). The Diagnostic Drawing Series and the Tree Rating Scale: An isomorphic representation of multiple personality disorder, major depression, and schizophrenia populations. *Art Therapy, 12*(2), 118–128.

Neale, E. L. (1994). The Children's Diagnostic Drawing Series. *Art Therapy, 11*(2), 119–126.

Rhyne, J. (1979). *Drawings as personal constructs: A study in visual dynamics.* Doctoral dissertation prepared for University of California, Santa Cruz, CA.

Rubin, J. A. (1978). *Child art therapy.* New York: Van Nostrand Reinhold.

---

*References marked with an asterisk are available from Barry M. Cohen, P. O. Box 9853, Alexandria, Virginia 22304.

Smitheman-Brown, V. (1998). *Survey of assessments taught in AATA-approved programs*. Unpublished manuscript.

Turkington, C. (1985). Therapist seeks correlation between diagnosis, drawings. *APA Monitor, 16*(4), 34–36.

Ulman, E. (1965). A new use of art in psychiatric diagnosis. *Bulletin of Art Therapy, 4*, 91–116.

Ulman, E., & Levy, B. I. (1968). An experimental approach to the judgement of psychopathology from paintings. *Bulletin of Art Therapy, 8*, 3–12.

Wadeson, H. (1971). Characteristics of art expression in depression. *Journal of Nervous and Mental Disease, 153*, 197–204.

Woodward, S. (1998). Usefulness of the Child Diagnostic Drawing Series within the child witness to domestic violence population. *Canadian Journal of Art Therapy, 12*(1), 11–33.

Yahnke, L. (2000). *The Diagnostic Drawing Series as an assessment for children who have witnessed marital violence*. Doctoral dissertation, Minnesota School of Professional Psychology, Minneapolis, MN.

Yamashita, Y. (Speaker). (1989). Analysis of Japanese general psychiatric population, in The Diagnostic Drawing Series: Its use in clinical practice. *Proceedings of the Twentieth Annual Conference of the American Art Therapy Association* (p. 21). Mundelein, IL: American Art Therapy Association.

Zeki, S. (1999). *Inner vision: An exploration of art and the brain*. Oxford: Oxford University Press.

The Silver Drawing Test of Cognition and Emotion

Rawley A. Silver

This chapter describes the Silver Drawing Test (SDT) and summarizes two new studies from its 2001 and 2002 updates: cross-cultural studies and the uses of humor in responses to the drawing tasks. The purpose of the SDT is to bypass an individual's language deficiencies which can mask the intelligence of a child or adult, assess cognitive skills and emotional strengths, and provide access to fantasies and concepts of self and others. The SDT is based on the premise that drawings can take the place of words as the primary channel for receiving and expressing ideas. Drawing can serve as a language parallel to the spoken or written word; can reflect emotion; and can help identify, assess, and develop cognitive skills.

The SDT uses "stimulus drawings" to prompt responses that solve problems and represent concepts. These stimulus drawings consist of line drawings of people, animals, places, and things. Some are explicit, while others are ambiguous to encourage associations (see Figure 1). The SDT includes two sets of 15 stimulus drawings. Form A is reserved for testing; Form B is provided for use in therapeutic or developmental programs. There are three subtests: Drawing from Imagination, Predictive Drawing, and Drawing from Observation. Responses to drawing tasks are scored on rating scales that range from 1 to 5 points, with 5 the highest score. The cognitive scales assess ability to represent concepts of space, sequential order, and class inclusion, the three independent structures that have been identified as fundamental in mathematics (Piaget, 1970) and reading (Bannatyne, 1971). Other scales assess emotional content, self-images, and humor.

This section presents each of the subtests; why and how the test items were selected and field-tested; a review of reliability, validity, and normative data; and summaries of studies that used the SDT with clinical and nonclinical populations. More detailed information can be obtained in *Three Art Assessments* (Silver, 2002).

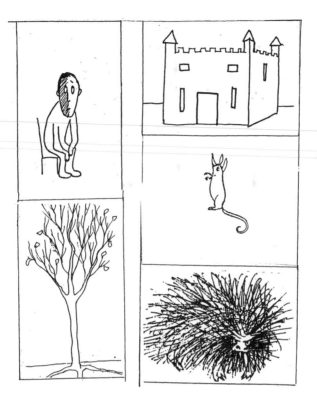

FIGURE 1. Stimulus drawing images. Copyright 1996 by Rawley Silver. Reprinted by permission.

HOW THE STIMULUS DRAWINGS AND SDT WERE DEVELOPED

I had volunteered to work with deaf children who could not lipread, speak, or communicate manually after I was deafened temporarily in an accident during the 1960s. Previously, painting had been my vocation, and I wanted to introduce the children to the pleasures of studio art experiences after visiting several schools which provided little or no art education for deaf students.

At first I used gestures, but sketching was much more effective. For example, a quick sketch of my family prompted sketches of their families, and soon we were sharing other experiences through drawing. It became evident that most of the children were highly intelligent, even though they performed poorly on traditional tests of intelligence. It seemed to me that art procedures could be used to bypass verbal deficiencies and develop the concepts cited by Piaget (1970) and others as fundamental in mathematics and reading. I asked the children to draw, paint, and model clay into sequences and reversals, as well as from observation and imagination. Children who needed help in getting started were asked to choose some of my sketches and use them in drawings of their own. Eventually, my most popular sketches became stimulus drawings in the SDT and two other assessments. The SDT was first published in 1983 (Silver, 1983), then revised in 1990 and 1996 (Silver, 1990/1996), and updated in Silver (2001, 2002).

THE DRAWING FROM IMAGINATION SUBTEST

Respondents are asked to choose two or more stimulus drawings and to imagine something happening between the subjects they choose; they then are asked to draw what they imagine. They are encouraged to change the stimulus drawings, adding their own subjects and ideas. When they finish drawing, they are asked to add titles or stories and, finally, when appropriate, discuss their responses to clarify meanings. The task is based on the observation that different individuals perceive the same stimulus drawings differently, and that responses reflect feelings about self and others, as well as cognitive skills, in ways that can be quantified.

The Drawing from Imagination subtest is used to assess the emotional content of responses, concepts of self and others, and three cognitive skills: ability to select, combine, and represent. These skills are fundamental in using language and forming concepts, as discussed next.

The Emotional Content Scale

This scale ranges from strongly negative to strongly positive themes or fantasies. Strongly negative themes, such as drawings about suicide or life-threatening relationships, receive the lowest score, 1 point. Moderately negative responses, such as drawings about angry subjects or stressful relationships, are scored 2 points. The intermediate score, 3 points, is used to characterize ambivalent, ambiguous, or unemotional themes (neither negative nor positive, or both negative and positive).

On the positive side, moderately positive themes, such as drawings about friendly relationships or fortunate but passive subjects, score 4 points, while strongly positive themes, such as drawings about caring relationships or effective individuals, score 5 points, the highest score.

The Self-Image Scale

This scale also ranges from strongly negative to strongly positive. A strongly negative self-image, such as identifying with a subject portrayed as sad, helpless, or in mortal danger, scores 1 point. A strongly positive self-image, such as identifying with a subject portrayed as beloved or achieving goals, scores 5 points. Unclear, ambivalent, unemotional, or invisible self-images score 3 points, and moderately negative or positive self-images score 2 and 4 points, respectively.

The Humor Scale

This scale ranges from Lethal humor (1 point) to Playful humor (5 points). Lethal humor seems to invite the viewer to laugh at subjects in mortal danger, as portrayed in responses to the Drawing from Imagination task. Disparaging humor (2 points) invites the viewer to laugh at unfortunate subjects, and may ridicule others or oneself.

On the positive side, Resilient humor (4 points) depicts or implies hopeful or favorable outcomes, while Playful humor (5 points) seems to have no hidden agenda but is meant to be amusing, motivated by feelings of good will. Humor that is both positive and negative, neither positive nor negative, or else unclear, scores 3 points.

The Cognitive Scale

There is evidence that language and thought develop independently, that language follows rather than precedes logical thinking, and that although language expands and facilitates thought, high-level thinking can and does proceed without it (Langer, 1951; Piaget, 1970; Schlain, 1998). The cognitive scale ranges between high and low levels of ability to deal with the concept of a class or category of objects which involves the ability to select and combine into a context. Selecting and combining are fundamental operations underlying verbal behavior. Disturbance in the ability to select words is evident in receptive language disorders. Disturbance in the ability to combine words into sentences is evident in expressive language disorders. Selecting and combining are also fundamental in creativity and the visual arts. Creative individuals make exceptional leaps in selecting, as well as combining and representing their selections, through images, words, or other media. Painters select colors and shapes, and if their work is figurative, they select and combine images into visual contexts.

Ability to Select (the Content of a Drawing)

Young children tend to select objects on the basis of perceptual attributes, such as color or shape, then begin to select on the basis of function—what subjects do or what is done to them. By early adolescence, they develop conceptual grouping based on invisible attributes or abstract ideas). As rated by the SDT, respondents who select stimulus drawings at a concrete or perceptual level, score 1 point. Those who select at the functional level, score 3 points, and those who select at the conceptual, abstract level, score 5 points. Intermediate levels score 2 and 4 points.

Ability to Combine (the Form of a Drawing)

Young children typically regard objects in isolation, then begin to consider objects in relation to neighboring objects and external frames of reference, such as drawing a line parallel to the bottom of their paper to represent the ground (Piaget & Inhelder, 1967). Adolescents and adults take into account distances, proportions, perspectives, and the dimensions of their paper. As rated by the SDT, respondents who relate their subjects on the basis of proximity score 1 point, 3 points if they combine subjects along a base line, and 5 points if the drawing shows overall coordination. Intermediate levels score 2 and 4 points.

Ability to Represent (the Creativity of a Drawing, Title, or Story)

It seems to be generally agreed that creative individuals share traits such as originality, fluency, flexibility, and playfulness. Torrance (1980) has cautioned against trying to separate creativity from intelligence because they interact and overlap.

As rated by the SDT, responses that are imitative, copying stimulus drawings or stereotypes, are characterized by the low score 1 point; responses that revise the stimulus drawings score 3 points, and responses that transform the stimulus drawings, or are original, expressive, playful, or suggestive, score 5 points, with intermediate levels scoring 2 and 4 points.

THE DRAWING FROM OBSERVATION SUBTEST

This subtest assesses concepts of space and the ability to represent spatial relationships in height, width, and depth. Respondents are asked to draw an arrangement in a standardized format of three different cylinders and a small stone. As observed by Piaget and Inhelder (1967), young children tend to regard objects in isolation. As they mature, they become aware of spatial relationships, and by adolescence, they arrive at a coordinated system embracing objects in three dimensions. On the SDT, responses that represent spatial relationships accurately receive the top 5-point score. Lower levels of ability receive lower scores. Details are provided in the SDT manual (Silver, 1990/1996, 2002).

THE PREDICTIVE DRAWING SUBTEST

This subtest evaluates ability to sequence and the ability to conserve; that is, to recognize constancy in spite of transformations in appearance. Most rational thought depends on this ability, which begins to develop around the age of 7. Participants are asked to predict changes in the appearance of objects by adding lines to outline drawings. The first task evaluates the ability to sequence. Individuals are asked to imagine taking sips of a soda until the glass is empty, then draw lines in a row of glasses to show how the liquid decreases as it is consumed. A response receives the highest rating if it represents the diminishing soda with a single series of lines without erasures or corrections, indicating a systematic approach. A descending series of line with erasures or corrections receives the intermediate rating (trial and error), and an incomplete sequence, or no sequence, receives the lowest rating.

Two additional tasks assess concepts of horizontality and verticality, as well as the ability to conserve. Respondents are asked draw lines in the stimulus drawings to show how water would appear in a tilted container, and how a house would appear if moved to a steep slope. Scores are based on observations by Piaget and Inhelder (1967), who devised these two tasks.

ADMINISTRATION

The SDT may be administered individually or in group settings to adults and children over age 5. It is not timed, but usually takes about 20 minutes and can be administered without prior training by art therapists, psychologists, and teachers.

RELIABILITY, VALIDITY, AND NORMATIVE DATA

To collect information about reliability and validity and to develop normative data, the SDT has been administered to 1,399 children, adolescents, and adults (Silver, 2002). The sample includes 849 presumably typical or unimpaired respondents, and 550 with brain injuries, hearing or language impairments, learning disabilities, or emotional disturbances. The SDT was administered and/or scored by 21 art therapists, psychologists, and teachers residing in California, Florida, Idaho, Nebraska, New Jersey, New York, Pennsylvania, Wisconsin, and Canada.

Scorer reliability was examined in six studies. In one, the correlation coefficients for seven judges ranged between .91 and .98 on the three SDT subtests. In another, the correlations between five judges ranged between .74 and .94 on the Self-Image and Emotional Content scales.

Retest reliability was examined in two studies. In one, the SDT was administered twice to 12 adolescents with learning disabilities after an interval of approximately 1 month. In each of the three subtests, the correlations were significant at the .05 level of probability. In the other, the test was administered twice to 10 third-graders after a 1-month interval. The retest–test correlation of total test scores was .72, significant at the .02 level of probability.

To determine validity, differences between pretest and posttest scores, relationships with traditional tests of intelligence, and evidence of age and gender differences were examined. Pre- and posttest changes were found in six studies, including studies of children with and without learning disabilities, adolescents with multiple handicaps, children with visual–motor disabilities and auditory or language impairments, as well as children performing below grade level and incarcerated adolescents.

The original norms, reported in the 1996 SDT manual (Silver, 1990/1996), were based on the cognitive scores of 624 subjects; students ages 6 to 18 and 77 adults. Their scores increased gradually with age and grade level.

Additional norms (and standard deviations) as well as new findings of age and gender differences in emotional expression, self-image, humor, and cognitive skills are reported in *Three Art Assessments* (Silver, 2002). These respondents included 208 girls and boys in grades 1 to 8, as well as 219 male and 243 female high school students, 51 young adults, and 44 senior adults.

In the cognitive skills assessed by the SDT, the younger adults had higher scores than high school students in each subtest and higher scores than senior adults in Predictive Drawing, but lower scores than senior adults in Drawing from Imagination. As measured by the Emotional Content scale, the neutral, 3-point score predominated. Nevertheless, males tended to have lower, more negative scores in Emotional Content than females, but higher, more positive scores in Self-Image.

To assess the use of humor, 888 Drawings from Imagination were reexamined, and 142 were identified (16%) as humorous. As scored on the 5-point humor scale, their humor tended to be negative (68%), with more disparaging (44%) than lethal (24%). Among positive responses, 17% were playful and 7% were resilient. The remaining 8% were neutral, ambivalent, or ambiguous.

Analyses of variance were used to compare age and gender groups. Males produced significantly more humorous responses than females (chi square (1) = 37.3, p .01), as well as more negative humor, but this tendency reached only borderline significance at the .10 level. Nine males who used strongly negative humor scored 1 point. All were adolescents; 3 had emotional disturbances, 6 were not disturbed. No females portrayed cruelty or suffering.

CROSS-CULTURAL STUDIES

Studies of cultural differences and similarities in responses to the SDT are summarized in Silver (2001, 2002). In Brazil, the SDT was standardized on approximately 2,000 children and adults, ages 5 to 40, by Allessandrini, Duarte, Dupas, and Bianco (1998) who confirmed the dependence of cognitive scores on age and grade level across the two cultures. In emotional content, they found high rates of ambivalence, more negative than positive responses, and a tendency toward negative themes by students in the seventh and eighth grades. They also found strong scorer reliability (correlations coefficients were .94, .95, and .95), and retest reliability (from .62 to .87).

In Russia, Alexander Kopytin (2001, 2002) standardized the SDT on 702 children, adolescents, and adults, with the assistance of Russian psychologists. As in the United States and Brazil, cognitive scores increased with age. Although no differences were found between adults, the cognitive scores of Russian children and adolescents were often higher than scores of their American counterparts in Predictive Drawing, Drawing from Observation, and total test scores, whereas the American scores were higher on the Drawing from Imagination subtest. Kopytin also found differences in Emotional Content and Self-Images.

In Australia, Glenda Hunter (1992) found significant gender differences in the cognitive scores of college men and women, as measured by the SDT. She also observed that her findings were consistent with the theory that cognitive skills evident in verbal conventions also can be evident in visual conventions.

In Thailand, Dhanachitsiriphong (1999) used the SDT as a pre-post test to study the effectiveness of an art therapy program on the cognitive and emotional development of incarcerated male adolescents. After her experiment, the scores of the experimental group were significantly higher than the scores of the control group at the .01 level.

FIELD TESTS

Initial field testing occurred from 1970 to 1983 when the SDT was first published. Two pilot studies (Silver, 1971, 1973a) found gains in the cognitive skills of experimental groups of my art students while the control groups did not improve.

Encouraged by the pilot studies, I applied for a grant for a State Urban Education Project in a school for children with auditory and language impairments. Approval for the project arrived late, after the 1972 school year had started. Because a pretest was scheduled for October, and a project evaluator had not yet been assigned, I was obliged to design the pretest. The test items included Predictive Drawing and Drawing from Imagination, among other tasks, and used stimulus drawings to convey the tasks through images rather than words (Silver, 1973b).

In the developmental program, I worked with an experimental group of 34 children, ages 8 to 15 years, once a week for 11 weeks in the fall and 9 weeks in the spring. The children were a randomly selected 50% sample of 12 classes in the school. The remaining 34 children served as controls. To compare the children with children who had no known impairments, the tasks were presented once to 63 children in a suburban public school.

On the posttest, the experimental group had significantly higher scores than did the control group (at the .01 level) in the combined abilities of Selecting, Combining, and Representing in Drawing from Imagination. In Drawing from Observation, the experimental group improved at the .05 level of significance. The control group did not improve. In Predictive Drawing, the experimental group improved significantly at the .01 level. The control group did not improve. The experimental group also made significant gains in both creativity and art skills (Silver, 1973b).

As shown in Figures 2 and 3, the normal children were superior to the experimental group in the pretest Drawing from Imagination, but not significantly superior. On the posttest, the experimental group was significantly superior. In Drawing from Observation, no significant difference emerged between experimental and normal groups. In Predictive Drawing, the normal group had significantly higher scores on the pretest in both horizontal and vertical orientation. After the art program, no significant difference was found in horizontal orientation. In vertical orientation, the experimental group was significantly superior to the unimpaired group.

A subsequent study found the test items, stimulus drawings, and art programs useful in working with children who had visual–motor disabilities, an opposite constellation of strengths and weaknesses (Silver, 1975; Silver & Lavin, 1977). Eleven graduate students followed the same art program, working under supervision with 11 children. After 10 1-hour sessions, the children showed significant gains in Drawing from Imagination, Drawing from

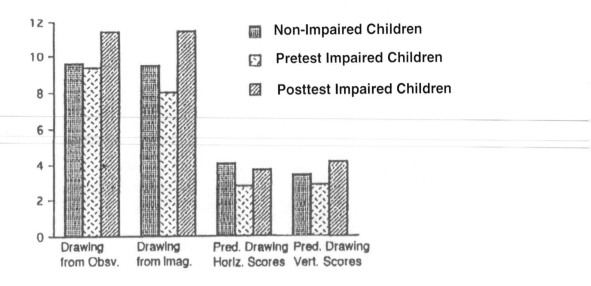

FIGURE 2. Comparing pretest–posttest scores of language/hearing impaired, control, and unimpaired children. Copyright 1996 by Rawley Silver. Reprinted by permission.

Observation, and the sequencing task of Predictive Drawing. The testing and developmental procedures were also tried with adolescents and adults who had suffered brain injuries with promising results (Silver, 1975).

A subsequent study, supported by a grant from the National Institute of Education, built on the previous studies, attempting to verify their results by using a more controlled research design, a wider variety of settings, and a more diverse population (Silver et al., 1980). It also

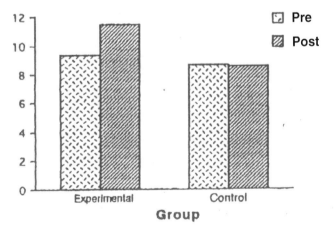

FIGURE 3. Comparing pretest–posttest scores of language/hearing impaired experimental and control groups. Copyright 1996 by Rawley Silver. Reprinted by permission.

examined the relationship of the SDT to traditional tests of intelligence or achievement. Five graduate students in art therapy worked with 84 children who performed at least 1 year below grade level in five schools, one school for children with learning disabilities and four schools for both normal children and those with special needs. A matched control group received no special treatment. Although the posttest scores showed significant gains, no significant differences were found between the posttest scores of experimental and control groups. Subsequently, however, a school-by-school analysis showed significant differences between experimental and control groups on the posttest in one of the schools, a school for children with learning disabilities.

The SDT has also been used in studies of age and gender differences in nonclinical populations. One such study examined differences in attitudes toward self and others. The subjects included 531 respondents in five age groups, ranging from children though senior adults (Silver, 1993). To a highly significant degree, they chose and fantasized about subjects the same gender as themselves. Males tended to express positive attitudes toward their solitary subjects and negative attitudes toward relationships, whereas females expressed positive attitudes toward solitary subjects and both positive and negative attitudes toward relationships. Although males drew assaultive relationships more frequently than females, age and gender differences interacted, resulting in significant age variability. A converse age and gender interaction was found for caring relationships.

Additional SDT studies and reports by other investigators also may be found in Silver (2001, 2002). The publications also include scored responses, scoring forms designed for files of individual students, patients, or clients; and developmental art programs.

REFERENCES

Allessandrini, C. D., Duarte, J. L., Dupas, M. A., and Bianco, M. F. (1998). SDT: The Brazilian standardization of the Silver Drawing Test of Cognition and Emotion. *Art Therapy: Journal of the American Art Therapy Association, 15*(2) 107–115.

Bannatyne, A. (1971). *Language, reading, and learning disabilities.* Springfield, IL: Charles C Thomas.

Dhanachitsiriphong, P. (1999). *The effects of art therapy and rational-emotive therapy on cognition and emotional development of male adolescents in Barn Karuna Training School of the Central Observation and Protection Center.* Unpublished master's thesis, Burapha University, Thailand.

Hunter, G. (1992). *An examination of some individual differences in information processing, personality, and motivation.* Unpublished master's thesis, University of New England, Armidale, Australia.

Kopytin, A. (2001). *The Silver Drawing Test standardization in Russia.* Presentation at the sixth annual conference of the European Consortium of Art Therapy Education (EcarTE).

Kopytin, A. (2002). The Silver Drawing Test of Cognition and Emotion: Standardization in Russia. *American Journal of Art Therapy, 40*(4), 223–237.

Langer, S. K. (1951). *Philosophy in a new key.* New York: Mentor.

Piaget, J. (1970). *Genetic epistemology.* New York: Columbia University Press.

Piaget, J., & Inhelder, B. (1967). *The child's conception of space.* New York: Norton.

Schlain, L. (1998). *The alphabet versus the goddess: The conflict between word and image.* New York: Penguin Putnam.

Silver, R. (1971). The role of art in the cognition, adjustment, transfer, and aptitudes of deaf children. In C. Deussen (Ed.), *Proceedings of the conference on art for the deaf* (pp. 15–26). Los Angeles: Junior Art Center.

Silver, R. (1973a). *A study of cognitive skills development through art experiences.* New York: City Board of Education. State Urban Education Project Number 147 232 101, pp. 3–4.

Silver, R. (1973b). *Cognitive skills development through art experiences: An educational program for language- and hearing impaired and aphasic children.* New York: State Urban Education Project (Report No. 147 232 101). ERIC (Document Reproduction Service No. ED 084 745).

Silver, R. (1975). *Using art to evaluate and develop cognitive skills: Children with communication disorders and children with learning disabilities.* (ERIC Document Reproduction Service No. ED 116 401).

Silver, R. (1983). *The Silver Drawing Test of Cognition and Emotion.* Seattle, WA: Special Child Publications.

Silver, R. (1990/1996). *The Silver Drawing Test of Cognition and Emotion.* Sarasota, FL: Ablin Press.

Silver, R. (1993). Age and gender differences expressed through drawings: A study of attitudes toward self and others. *Art Therapy: Journal of the American Art Therapy Association, 10*(3), 159–168.

Silver, R. (2001). *Art as language: Access to thoughts and feelings through stimulus drawings.* Philadelphia: Brunner-Routledge Psychology Press.

Silver, R. (2002). *Three art assessments: Silver drawing test of cognition and emotion, draw a story, screening for depression and stimulus drawings and techniques.* New York: Brunner-Routledge.

Silver, R., Boeve, E., Hayes, K., Itzler, J., Lavin, C., O'Brien, J., Terner, N., & Wohlberg, P. (1980). *Assessing and developing cognitive skills in handicapped children through art.* New York: College of New Rochelle. (National Institute of Education Project No. G 79 0081. ERIC Document Reproduction Service No. ED 209 878).

Silver, R., & Lavin, C. (1977). The role of art in developing and evaluating cognitive skills. *Journal of Learning Disabilities, 10*(7), 27–35.

Torrance, E. P. (1980). Creative intelligence and an agenda for the 1980s. *Art Education, 33*(7), 8–14.

The Formal Elements Art Therapy Scale and "Draw a Person Picking an Apple from a Tree"

Linda Gantt
Carmello Tabone

For more than 14 years, we have used a single-picture assessment with psychiatric patients and have developed a rating system to measure its variables. Using these tools we conduct both basic and applied art therapy research and clinical studies. The picture is one Lowenfeld employed while studying children's drawings (Lowenfeld, 1939, 1947). The instructions are simply "Draw a person picking an apple from a tree" (PPAT). By holding the content constant we can study the effects of a variety of demographic and psychological characteristics on the way people draw.

Our rating system is a set of 14 scales based on global, formal attributes which we call the Formal Elements Art Therapy Scale (FEATS) (see Table 1) and a set of Content Scales that code for specific colors, the gender of the drawn person, and additional items beyond a person, an apple, and a tree (Gantt, 2001; Gantt & Tabone, 1998).

Originally, we endeavored to measure diagnostic information using the PPAT and the FEATS. Subsequently, we expanded the number of possible applications to a variety of special populations as well as representative samples of both children and adults.

PICTURE COLLECTION

The art materials required are "Mr. Sketch"™ watercolor markers, and white drawing paper 12″ × 18″. The colors are black, brown, yellow, orange, red, purple, magenta, hot pink, turquoise, blue, green, and dark green.

420

TABLE 1. FEATS Scores on Two PPAT Drawings during ECT Treatment

	FEATS scores	
FEATS Scale	Figure 1	Figure 2
1. Prominence of color	1.0	3.0
2. Color fit	1.5	3.0
3. Implied energy	2.0	3.0
4. Space	1.5	2.5
5. Integration	1.5	3.5
6. Logic	1.5	3.5
7. Realism	0	3.0
8. Problem. solving	0	3.5
9. Developmental level	2.0	3.5
10. Details of objects and environment	0	1.5
11. Line quality	3.0	3.0
12. Person	0	2.5
13. Rotation	2.0	5.0
14. Perseveration	4.0	5.0
Total FEATS Score[a]	20.0	45.5

[a]One should exercise caution in comparing the total FEATS scores from other individuals with these above. There are several scales for which a score of 5 is associated with mania (e.g., Implied Energy and Details of Objects and Environment). However, until we can establish norms for a representative sample of nonpatients we cannot say which scores are correlated with specific diagnostic groups. At the time we do establish such norms we will be able to offer a conversion formula or a range of scores so that one can interpret a total score more easily.

We hand the artist the paper so that he or she decides the orientation of the paper and say simply, "Draw a person picking an apple from a tree." If the person asks whether it should be a man or a woman, we repeat the same words emphasizing the word "person." We do not place a time limit on doing the drawing. (Gantt & Tabone, 1998, p. 13)

We ask patients in our psychiatric hospital for a PPAT in the first art therapy session and at discharge. Collecting the drawings at these times is crucial. We assume the pictures reflect symptoms experienced at the time of the drawing (p. 16). For patients getting electroconvulsive therapy (ECT) we obtain a baseline drawing and one after each treatment.

The ease of obtaining PPATs allows us to study a large number of different groups. We currently have PPATs from over 5,000 psychiatric patients and approximately 1,000 adult and child nonpatients. We are working with others to get a representative normative sample of nonpatients for comparison.

THE ADVANTAGES OF USING THE PPAT AND THE FEATS

Lehmann and Risquez (1953) developed specific requirements for an art-based assessment: that it be repeatable; that it could be given to anyone regardless of "artistic ability, interest, cooperation, and intelligence"; that there be a "standardized method of rating"; and that information could be obtained directly from the picture (p. 39). Our methods meet those criteria. Yet, there are some limitations. We recognize that there can be no single art therapy assessment, only a variety of assessments suitable for use in specific situations. Single-picture assessments have the advantage of being easily repeated and are ideal for research. But one picture gives a circumscribed view of a person's art-making capacity and of that person's individuality. Nonetheless, we see the advantages of using the PPAT and the FEATS as follows:

- We can easily compare one group to another.
- Our scales are based on global artistic elements.
- Our scales are correlated with specific psychiatric symptoms and diagnostic information.
- We can apply these methods to both children and adults.
- We can measure changes over time.

Group Comparisons

If there are differences between two or more groups (whatever the group membership criteria), we contend that these differences will be found in the *way* the group members draw rather than *what* they draw. Given that the possible subject matter for art is vast, one would have considerable difficulty testing for measurable differences in content between groups. Furthermore, because much symbolism is often culture-bound, cross-cultural studies would be problematic if the focus were only on content.

Granted, there are individual differences within any group. But, using descriptive statistics (distributions and mean scores), we can arrive at a description of the group *as a group*. Then, we can determine whether there are statistically significant differences between groups that are unlikely to be by chance alone. For example, most art therapists working with hospitalized depressed patients would probably agree that such patients frequently make drawings with few details and little color. Using the PPAT and the FEATS one can easily test this assertion and compare that group to a group of nonpatients or to another group of patients.

Global Artistic Elements

The majority of the FEATS variables are those formal elements of great concern to artists. We feel the research on projective drawings bogged down in a search for details that infrequently occur and are difficult to rate. Many such details are either present or absent and are measured on nominal scales. Subtle differences are hard to capture. Global attributes such as the use of color, integration, and implied energy can be measured on ordinal or interval scales, making degrees of a variable easy to determine. These attributes are among the first things we notice about a work of art. But more than that, artists are accustomed to taking in the entire piece at a glance. As we tried to tease out measurable variables in the PPATs, we realized that we seemed to know more than we could put into words. No doubt, many art therapists have experienced a similar phenomenon—that they have a seemingly intuitive sense of the information a picture conveys. We have come to recognize that this "intuition" is actually a process of *pattern matching* that seemed to occur without verbal mediation (Gantt & Tabone, 1998, pp. 21–22, 52–59). Once we recognized the essential pattern we realized that it was contained in the global formal elements.

Correlation with Symptoms and Diagnosis

The majority of the FEATS scales can be related to specific psychiatric symptoms. This is what we call the *graphic equivalent of symptoms* (Gantt & Tabone, 1998, pp. 22–27). As we developed the FEATS we combed the literature for characteristics others associated with particular diagnostic groups. Then, using our own clinical observations we searched the *Diagnostic and Statistical Manual of Mental Disorders* (DSM) for symptoms that could be logically expressed in pictures. For example, if a person is severely depressed with psychomotor retardation, depressed mood, loss of energy, and a diminished ability to think or concentrate (American Psychiatric Association, 1994, p. 327), an art therapist could reasonably expect the persons's PPAT to have lower scores on the scales for Details of Objects and Environment, Prominence of Color, Implied Energy, and Space than the PPATs of a nonpatient sample.

Useful for Children as Well as Adults

We collected PPATs from 322 children in a suburban elementary school in a metropolitan area. We applied the FEATS just as easily to these drawings as to those of adults. It is a distinct advantage to have a rating system that applies to all ages. This makes it possible to study age-related changes and compare our statistical results to Viktor Lowenfeld's descriptions of developmental stages (Lowenfeld & Brittain, 1975).

Measuring Change

An advantage of the FEATS is that we can measure small changes (½ point). We can collect a PPAT as part of a study on treatment response (e.g., before and after prescribing antidepressants, antipsychotics, or Ritalin), during ECT monitoring, or in a research design involving pre- and posttesting. With patients undergoing ECT we have observed subtle changes for the better on some FEATS variables, but these changes are not uniform. For instance, a person's drawing may be rated higher or the Person scale but lower on the Integration scale. Further studies will help us tease out the most important FEATS scales for gauging improvement.

AN EXAMPLE OF CHANGE USING THE PPAT AND THE FEATS

Figure 1 shows an admission PPAT of a 40-year-old man, John, with a history of multiple hospital admissions for schizophrenia over a 14-year period. We have followed changes in his PPATs over this period and have more than 20 PPATs in his file. During most of his hospital stays he was given antipsychotic medication. His usual reason for being hospitalized has been not taking his medicine.

During one stay, John's psychiatrist decided to give him ECT. John did a PPAT (Figure 1) 1 day before the first treatment. He selected the colors turquoise (top right-hand corner), yellow (small dot-like forms, purple (vertical lines), and red (two lines at right angles). John drew most of the PPAT with the paper in a horizontal orientation and then rotated the paper vertically to add the red lines. Figure 2 is John's PPAT after one ECT session 2 days later. It has an orange sun, a blue person, a dark green tree, and red apples. Table 1 presents the FEATS scores on each drawing.

One year and 5 months later, John returned to the hospital. His admission PPAT was a multicolored drawing that filled the paper, but there was no discernible person, tree, or apple (Figure 3). After one ECT treatment John's PPAT (Figure 4) looked similar to Figure 2. Less

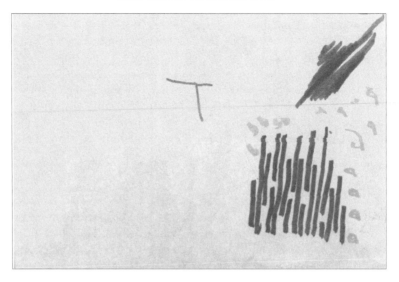

FIGURE 1. Admission PPAT.

than 1 month later John returned to the hospital. His first PPAT resembled Figure 2. After one ECT treatment John changed the colors of the tree to a brown trunk and green leaves and showed the person with the apple in hand. He moved the sun to the opposite corner of the page and made it larger.

The total FEATS scores for these last two drawings (not shown) were 39.5 and 45.5, respectively. Because the hospital added other measures to its protocol for ECT monitoring we can compare them with the FEATS scores. One day after the most recent admission John scored 40 on the Beck Depression Inventory and 29 on the Mini-Mental Status Exam

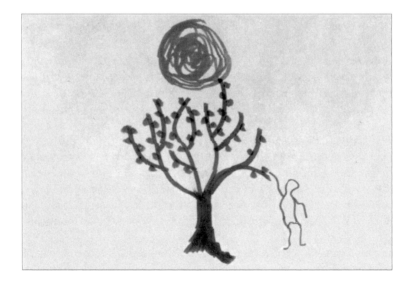

FIGURE 2. John's PPAT after one ECT session 2 days later.

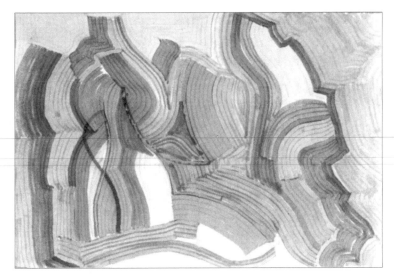

FIGURE 3. Admission PPAT, 1 year and 5 months later.

(MMSE). A score of 14 or higher indicates depression (Beck & Beamesderfer, 1974). The expected score for nonpatients on the MMSE is 30 (Folstein & McHugh, 1975). A day after one ECT treatment John scored 0 on the Beck (no depression) and 28 on the MMSE (a slight decline). John refused any additional ECT treatments.

Because the Beck Depression Inventory is a well-known test we could conduct a correlation study to see if the FEATS scores for other patients are correlated with the Beck. If the two measures are correlated we could claim validity for the FEATS in measuring depression.

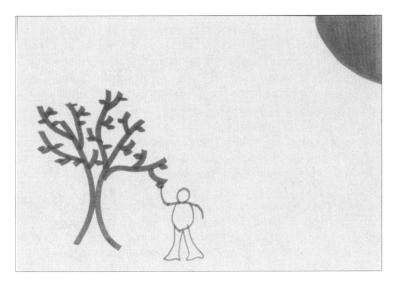

FIGURE 4. John's PPAT after one ECT treatment.

ADDING CONTENT SCALES

Although the FEATS provides much useful information it does not answer all the questions we have about the PPATs. For instance, two FEATS scales measure color use. The Prominence of Color scale is concerned with the amount of color and the Color Fit scale determines whether the artist has used colors based on the items in the task. Both are equal interval scales and therefore are concerned with the *degree* of the particular attribute. Of equal interest is which specific colors are used both for the drawing as a whole and for individual elements. For example, *as a group* our control group members color the tree with a brown trunk, a green top, and red apples. Black trunks and green or yellow apples are statistically rare. The controls also draw the person with three or more colors. But we have many patients' drawings with the person done in only one color. Because we have seen a number of all-blue and all-yellow people we want to know whether such color use is associated with a particular group. We added a number of Content Scales (nominal or categorical scales) to measure such variables (Gantt & Tabone, 1998, pp. 47–51).

RELIABILITY AND VALIDITY

A cardinal principle of any assessment is that it be both reliable and valid. Most projective drawings fail to meet scientific muster because they cannot meet this requirement. Groth-Marnat (1990) discusses the problems of reliability and validity in projective drawings (pp. 367–369) as well as the tendency for raters to project their own attitudes into the work (p. 370). But it is clear that he assumes, as do many researchers, that the art mirrors enduring personality traits. We do not make that assumption. Rather, because we have seen such drastic changes in PPATs in short order, we consider these drawings a barometer of psychological state. Few others seem to agree implicitly or explicitly with us. Treating the PPATs (or any other art) as a reflection of the moment demands different hypotheses and imposes a specific type of research design than has been customary.

In determining reliability we deal strictly with interrater reliability. Because we focus on changes in state, we are not concerned with test–retest reliability. In our studies we ask whether three raters blind to our hypotheses rate pictures in essentially the same way. Unless a researcher can demonstrate that his or her rating method can be applied in the same way by others all further investigation grinds to a halt. In several studies (Gantt, 1990; Williams, Agell, Gantt, & Goodman, 1996) we demonstrated that the majority of our scales have excellent interrater reliability, generally ranging from .88 and up. The two scales with which we have struggled to obtain acceptable interrater reliability are Rotation and Perseveration. This difficulty may be explained by the fact that they are not normally distributed and are rare, even in the drawings of patients. However, we are not yet ready to discard them as both variables appear in the work of very young children and some patients with dementia.

We are in the process of repeating the original validity study (Gantt, 1990) on a larger sample. That research demonstrated that on 10 FEATS scales there was a statistically significant difference between two or more groups (four diagnostic groups and a control group). Because we contend the FEATS scores can measure changes of psychological state, we will need to do validity studies confirming the correlation of those scores with an independent measure of clinical condition.

REFERENCES

American Psychiatric Association. (1994). *Diagnostic and statistical manual of mental disorders* (4th ed.). Washington, DC: Author.

Beck, A., & Beamesderfer, A. (1974). Assessment of depression: The depression inventory: Psychological measurements in psychopathology. In P. Pichot (Ed.), *Modern problems in pharmacopsychiatry* (pp. 151–169). Basel: S. Karger.

Folstein, M., & McHugh, P. (1975). "Mini-mental state": A practical method for grading the cognitive state of patients for the clinician. *Journal of Psychiatric Research, 12,* 189.

Gantt, L. (1990). *A validity study of the Formal Elements Art Therapy Scale (FEATS) for diagnostic information in patients' drawings.* Unpublished doctoral dissertation, University of Pittsburgh, Pittsburgh, PA.

Gantt, L. (2001). The Formal Elements Art Therapy Scale: A measurement system for global variables in art. *Art Therapy: Journal of the American Art Therapy Association, 18*(1), 50–55.

Gantt, L., & Tabone, C. (1998). *The Formal Elements Art Therapy Scale: The rating manual.* Morgantown, WV: Gargoyle Press.

Groth-Marnat, G. (1990). *Handbook of psychological assessment* (2nd ed.). New York: Wiley.

Lehmann, H., & Risquez, F. (1953). The use of finger paintings in the clinical evaluation of psychotic conditions: A quantitative and qualitative approach. *Journal of Mental Science, 99,* 763–777.

Lowenfeld, V. (1939). *The nature of creative activity.* New York: Harcourt, Brace.

Lowenfeld, V. (1947). *Creative and mental growth.* New York: Macmillan.

Lowenfeld, V., & Brittain, W. (1975). *Creative and mental growth* (6th ed.). New York: Macmillan.

Williams, K., Agell, G., Gantt, L., & Goodman, R. (1996). Art-based diagnosis: Fact or fantasy? *American Journal of Art Therapy, 35,* 9–31.

The MARI Assessment

Carol Thayer Cox

Joan Kellogg, a pioneer in the art therapy field, developed a therapeutic and projective instrument called the MARI® Card Test© which evolved from her experience with mandala art. She worked from 1969 to 1971 as an art therapist in psychiatric facilities, and thereafter in the 1970s as an art therapy consultant to a number of treatment programs and research projects that incorporated art therapy. Drawn to Carl Jung's concept of archetypes, she always requested a mandala drawing of her patients.

"Mandala" is a Hindi word derived from Sanskrit meaning circle or center. Jung considered the mandala to be an archetypal symbol representing the self, the center of personality striving for wholeness in the individuation process. During Jung's many years as a psychotherapist (some might consider him one of the first art therapists), mandalas were not only described to him as dream images but were often drawn, painted, modeled, or danced by his patients as well, usually in times of crisis or transformation (Jung, 1963). Although Jung believed in the significance of a spontaneously created mandala (Jung, 1973), later in his career it is possible that he may have encouraged his clients to create in a circular form, particularly when he determined that it might assist in providing a container or safe boundary within which chaos could be potentially transformed into order, balance, and wholeness (Jung, 1933; Slegelis, 1987).

While working as a consultant for the Maryland Psychiatric Research Center (1972–1978), Kellogg standardized the materials for mandala drawings, offering a box of Holbein oil pastels, either the 36 or 48 set, and a piece of 12″ × 18″ white drawing paper with a 10½″ circle in the center, predrawn in pencil. The directions are simply to use the space in any way you wish, allowing images or shapes to spontaneously evolve, starting in the center if it feels right to do so, and using the boundary of the circle as a guide, not a barrier.

In 1977, after spending 8 years collecting, observing, and classifying thousands of patients' mandala drawings, Kellogg developed a system based on form, symbol, movement, and color for understanding patterns and shapes in a circular design. Drawing from her vast knowledge of psychology, mythology, anthropology, religion, and cross-cultural studies, she

428

organized into a circular format 12 constructs that symbolize the basic stages of the life cycle (in 1984, she added an additional category—stage 0), which she calls the "Archetypal Stages of the Great Round of Mandala" (Kellogg, 1978, 2002). Her theoretical model provides a symbolic way to map stages of psychological growth represented by different states of consciousness from before birth to after death. It incorporates psychosocial, physiological, and spiritual aspects of human development.

A unique art therapy theory to comprehend patients' art is a major contribution to the field of art therapy; however, the depth and breadth of this extraordinary concept goes far beyond art therapy. Kellogg's life-cycle theory can be applied to enhance the understanding of just about anything, from the evolution of man, to the development of an idea, to the stages of a relationship. "If what Joan Kellogg had discovered about human ideation was true, she may well have stumbled upon the schema for the hard wiring of the human mind. If this is so . . . then every emanation of our brains, from childhood play toy to schemes for city planning, coming as it would from the same hardware, will bear unmistakable characteristics which can be traced back to the same mainframe architecture" (Thayer, 1994, p. 201).

Be that as it may, Kellogg's intent was to create a reliable graphic assessment theory for determining states of consciousness. Because evaluating drawings can sometimes be subjective and difficult to quantify for purposes of research, Kellogg introduced the MARI Card Test in 1980 as an assessment tool for clinical and research settings. MARI is the registered trademark for Mandala Assessment and Research Institute, which Kellogg directed for the next 10 years. It is a legal entity which she established for the development, production, and teaching of the appropriate use of the MARI Card Test. In 1989, she formed a contractual alliance with a new corporation, The Association of Teachers of Mandala Assessment, to teach her work.

The MARI Card Test has undergone several revisions since its first edition (Kellogg, 2002), and in its present state, each of the 13 stages is represented by three archetypal designs (Figure 1). These 39 designs are embossed in black on clear, $3'' \times 5''$ plastic cards. The test includes 40 color cards on paper stock of the same size. A test subject is usually asked to draw a mandala first, according to the standards outlined previously, and is then asked to select six design cards to which he or she is attracted. Proper orientation of the cards is essential. The next instruction is to choose a color card that seems most appropriate for each of the six selected design cards and finally to rank-order the choices. The colors were derived by Kellogg from the Holbein set of pastels used for the mandala drawing. An additional directive has been suggested by MARI teacher Phyllis Frame (2002) and is considered optional for administration: to choose one design card the subject is attracted to least of all (the reject card) and to select a corresponding color for it, as well as a second color that makes it more acceptable (the healing color). I suggest another directive when using this assessment clinically—to include an inquiry after all the selections have been made to ensure that the subject's personal associations to design and color can be taken into consideration.

Kellogg's life cycle is represented by Figure 1, which includes all the design cards of the MARI Card Test. The lower half of this circle symbolizes the unconscious, whereas the upper half denotes conscious realms. Stage 0 (Clear Light), at the center of the circle, is a transpersonal space that is considered the source of all existence. The lower left quadrant encompasses prenatal and/or deeply unconscious material. Within this quadrant, Stage 1 (The Void) has to do with attachment, trust, and safety issues; Stage 2 (Bliss) is a passive, receptive, generative state; and Stage 3 (Labyrinth, Spiral) introduces a focused movement of energy. The upper left quadrant developmentally parallels the years from birth to adolescence, which includes Stage 4 (Beginning), reflecting oral dynamics and nurturance needs; Stage 5 (The Target), anal dynamics and boundary setting; and Stage 6 (The Dragon Fight), Oedipal dynamics

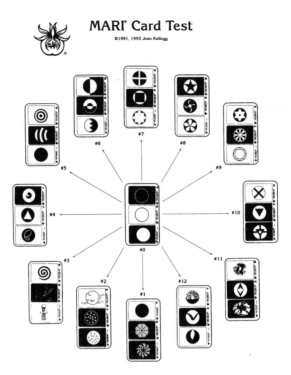

FIGURE 1. Life cycle of mandala. Copyright 1991, 1993 by Joan Kellogg. Reprinted by permission.

and dealing with the shadow. The upper right quadrant correlates with adulthood and its many challenges. Stage 7 (Squaring the Circle) is a place of integration, readiness, and commitment; Stage 8 (The Functioning Ego) has to do with self-identity and autonomy; and Stage 9 (Crystallization) concerns completion of goals and relationship to others. The final quadrant in the lower right addresses the return to the unconscious resulting in a change of consciousness. Stage 10 (Gates of Death) marks endings and loss; Stage 11 (Fragmentation) signifies disintegration and chaos; and Stage 12 (Transcendent Ecstasy) heralds transformation (Cox & Cohen, 2000; Cox & Frame, 1993; Kellogg, 1978, 2002).

The following is a case example to illustrate a MARI assessment. A 54-year-old divorced woman, whom I will call Karen, had a stable job for 10 years in a counseling department for a university, but she was beginning to feel restless and unfulfilled. Although she loved where she lived, she was experiencing dissatisfaction at work, particularly with her immediate supervisor. She decided to attend a MARI Course in Mandala Assessment to learn about a field that was unfamiliar to her, thinking that it might inspire her to develop her creativity. Her mandala drawing (Figure 2) is a Stage 3 spiral composed of all three primary colors, red, yellow, and blue, rendered with heavy pressure. Each primary color represents an essential energy (i.e., creating, preserving, and letting go) vital to healthy functioning, according to Kellogg's hypotheses regarding color (Kellogg, 1992). This drawing reflects the intense stirrings of movement toward growth and change, with all the energies necessary for such transition to take place.

Karen's MARI card choices are listed and shown in Figure 3. The cards are well distrib-

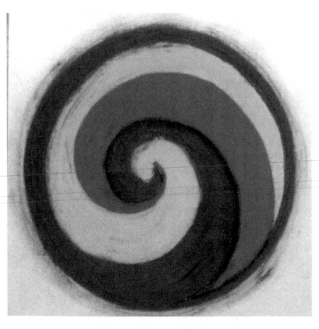

FIGURE 2. Karen's spiral mandala drawing.

uted throughout Kellogg's life-cycle chart, with stages chosen in each quadrant, though there are more cards in the unconscious than the conscious area. The selection of Stages 0 and 1 offers clues to early dynamics that can have long-lasting effects. Two axes are in evidence. The axis of Stages 3 and 9 has to do with generating energy toward something new and completion of a cycle. Stages 5 and 11 form another axis that reflects control versus lack of control, especially highlighted with Stage 11 as the rejected card. The combination of Stages 1, 5, and 9 indicates a well-constructed defense system, sometimes bordering on rigidity. However, the selection and drawing of Stage 3, symbolizing motion, counteracts the extreme interpretation of this triangle combination.

- *Card A (Stage 0) with 000G (gold foil).* Drawn to the "simplicity" of this design, Karen reveals by this choice a deeply transpersonal nature that is inclined toward transformation on a spiritual level, though it would not be apparent to most who know her. Not a frequently chosen card, it tends to resonate with those who have a steadfast longing for something that is indefinable.
- *Card c–d (Stage 1) with #900 (white) and Card D (Stage 1) with #103 (magenta).* These two choices of Stage 1 indicate issues regarding trust and safety that originated early in Karen's history, possibly during prenatal experiences. She may have encountered a crisis of basic survival, which may have been on a transpersonal level, considering Karen's Stage 0 selection. Karen is most likely a person who proceeds carefully, checking out a situation thoroughly before making a decision. Bonding with others may raise her anxiety. The impending change depicted in her Stage 3 drawing could be the impetus for reawakening these unconscious fears.
- *Card G (Stage 3) with 800 (grey).* The same design as her drawing, the "fluidity" of this card is what Karen found appealing. Unlike her previous card selections, this one indi-

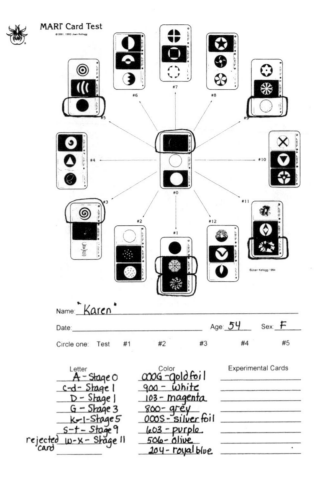

FIGURE 3. Chart showing Karen's selections from the MARI Cards.

cates flowing movement. It is often chosen when there is a quest or seeking for an inner journey. However, Karen's color for this card is surprising compared to the bright hues in her picture. It is almost as if this choice reveals a shadow side of her journey, possibly guilt, maybe
some depression.

• *Card k–l (Stage 5) with 000S (silver foil)*. Karen liked the "repetition" of this design,
which epitomizes predictability and perfectionism. It also reflects the need for boundaries
when encountering a power struggle, which may have been what Karen was experiencing at
work. The silver foil on Stage 5 may indicate a tendency to fantasize that reality is better than
it is, or it may, in Karen's case especially, reflect her wish to transform the situation.

• *Card s–t (Stage 9) with 603 (purple)*. It is interesting that Karen was attracted to the
"stability" of this card, a design symbolizing a state of completion and homeostasis with others, which probably reflected Karen's university position where she interacted successfully
with colleagues and students. Kellogg (2002) says, "It speaks of present harmony and status,
such as a full-blown rose might display seconds before all the petals fall" (p. 79). This is usually the case with the color purple, which can denote a sense of imminent mourning over ending and loss, calling for change and renewal.

• *Rejected Card w–x (Stage 11) with 506 (olive), healing color 204 (royal).* It is not surprising that Karen would find the "broken" quality of Stage 11 unappealing, as she selected Stages 5 and 9, both symmetric and orderly. The chaos of Stage 11 can be uncomfortable for many people. The muddy olive green color is reminiscent of toxicity that can cause illness, either physiological or psychological, when held within the system. Stage 11 invites the appropriate release of all toxic material. The compelling pull toward letting go was probably frightening to Karen, who more than likely knew on some level that she ran the risk of getting sick if she did not follow her intuition (the healing royal blue) to start on the path toward change, which would require her to encounter the temporary quality of disorientation and confusion of Stage 11.

Karen's final drawing on black paper is a rainbow-colored, luminescent Stage 12, seen as a bird's-eye view of the fountain image (Figure 4). This picture exemplifies transcendence, coming from a center point and breaking beyond the border of the circle with a gradual gradation of color from dark to light. There is evidence of Karen's need for control in this picture, but it reflects a breakthrough for her, as she had begun on the path toward transformation. During the next 6 months she journaled and drew mandalas every day, which helped her to decide to apply for a position in a university in another state. She got the job, bought a house in her new location, has since been promoted, and at this writing, several years later, is happy to have embraced the challenge.

The MARI Card Test is a relatively new assessment and is still undergoing rigorous research to test its reliability and validity with various populations. It is an excellent tool to use

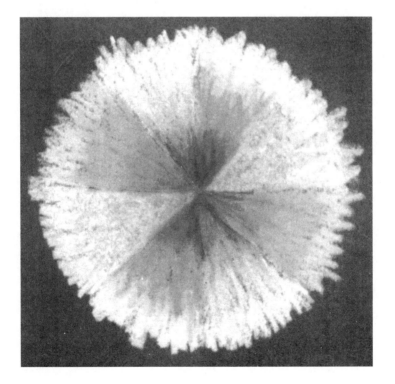

FIGURE 4. Karen's mandala drawing on black paper.

for pre- and posttesting of subjects undergoing a particular type of treatment. Clinicians have also found it beneficial as a tool for monitoring a client's progress over time. There are many advantages to using the MARI assessment: It is easy to administer, does not require verbal feedback, and tends to be a procedure that is nonthreatening and enjoyable.

The beauty of this assessment is that it is theory based, so there is a cohesive and logical means of interpreting the Card Test along with the drawings. And the theory itself can be applied to enhance the evaluation of any artwork, not just mandalas. However, to use Kellogg's assessment appropriately, it is necessary to be thoroughly trained in the life-cycle theory and the proper administration and interpretation of the MARI Card Test, which is best done by therapists who are good at intuiting and integrating multileveled information.

REFERENCES

Cox, C. T., & Cohen, B. (2000). Mandala artwork by clients with DID: Clinical observations based on two theoretical models. *Art Therapy: Journal of the American Art Therapy Association, 17*(3), 195–201.

Cox, C. T., & Frame, P. (1993). Profile of the artist: MARI® Card Test© research results. *Art Therapy: Journal of the American Art Therapy Association, 10*(1), 23–29.

Frame, P. (2002). The value of the rejected card choice in the MARI® Card Test©. *Art Therapy: Journal of the American Art Therapy Association, 19*(1), 28–31.

Jung, C. G. (1933). *Modern man in search of a soul* (W. S. Dell & C. F. Baynes, Trans.). New York: Harcourt Brace.

Jung, C. G. (1963). *Memories, dreams, and reflections* (A. Jaffe, Ed.; R. Winston & C. Winston, Trans.). New York: Pantheon.

Jung, C. G. (1973). *Mandala symbolism* (3rd printing) (R. F. C. Hull, Trans.) (Bollingen Series). Princeton, NJ: Princeton University Press.

Kellogg, J. (1978). *Mandala: Path of beauty.* Baltimore: MARI.

Kellogg, J. (1992). Color theory from the perspective of the great round of mandala. *The Journal of Religion and Psychical Research, 15*(3), 139–146.

Kellogg, J. (2002). *Mandala: Path of beauty* (3rd ed., 2nd printing). Belleair, FL: Association for Teachers of Mandala Assessment.

Slegelis, M. H. (1987). The study of Jung's mandala and its relationship to art psychotherapy. *The Arts in Psychotherapy, 14*(4), 301–311.

Thayer, J. A. (1994). An interview with Joan Kellogg. *Art Therapy: Journal of the American Art Therapy Association, 11*(3), 200–205.

APPENDIX II

Scope of Practice, Education, Supervision, Standards of Practice, and Ethics

The following appendix contains a brief overview of the scope of practice, educational standards, supervision standards and issues relevant to art therapy, standards of practice, and ethical standards. It is intended to give the reader information on the profession with regard to accountability and competency in the field of art therapy.

SCOPE OF PRACTICE*

In 1997, the American Art Therapy Association drafted the following *Scope of Practice* for its members and the general public, defining the nature of professional art therapy services.

A professional art therapist has completed the requirements for professional membership set forth by the American Art Therapy Association, Inc. (AATA). These requirements include the successful completion of a graduate art therapy educational program and supervised art therapy practicum.

A registered art therapist has successfully completed the requirements for Art Therapist Registered (ATR) set forth by the Art Therapy Credentials Board, Inc. (ATCB). Only those individuals who meet the ATCB requirements may use the initials "ATR."

A board-certified art therapist has completed the requirements for ATR and has passed a certification examination administered by the ATCB. Only those individuals who have passed the examination may use the initials "ATR-BC."

Professional art therapists may provide art therapy services as primary, parallel, or adjunctive treatment within clinical, educational, rehabilitative, and mental health settings.

---

*From *Title and Scope of Practice*. Copyright 1997 by the American Art Therapy Association, Inc. All rights reserved. Reprinted by permission.

These services may be provided independently or as a member of a treatment team. The duties of an art therapist may include, but are not limited to, diagnostic art assessments and/or implementation of treatment according to developed treatment plans with individuals, families, and groups.

Professional art therapists assist their patients/clients in alleviating distress and reducing physical, emotional, behavioral, and social impairment while supporting and promoting positive development through the use of art media and imagery. Within agency guidelines and professional standards, professional art therapists may provide any or all of the following: assessments, development of patient treatment plans, goals, and objectives; case management services; and direct therapeutic interventions and treatment. Professional art therapists also maintain appropriate charting records and regular reports on patient/client progress, participate in professional staff meetings and conferences, and provide information and consultation regarding the patient's/client's clinical progress in the art therapy setting. Professional art therapists in independent practice maintain appropriate records and provide information and consultation, but only with the consent of the patient (except as required by law). Professional art therapists may also function as supervisors, administrators, consultants, researchers, and expert witnesses.

Professional art therapists use drawings and other art media and imagery to assess, treat, and rehabilitate patients with mental, emotional, physical, and/or developmental impairments.

Professional art therapists are trained to use and facilitate art processes by providing materials, interventions, instruction, and structuring of tasks tailored to the individual and group needs of patients/clients.

Professional art therapists plan and understand the appropriate use of materials in relation to the therapeutic needs of patients/clients while calling on their skills and education for interpretation of images within the context of assessment and treatment.

While the art therapy process utilizes the creative process and symbolic representation as a means of nonverbal communication and expression, the professional art therapist utilizes verbal expression in conjunction with the nonverbal expressions to facilitate assessment and treatment.

Professional art therapists in agency settings are active participants in the therapeutic milieu and work with other treatment team members in promoting and maintaining health and well-being.

The scope of practice for art therapists is limited in accordance with any and all applicable state laws and licensure restrictions regarding the provision of such services.

EDUCATION*

As defined in the *Scope of Practice*, the AATA has established educational standards for graduate programs at the master's level. Like other mental health professions art therapy education includes courses in psychopathology and diagnostic categories, assessment, therapeutic approaches with various populations, group dynamics, human development, cultural diversity, ethics, legal issues, and research. Supervised practicum experiences with various populations are also required. Many educational programs include additional coursework in counseling theory and practice because many art therapists eventually seek state licensure as professional counselors, clinical mental health counselors, or marriage and family therapists. Other pro-

*Adapted from the *Art Therapy Education: Preparation for the Profession* brochure. Copyright 1999 by the American Art Therapy Association, Inc. All rights reserved. Adapted by permission.

grams offer courses in related subjects such as play therapy, sandtray work, or expressive arts therapies. Currently, doctoral programs are being developed to meet the need for both advanced art therapy training and research.

Although goals are similar to those in psychology and counseling, art therapy education distinguishes itself through several unique competencies:

- *Materials.* Art therapists are familiar with a variety of materials and art processes that can be used in therapy. These include a wide range of two- and three-dimensional media such as drawing tools, paints, clay, and collage. Specific qualities and capacities of materials, such as those described in the expressive therapies continuum discussed in Chapter 9 (this volume), are an important component of training. Art therapists are also cognizant of any hazards involved in using specific materials or equipment used in art therapy.

  Because most art therapists are also artists, most have had personal experiences with the art process and media. For those individuals who have not had extensive experience with art, additional studio courses are required to develop competency with materials and a variety of art processes. Basic competency in drawing, painting, and clay sculpture along with an understanding of the creative process is standard.

- *Art expression.* Art therapists have an understanding of and respect for the content and meaning of client-produced art. This includes familiarity with the normal developmental levels of artistic expression; possible indicators of mental illness, developmental and neurological disorders, and trauma in artistic expression; and the uses and limitations of art-based assessments. Art therapists are also familiar with the specific ethical considerations that apply to confidentiality and disposition of art expressions created in therapy (see section, "Ethical Standards").

- *The art therapeutic relationship.* Art therapy involves not only a client and a therapist but also art materials and the creative process of art making. Facilitating expression, creating a safe space for art making, and understanding the integration of art materials into therapy define the art therapeutic relationship between client and therapist. These unique dimensions are emphasized in education in addition to psychotherapeutic skills and knowledge areas common to other mental health professions.

Upon completion of required master's-level coursework in art therapy and a supervised postgraduate internship, an individual is eligible to apply to become a Registered Art Therapist from the Art Therapy Credentials Board (for contact information, see the end of this appendix). The ATCB also administers an art therapy board certification exam for those who wish to become a board-certified art therapist. Several states currently use this examination to qualify art therapists for licensure as professional art therapists.

There are now numerous training opportunities for counselors, social workers, and psychologists to take coursework in art therapy leading to either certification as an art therapist, specialization in art therapy, or learning a clinical application to a specific population. For non-art therapist professionals, the question becomes, "How much education does one needs to do art therapy?" There is no simple answer to this question because of the diversity of how art therapy is used in treatment. While art therapy is considered a profession and its practice defined and restricted by law in some states, it is also a modality that is incorporated in therapeutic work by many non-art therapist clinicians. All mental health professions' codes of ethics encourage clinicians not to practice beyond the scope of their experience or training. Clinicians not specifically trained in art therapy should consider the importance of additional education to enhance their skills in art therapy if they feel they have not had adequate training.

SUPERVISION*

Supervision in art therapy is an important aspect of both education and postgraduate work. To date, only one book on art therapy has been published, *Supervision and Related Issues* (1996), by Cathy Malchiodi and Shirley Riley. The authors proposed the following guidelines for art therapy supervision.

Supervision of art therapists is a distinct field of preparation and practice. The following suggested guidelines describe the training, knowledge, and competencies that characterize effective art therapy supervisors.

I. Supervisor's Qualifications

A. General

A supervisor shall have been a Registered Art Therapist (ATR) for at least 2 years prior to acting as a supervisor; will not be under censure for any ethical malfeasance; and should not be related by blood or marriage to the supervisee or have a personal relationship with the same that may undermine the effectiveness of the supervision.

B. Training

A supervisor will have a graduate degree and training that includes the core curriculum and practicum hours suggested in the AATA Education Standards (AATA, 1994). In addition, the supervisor will have a current credential plus 2 additional years of active practice and is currently an active clinician. The supervisor will have had postgraduate training in supervision including courses/seminars.

C. Experience

A supervisor will have had supervised experience in an approved agency that provides health care to the public. The supervisor will have trained for at least 1 year in an institution serving a population similar to that of the supervisee's current placement/employment. The supervisor will also have a broad understanding and education in art therapy theory and practice that is compatible with the supervisee's current placement/employment.

D. Additional Qualifications

The supervisor demonstrates a knowledge of differences with regard to gender, race, ethnicity, culture, and age, understanding the importance of these characteristics in clients and in the supervisory relationship; is sensitive to the evaluative nature of supervision; understands the developmental nature of supervision and uses supervisory methods and materials appropriate to

---

* Copyright 1996 by Cathy A. Malchiodi and Shirley Riley. Adapted by permission.

the supervisee's level of conceptual development, training and experience; and can identify learning needs of supervisee and adjusts consultation to best meet these needs.

II. Continuing Education

Continuing education is recommended for all supervisors. The focus of the continuing education courses should be on improving skills in supervision and evaluation and should assist the supervisor in acquiring additional knowledge of theory and practice in which supervisees are training.

III. Responsibilities of Supervisors

A. General

The supervisor will be responsible for the extent, type, and quality of the art therapy performed by the supervisee. Supervisors will be compliant with all laws, rules, and regulations governing the practice of art therapy with clients and consumers: knowledge of AATA ethical codes and related codes of ethics, knowledge of regulatory documents that affect the profession (certification, licensure, standards of practice, etc.), and knowledge of ethical considerations that pertain to the supervisory relationship (dual relationships, evaluation, due process, confidentiality, and vicarious liability).

B. Knowledge of Supervisory Methods and Techniques

The supervisor:

- Is clear about the purpose of supervision and the methods to be used;
- Works with the supervisee to decide direction of supervisory experiences;
- Uses appropriate supervisory interventions such as art tasks, role-play, modeling, live supervision, homework, suggestions and advice, review of audio- and videotapes;
- Makes every effort to observe the supervisee in the practice of art therapy with clients (e.g., audiotape, videotape, or live supervision);
- Uses media to enhance learning (printed material, tapes, art process);
- Understands how to facilitate the supervisor's self-exploration and problem-solving;
- Devises a method of evaluation which will inform the person being supervised of the quality of his or her clinical abilities and learning experience, and
- Can serve as an evaluator and can identify the supervisee's professional and personal strengths as well as weaknesses.

C. Case Management

The supervisor:

- Recognizes that the primary focus of supervision is the client of the supervisee;
- Assists the supervisee in choosing assessment procedures and interventions;
- Assists in planning therapy and prioritizing client goals and objectives;
- Assists the supervisee in providing rationale for art therapy interventions;
- Assists with the referral process, when appropriate;

- Assists the supervisee in effectively documenting interactions with clients and identifying appropriate material to include in verbal or written reports;
- Assists the supervisee in areas of confidentiality of client and supervisory records;
- Is cognizant of the roles of other professionals at the supervisee's placement/employment; and
- Requires the supervisee to keep an accurate record of client contact and signs these records monthly.

IV. Other

1. Supervision is conducted in a ratio of 1 hour of supervision to every 10 hours of the supervisee's client contact, or as required by certifying agencies and/or licensure boards. Graduate-level trainees' supervision also conforms to any additional program requirements of the educational program.
2. Supervision is a confidential contract between supervisor and supervisee. Both the supervisee and the supervisor will not breach client confidentiality unless there is a question of danger to the client or unethical performance on the part of the trainee.
3. The supervisor will advise the supervisee that all client artwork is part of confidential clinical records. If client artwork is to be used for display or reproduced for clinical or educational presentations, a written release must be obtained from the client. Any identifying marks should be disguised or removed prior to presentation or display.
4. If the supervisor has concerns about the ability of the supervisee to do art therapy, it is the supervisor's responsibility to share these concerns with the supervisee. The supervisor should decide how to best help the supervisee, and, if this is not possible, the supervisor will not sign for hours and will terminate supervision. The supervisor should encourage the trainee to acquire additional training before resuming work as an art therapist with clients.

Because these guidelines are suggested standards and have not been formally adopted, please contact the AATA, ATCB, and/or other professional organizations and licensure boards for current standards of practice regarding supervision.

Art therapy supervision uses not only verbal methods of evaluation but also art. For example, supervisors may use directives such as "draw your reaction to your client," "draw yourself in relationship to your client," or "draw a difficulty you are having in your work." While supervision emphasizes sound clinical practice and self-awareness on the part of the therapist, many art therapy supervisors stress continuing development of flexibility, inventiveness, and creativity in clinical work.

STANDARDS OF PRACTICE

Like most professions, art therapy has established standards of practice for its practitioners. The AATA sets forth clear guidelines for therapists and for programs. Standards for conducting art therapy during referral, intake/acceptance, assessment, documentation, planning, and termination and standards for accountability and the art therapy environment are included. Because art therapy involves the use of art materials and tools, attention is given to issues of safety and toxicity in carrying out treatment plans. These standards are available from the AATA (see contact information at the end of the appendix).

ETHICAL STANDARDS

Like other mental health professions, art therapy has developed a specific set of ethical standards for practitioners. The AATA document reflects ethical areas common to counseling and psychology, such as patient welfare, confidentiality, research, and professional character and behavior. The AATA ethics document differs from other professional codes in its inclusion of standards for disposition, use, and ownership of client-created art expressions (see Section 4.0). The role of art making in therapy poses unique ethical dilemmas and concerns for the therapist and all therapists should be cognizant of these in introducing art to therapy. The most important of these include the following:

- *Confidentiality.* Art expressions must be recognized as confidential communications, just as verbal statements or videotapes are. Permission to display, exhibit, publish, or share art expressions must be obtained from either the client or, in the case of a child, the parent or guardian. If a client agrees to display of art expressions in any form, the therapist must be careful to consider if this is in the best interest of the client based on the context and relevant factors in the client's treatment or status. Art therapists generally agree that the client's identity must be protected; this may include disguising any signatures or revealing information found on the art product before displaying, publishing it, or sharing it in clinical or educational settings.
- *Ownership.* Most art therapists believe that the client—the art maker—owns the art created in art therapy. In most cases, there is no question about this belief. Art therapists generally keep cases notes on artwork created in therapy and either make photocopies, photographs, or, with the newer technologies, digital images of client work for recordkeeping purposes. Because art making is usually an enjoyable activity, it makes sense that part of the therapy for the client is in the art products created.

However, it becomes necessary for the therapist to retain art expressions in cases in which there is an indication of suicide, harm to others, or possible physical or sexual abuse. Chapter 13 (this volume), which covers forensic art evaluation, provides a good example of this ethical practice. In these cases, art expressions are treated similarly to medical records which are retained for an extended period.

Ethical Standards for Art Therapists*

The Board of Directors of the American Art Therapy Association (AATA) hereby promulgate, pursuant to Article 8, Sections 1, 2, and 3 of the Association Bylaws, a Revised Code of Ethical Standards for Art Therapists. Members of AATA abide by these standards and by applicable state laws and regulations governing the conduct of art therapists and any additional license or certification which the art therapist holds.

1.0 Responsibility to Clients

Art therapists shall advance the welfare of all clients, respect the rights of those persons seeking their assistance, and make reasonable efforts to ensure that their services are used appropriately.

* From *Ethics Document* brochure. Copyright 1999 by the American Art Therapy Association, Inc. All rights reserved. Reprinted by permission. Certain portions of these Ethical Standards are adapted from the American Association for Marriage and Family Therapy Code of Ethics (1991) with their permission. Effective date: 11/27/00. As of this writing, the Ethical Standards are undergoing a revision; please contact the American Art Therapy Association for the most recent version.

1.1 Art therapists shall not discriminate against or refuse professional service to anyone on the basis of race, gender, religion, national origin, age, sexual orientation, or disability.

1.2 At the outset of the client–therapist relationship, art therapists shall discuss and explain to clients the rights, roles, expectations, and limitations of the art therapy process.

1.3 Where the client is a minor, any and all disclosure or consent required hereunder shall be made to or obtained from the parent or legal guardian of the minor client, except where otherwise provided by state law. Care shall be taken to preserve confidentiality with the minor client and to refrain from disclosure of information to the parent or guardian which might adversely affect the treatment of the client.

1.4 Art therapists shall respect the rights of clients to make decisions and shall assist them in understanding the consequences of these decisions. Art therapists advise their clients that decisions on the status of therapeutic relationships is the responsibility of the client. It is the professional responsibility of the art therapist to avoid ambiguity in the therapeutic relationship and to ensure clarity of roles at all times.

1.5 Art therapists shall not engage in dual relationships with clients. Art therapists shall recognize their influential position with respect to clients, and they shall not exploit the trust and dependency of persons. A dual relationship occurs when a therapist and client engage in separate and distinct relationship(s) or when an instructor or supervisor acts as a therapist to a student or a supervisee either simultaneously with the therapeutic relationship, or less than two (2) years following termination of the therapeutic relationship. Some examples of dual relationships are borrowing money from the client, hiring the client, engaging in a business venture with the client, engaging in a close personal relationship with the client, or engaging in sexual intimacy with a client.

1.6 Art therapists shall take appropriate professional precautions to ensure that their judgment is not impaired, that no exploitation occurs, and that all conduct is undertaken solely in the client's best interest.

1.7 Art therapists shall not use their professional relationships with clients to further their own interests.

1.8 Art therapists shall continue a therapeutic relationship only so long as it is reasonably clear that the client is benefiting from the relationship. It is unethical to maintain a professional or therapeutic relationship for the sole purpose of financial remuneration to the art therapist or when it becomes reasonably clear that the relationship or therapy is not in the best interest of the client.

1.9 Art therapists shall not engage in therapy practices or procedures that are beyond their scope of practice, experience, training and education. Art therapists shall assist persons in obtaining other therapeutic services if the therapist is unable or unwilling, for appropriate reasons, to provide professional help, or where the problem or treatment indicated is beyond the scope of practice of the art therapist.

1.10 Art therapists shall not abandon or neglect clients in treatment. If the art therapist is unable to continue to provide professional help, the art therapist will assist the client in making reasonable, alternative arrangements for continuation of treatment.

2.0 Confidentiality

Art therapists shall respect and protect confidential information obtained from clients in conversation and/or through artistic expression.

2.1 Art therapists shall treat clients in an environment that protects privacy and confidentiality.

2.2 Art therapists shall protect the confidentiality of the client therapist relationship in all matters.

2.3 Art therapists shall not disclose confidential information without client's explicit written consent unless there is reason to believe that the client or others are in immediate, severe danger to health or life. Any such disclosure shall be consistent with state and federal laws that pertain to welfare of the client, family, and the general public.

2.4 In the event that an art therapist believes it is in the interest of the client to disclose confidential information, he/she shall seek and obtain written authorization from the client or client's guardian(s), before making any disclosures.

2.5 Art therapists shall disclose confidential information when mandated by law in a civil, criminal, or disciplinary action arising from the art therapy. In these cases client confidences may only be disclosed as reasonably necessary in the course of that action.

2.6 Art therapists shall maintain client treatment records for a reasonable amount of time consistent with state regulations and sound clinical practice, but not less than 7 years from completion of treatment or termination of the therapeutic relationship. Records are stored or disposed of in ways that maintain confidentiality.

3.0 Assessment Methods

Art therapists develop and use assessment methods to better understand and serve the needs of their clients. They use assessment methods only within the context of a defined professional relationship.

3.1 Art therapists who use standardized assessment instruments are familiar with reliability, validity, standardization, error of measurement, and proper application of assessment methods used.

3.2 Art therapists use only those assessment methods in which they have acquired competence through appropriate training and supervised experience.

3.3 Art therapists who develop assessment instruments based on behavioral science research methods follow standard instrument development procedures. They specify in writing the training, education, and experience levels needed to use the assessment appropriately.

3.4 Art therapists obtain informed consent from clients regarding the nature and purpose of assessment methods to be used. When clients have difficulty understanding the language or procedural directives used, art therapists arrange for a qualified interpreter.

3.5 In choosing assessment methods and reporting the results, art therapists consider any factors potentially influencing outcomes, such as culture, race, gender, sexual orientation, age, religion, education, and disability. They take special care so that the results of their assessments are not misused by others.

3.6 Art therapists ensure that all assessment artwork and related data are kept confidential according to the policies and procedures of the professional setting in which these assessments are administered.

4.0 Public Use and Reproduction of Client Art Expression and Therapy Sessions

Art therapists shall not make or permit any public use or reproduction of the clients' art therapy sessions, including dialogue and art expression, without express written consent of the client.

4.1 Art therapists shall obtain written informed consent from the client or, where applicable, a legal guardian before photographing clients' art expressions, videotaping, audio recording, or otherwise duplicating, or permitting third-party observation of art therapy sessions.

4.2 Art therapists shall only use clinical materials in teaching, writing, and public presentations if a written authorization has been previously obtained from the clients. Appropriate steps shall be taken to protect client identity and disguise any part of the art expression or videotape which reveals client identity.

4.3 Art therapists shall obtain written, informed consent from the client before displaying client's art in galleries, mental health facilities, schools, or other public places.

4.4 Art therapists may display client art expression in an appropriate and dignified manner only when authorized by the client in writing.

5.0 Professional Competence and Integrity

Art therapists shall maintain high standards of professional competence and integrity.

5.1 Art therapists shall keep informed and updated with regard to developments in their field through educational activities and clinical experiences. They shall also remain informed of developments in other fields in which they are licensed or certified, or which relate to their practice.

5.2 Art therapists shall diagnose, treat, or advise on problems only in those cases in which they are competent as determined by their education, training, and experience.

5.3 Art therapists shall not provide professional services to a person receiving treatment or therapy from another professional, except by agreement with such other professional, or after termination of the client's relationship with the other professional.

5.4 Art therapists, because of their potential to influence and alter the lives of others, shall exercise special care when making public their professional recommendations and opinions through testimony or other public statements.

5.5 Art therapists shall seek appropriate professional consultation or assistance for their personal problems or conflicts that may impair or affect work performance or clinical judgment.

5.6 Art therapists shall not engage in any relationship with clients, students, interns, trainees, supervisees, employees, or colleagues that is exploitive by its nature or effect.

5.7 Art therapists shall not distort or misuse their clinical and research findings.

5.8 Art therapists shall be in violation of this Code and subject to termination of membership or other appropriate actions if they: (a) are convicted of a crime substantially related to or impacting upon their professional qualifications or functions; (b) are expelled from or disciplined by other professional organizations; (c) have their license(s) or certificate(s) suspended or revoked or are otherwise disciplined by regulatory bodies; (d) continue to practice when impaired due to medical or mental causes or the abuse of alcohol or other substances that would prohibit good judgment; or (e) fail to cooperate with the American Art Therapy Association or the Ethics Committee, or any body found or convened by them at any point from the inception of an ethical complaint through the completion of all proceedings regarding that complaint.

6.0 Multicultural Competence

Cultural competence is a set of congruent behaviors, attitudes, and policies that enable art therapists to work effectively in cross-cultural situations. Art therapists acknowledge and incorporate into their professional work the importance of culture; variations within cultures;

the assessment of cross-cultural relations; cultural differences in visual symbols and imagery; vigilance toward the dynamics that result from cultural differences; the expansion of cultural knowledge; and the adaptation of services to meet culturally unique needs.

6.1 Art therapists are sensitive to differences that exist between cultures. They must be earnest in their attempts to learn about the belief systems of people in any given cultural group in order to provide culturally relevant interventions and treatment.

6.2 Art therapists are aware of their own values and beliefs and how they may affect cross-cultural therapy interventions.

6.3 Art therapists obtain education about and seek to understand the nature of social diversity and oppression with respect to race, ethnicity, national origin, color, gender, sexual orientation, age, marital status, political belief, religion, and mental or physical disability.

6.4 Art therapists acquire knowledge and information about the specific group(s) with whom they are working, the strengths inherent in that group, and understand that individuals respond differently to group norms.

6.5 While working with people from cultures different from their own, when necessary, art therapists will seek supervision, assistance from members of that culture, or make an appropriate referral.

6.6 Art therapists are able and willing to exercise institutional, group, and individual intervention skills on behalf of people who are from a different culture.

7.0 Responsibility to Students and Supervisees

Art therapists shall instruct their students using accurate, current, and scholarly information and will, at all times, foster the professional growth of students and advisees.

7.1 Art therapists as teachers, supervisors, and researchers shall maintain high standards of scholarship and present accurate information.

7.2 Art therapists shall be aware of their influential position with respect to students and supervisees and they shall avoid exploiting the trust and dependency of such persons. Art therapists, therefore, shall not engage in a therapeutic relationship with their students or supervisees. Provision of therapy to students or supervisees is unethical.

7.3 Art therapists shall not permit students, employees or supervisees to perform or to hold themselves out as competent to perform professional services beyond their education, training, level of experience or competence.

7.4 Art therapists who act as supervisors shall be responsible for maintaining the quality of their supervision skills and obtain consultation or supervision for their work as supervisors whenever appropriate.

8.0 Responsibility to Research Participants

Researchers shall respect the dignity and protect the welfare of participants in research.

8.1 Researchers shall be aware of federal and state laws and regulations and professional standards governing the conduct of research.

8.2 Researchers shall be responsible for making careful examinations of ethical acceptability in planning studies. To the extent that services to research participants may be compromised by participation in research, investigators shall seek the ethical advice of qualified professionals not directly involved in the investigation and shall observe safeguards to protect the rights of research participants.

8.3 Researchers requesting participants' involvement in research shall inform them of all aspects of the research that might reasonably be expected to influence willingness to participate. Investigators shall be especially sensitive to the possibility of diminished consent when participants are also receiving clinical services and have impairments which limit understanding and/or communication or when participants are children.

8.4 Researchers shall respect participants' freedom to decline participation in or to withdraw from a research study at any time. This obligation requires special thought and consideration when investigators or other members of the research team are in positions of authority or influence over participants. Art therapists, therefore, shall avoid dual relationships with research participants.

8.5 Information obtained about a research participant during the course of an investigation shall be confidential unless there is an authorization previously obtained in writing. When there is a risk that others, including family members, may obtain access to such information, this risk, together with the plan for protecting confidentiality, is to be explained as part of the procedure for obtaining informed consent.

9.0 Responsibility to the Profession

Art therapists shall respect the rights and responsibilities of professional colleagues and participate in activities which advance the goals of art therapy.

9.1 Art therapists shall adhere to the standards of the profession when acting as members or employees of organizations.

9.2 Art therapists shall attribute publication credit to those who have contributed to a publication in proportion to their contributions and in accordance with customary professional publication practices.

9.3 Art therapists who author books or other materials which are published or distributed shall appropriately cite persons to whom credit for original ideas is due.

9.4 Art therapists who author books or other materials published or distributed by an organization shall take reasonable precautions to ensure that the organization promotes and advertises the materials accurately and factually.

9.5 Art therapists shall recognize a responsibility to participate in activities that contribute to a better community and society, including devoting a portion of their professional activity to services for which there is little or no financial return.

9.6 Art therapists shall assist and be involved in developing laws and regulations pertaining to the field of art therapy which serve the public interest and with changing such laws and regulations that are not in the public interest.

9.7 Art therapists shall cooperate with the Ethics Committee of the American Art Therapy Association, Inc. and truthfully represent and disclose facts to the Ethics Committee when requested or when necessary to preserve the integrity of the art therapy profession.

9.8 Art therapists shall endeavor to prevent distortion, misuse, or suppression of art therapy findings by any institution or agency of which they are employees.

10.0 Financial Arrangements

Art therapists shall make financial arrangements with clients, third-party payers, and supervisees that are understandable and conform to accepted professional practices.

10.1 Art therapists shall not offer or accept payment for referrals.

10.2 Art therapists shall not exploit their client financially.

10.3 Art therapists shall disclose their fees at the commencement of services and give reasonable notice of any changes in fees.

10.4 Art therapists shall represent facts truthfully to clients, third-party payers, and supervisees regarding services rendered and the charges therefore.

11.0 Advertising

Art therapists shall engage in appropriate informational activities to enable laypersons to choose professional services on an informed basis.

11.1 Art therapists shall accurately represent their competence, education, training, and experience relevant to their professional practice.

11.2 Art therapists shall ensure that all advertisements and publications, whether in directories, announcement cards, newspapers, or on radio or television, are formulated to accurately convey, in a dignified and professional manner, information that is necessary for the public to make an informed, knowledgeable decision.

11.3 Art therapists shall not use a name which is likely to mislead the public concerning the identity, responsibility, source, and status of those under whom they are practicing, and shall not hold themselves out as being partners or associates of a firm if they are not.

11.4 Art therapists shall not use any professional identification (such as a business card, office sign, letterhead, or telephone or association directory listing) if it includes a statement or claim that is false, fraudulent, misleading, or deceptive. A statement is false, fraudulent, misleading, or deceptive if it: (a) fails to state any material fact necessary to keep the statement from being misleading; (b) is intended to, or likely to, create an unjustified expectation; or (c) contains a material misrepresentation of fact.

11.5 Art therapists shall correct, whenever possible, false, misleading, or inaccurate information and representations made by others concerning the therapist's qualifications, services, or products.

11.6 Art therapists shall make certain that the qualifications of persons in their employ are represented in a manner that is not false, misleading, or deceptive.

11.7 Art therapists may represent themselves as specializing within a limited area of art therapy only if they have the education, training, and experience which meet recognized professional standards to practice in that specialty area.

11.8 AATA credentialed professional, professional, associate, and other members in good standing may identify such membership in AATA in public information or advertising materials, but they must clearly and accurately represent the membership category to which they belong.

11.9 Art therapists shall not use the ATR® and/or ATR-BC following their name unless they are officially notified in writing by the Art Therapy Credential Board, Inc. that they have successfully completed all applicable registration or certification procedures. Art therapists may not use the initials "AATA" following their name like an academic degree.

11.10 Art therapists may not use the AATA initials or logo without receiving written permission from the Association.

12.0 Independent Practitioner

Definition: The Independent Practitioner of Art Therapy is a Credentialed Professional Member of the American Art Therapy Association, Inc. who is practicing art therapy independently and who is responsible for the delivery of services to clients where the client pays the clinician directly or through insurance for art therapy service rendered.

Guidelines

12.1 Independent practitioners of art therapy shall maintain Registration with Art Therapy Credentials Board, Inc. and shall have in addition to their Registration at least 2 full years of full-time practice or 3,000 hours of paid clinical art therapy experience.

12.2 Independent practitioners of art therapy shall obtain qualified medical or psychological consultation for cases in which such evaluation and/or administration of medication is required. Art therapists shall not provide services other than art therapy unless licensed to provide such other services.

12.3 Independent practitioners of art therapy must conform to relevant federal, state, and local government statutes which pertain to the provision of independent mental health practice. (Laws vary from state to state.) It is the sole responsibility of the independent practitioner to conform to these laws.

12.4 Independent practitioners of art therapy shall confine their practice within the limits of their training. The art therapist shall neither claim nor imply professional qualifications exceeding those actually earned and received by them. The therapist is responsible for avoiding and/or correcting any misrepresentation of these qualifications. Art therapists must adhere to state laws regarding independent practice and licensure, as applicable.

Environment

13.0 Independent practitioners of art therapy must provide a safe, functional environment in which to offer art therapy services. This includes:

a. Proper ventilation.
b. Adequate lighting.
c. Access to water supply.
d. Knowledge of hazards or toxicity of art materials and the effort needed to safeguard the health of clients.
e. Storage space for art projects and secured areas for any hazardous materials.
f. Monitored use of sharps.
g. Allowance for privacy and confidentiality.
h. Compliance with any other health and safety requirements according to state and federal agencies which regulate comparable businesses.

Referral and Acceptance

14.0 Independent practitioners of art therapy, upon acceptance of a client, shall specify to clients their fee structure, payment schedule, session scheduling arrangements, and information pertaining to the limits of confidentiality and the duty to report.

Treatment Planning

15.0 Independent practitioners of art therapy shall design treatment plans:

a. To assist the client in attaining maintenance of the maximum level of functioning and quality of life appropriate for each individual.
b. In compliance with federal, state, and local regulations and any licensure requirements governing the provision of art therapy services in the state.
c. That delineate the type, frequency, and duration of art therapy involvement.
d. That contain goals that reflect the client's current needs and strengths. When possible, these goals are formulated with the client's understanding and permission.
e. Provide for timely review, modification, and revision.

Documentation

16.0 Independent practitioners of art therapy shall document activity with clients so that the most recent art therapy progress notes reflect the following:

a. Current level of functioning.
b. Current goals of treatment plan.
c. Verbal content of art therapy sessions relevant to client behavior and goals.
d. Graphic images relevant to client behavior and goals.
e. Changes in affect, thought process, and behavior.
f. No change in affect, thought process, and behavior.
g. Suicidal or homicidal intent or ideation.

16.1 Upon termination of the therapeutic relationship, independent practitioners of art therapy shall write a discharge/transfer summary that includes the client's response to treatment and future treatment recommendations.

Termination of Services

17.0 Independent practitioners of art therapy shall terminate art therapy when the client has attained stated goals and objectives or fails to benefit from art therapy services.

17.1 Independent practitioners of art therapy shall communicate the termination of art therapy services to the client.

For more information:

American Art Therapy Association
1202 Allanson Road
Mundelein, IL 60060-3808
Phone: 888-290-0878
Fax: 847-566-4580
E-mail: arttherapy@ntr.net
Web site: www.arttherapy.org

Art Therapy Credentials Board
P.O. Box 30428
Charlotte, NC 28230
Phone: 877-213-2822
Fax: 336-482-2852
E-mail: atcb@nbcc.org
Web site: www.atcb.org

Index

Page numbers in boldface refer to pages with artwork; "t" indicates a table.

451

sexual abuse, 341–343, 346–348
themes in groupwork, 327
treatment with older adults, 299–300
Treatment structure
    AD/HD, **185–188**
    adolescent depression, 225–227
    adult art therapy, 245–250
    autism, 195–196, 199
    children, 120, 136–137
    cognitive-behavioral therapy, 75–76
    couple therapy, **388–392**
    Diagnostic Drawing Series administration,
        402
    expressive arts therapy, 112–113
    interactive group psychotherapy, 315–317
    MARI Card Test administration, 429–430
    medical art therapy group, **355–360**
    multicultural case example, **380–384**
    narrative therapy, 90
    older adults, 298–301
    sandplay, 255, 256–257
    severe mental illness, **271–277**
    sexual abuse, 153–155, 343–346
    shame reduction in addiction, **284–291**
    solution-focused therapy, **83–88**
    themes in groupwork, 327–329, 329–331
    violent imagery, **233–236**
Twelve-step model
    See also Addiction
    denial, 283
    Higher Power, 289–290
    powerlessness, 286, **287**

supporting, 289
treatment structure, **284–291**

U

Unbalancing, case example, **369–371**
Unconsciousness
    adult art therapy, 243
    analytical psychology, 42–43
    dynamically oriented art therapy, 43
    expressive arts therapy, 107
    medically ill children, 209
    psychoanalytic personality theory, 42
    spontaneous expression, **46–49**
    violent imagery, 232–233

V

Violence
    adolescence, 123, **222–224**
    art expression as an indicator of, 231–232
    PTSD in children, 140
Violent imagery
    adolescent development, 229–230
    censorship issues, 237
    encouraging sublimation, 232–233
    meaning, 230–231
    treatment structure, **233–236**

W

Writing, creative, 114
    See also Expressive arts therapy